Pharmaceutical Statistics

DRUGS AND THE PHARMACEUTICAL SCIENCES

A Series of Textbooks and Monographs

Edited by
James Swarbrick
School of Pharmacy
University of North Carolina
Chapel Hill, North Carolina

Pharmaceutical Statistics

PRACTICAL AND CLINICAL APPLICATIONS

Second Edition, Revised and Expanded

Sanford Bolton

College of Pharmacy and
Allied Health Professions
St. John's University
Jamaica, New York

MARCEL DEKKER, INC.   New York and Basel

Library of Congress Cataloging-in-Publication Data

Bolton, Sanford.
    Pharmaceutical statistics : practical and clinical applications /
Sanford Bolton. -- 2nd ed., rev. and expanded.
        p.   cm. -- (Drugs and the pharmaceutical sciences ; v. 44)
    Includes bibliographical references.
    ISBN 0-8247-8267-4
    1. Pharmacy--Statistical methods. I. Title. II. Series.
    [DNLM: 1. Pharmacy. 2. Statistics. W1 DR893b v. 44 / QV 25
B694p]
    RS57.B65   1990
    615'.1'072--dc20
    DNLM/DLC
    for Library of Congress   90-2706
                                                CIP

This book is printed on acid-free paper.

MARCEL DEKKER, INC.
270 Madison Avenue, New York, New York 10016

Current printing (last digit):
10 9 8 7 6 5 4 3 2

PRINTED IN THE UNITED STATES OF AMERICA

To my wife, Phyllis

always present,
always sensitive,
always inspirational

Preface

While writing the first edition of this book — which is still, to the best of my knowledge, the only textbook on statistical applications in the pharmaceutical sciences — I thought of Brownlee's definition of statistics as "the science of making wise decisions in the presence of uncertainty," for I had to make many decisions in the presence of uncertainty. Answers to my own questions of which topics to include and the depth of coverage required were not always obvious.

The first edition has now had more than five years of exposure, and it has been well received. Thus, I have had the good fortune to receive much instructive feedback from students, teachers, readers, and reviewers that has been extremely helpful to me in revising the book for this second edition. The challenge was to make this book as good as possible while encompassing a wide variety of subject matter and serving a wide variety of readers with specific interests.

This is a book for pharmacists and health science-related scientists who want to learn statistics. A basic knowledge of procedures used in the pharmaceutical sciences is implied. I have tried to include material that has practical utility, most of it based on real problems that I have personally experienced. This new edition has more detailed information on graphics, sampling, statistical inference, regression, factorial designs, clinical studies, quality control, and nonparametric methods. References, exercises, and tables have been updated and expanded. An important new chapter has been added on statistical techniques and examples in process and assay validation.

This volume retains the structure of the original. The first chapters contain basic introductory statistics, whereas the latter chapters deal with more specific applied topics.

Most of Chapters 1 through 8, and Chapters 10 and 15 can be used for an introductory college-level course. More information or less may be included in a course, depending on the background of the students. The remaining chapters cover specialized topics and are often more advanced. Those sections and chapters that cover material of a more advanced nature are designated by a double asterisk (**). Every effort has been made to present these ideas as simply as possible.

No previous statistical education or extensive mathematical background is required. All that is needed is effort and an ability to perform arithmatical calculations (adding, subtracting, multiplying, dividing, etc.). The use of a pocket calculator or a home computer is highly recommended.

The exercises are an integral part of the book; most of them are meant to give the student practice with the material presented herein. Some exercises, also identified by double asterisks, make use of the material presented but also attempt to bring forth ideas not explicitly or completely presented in the text. These more difficult exercises should expand the scope of the book.

As before, theory is kept to a minimum and, whenever possible, a numerical example accompanies each practical statistical application and problem.

It is with high hopes and some measure of certainty that I feel readers will find this second edition more useful in relevant aspects of their research. If this be so, I have succeeded in my aim and efforts.

Sanford Bolton

Introduction

Statistical techniques have been widely used in many diverse areas of scientific investigation. Although the need for statistical input in the pharmaceutical sciences has always been evident, 20 or 30 years ago its absence posed no immediate or tangible problems. There was no review process to criticize possible poor design or possible lack of optimality. The consumer or the "marketplace" was the final judge of product development. Also, to assign a cost/benefit parameter in terms of dollars to the "abstract" contribution of statistics and statisticians to pharmaceutical development is a difficult concept.

Before proceeding, a few words are needed to describe what is meant by "statistics" in the context of this book. Statistics mean different things to different people. Some persons visualize a statistician as a type of accountant—a caretaker and manipulator of figures. Others think of statisticians as spending their time compiling tables of numbers—as actuaries. Still others view statistics as a way of helping to make decisions, creating order out of a chaos of numbers, often a savior of otherwise uninterpretable data. Actually, all of these concepts contain some truth. Statistics encompass a wide range of endeavors and applications. We will restrict our presentation to a limited view of this field, concentrating on topics which find particular application to pharmaceutical research. These topics include estimation and decision making, and testing of hypotheses. Also, we will describe frequently used statistical experimental designs. Another somewhat advanced topic which will be introduced is formulation optimization.

The statistical process depends on the degree to which uncertainty follows laws of probability. We call the uncertainty "variability." When a new drug is said to be proven superior to previous treatments, based on a series of clinical studies, we have our "fingers crossed." What is meant by "proven" is really based on a belief. The "belief" is not founded on intuition, but is based on objective statistical criteria, which are based on probability. Thus, when we say that the new drug is more effective than previous treatments, we are really saying that the new drug is "most probably" more effective. The drug development process consists of many separate steps, which eventually lead to the use of the drug in many patients in many clinical locations. The slow and methodical development of new drug entities in today's consumer-oriented environment ensures that the probability is very high that the final product is safe and effective. The process of making predictions based on observations of a small portion of the population (a sample) and applied to a larger population is known as statistical inference. It is this aspect of statistics which will concern us to a great extent.

Statistical applications have gradually become integrated in diverse areas of the great "diversity" of the drug development process. Pharmaceutical research, in its broadest sense, provides one of the most fertile areas for statistical research and applications. The development of drugs is eventually dependent on their safety and effectiveness in living material, particularly in humans. The incredible variability of human response, including the well-known placebo effect, makes the use of statistical input a necessity when assessing drug efficacy and safety in the present scientific environment. Applications of statistical methods are now routinely found not only in clinical studies, but also in the endeavors of pre-clinical, quality control, and pharmaceutical development laboratories, as previously noted. The scientific personnel in these areas are those who now confront and use statistical techniques every day in the pharmaceutical industry.

To precisely identify the reasons for the relatively recent surge and popularity of statistics in the drug development process, as well as to account for the respect which it now commands, is difficult. One could easily pinpoint one major impetus, the close connection between industry and government, particularly the FDA. The FDA now has a well-established statistical group which has made its voice heard loud and clear. No longer are "testimonials" sufficient to get a drug to market. Results from clinical trials, quality control, and pre-clinical studies are usually statistically designed, analyzed, and documented, as evidence of good scientific practice.

With regard to clinical studies, Dr. S. Dubey of the FDA has discussed the statistical documentation for protocols, which include the design, the "hypothesis" to be tested and the patient sample size [1]. He notes that "quantitative" measurements should be used whenever possible and that less objective measurements deserve to be clearly specified. Dr. Dubey states that design factors should be accounted for, and pooling of data from different sources justified, particularly when combining data from multiclinic studies. Statistical methods to be used in data analysis should be documented and clearly presented, and should include a statement of the assumptions necessary for the validity of the analysis. A power analysis, useful for determining sample size, is also desirable. Finally, he emphasizes the use of summary tables and graphs as an aid in explaining and presenting the experimental results. This attests to the FDA's concern for the quality of data and analysis in FDA submissions.

Although the need for a lucid presentation of data may seem self-evident and, perhaps, not such a great challenge, it is a crucial part of transmitting the message culled from any experiment to a third party. How to best present summaries and "pictures" of the data which clearly relay the intended message is not always immediately apparent. FDA statisticians have made some recommendations in this respect. They also understand the importance and challenges of presenting well-thought-out, clear data displays [2].

The proper statistical analysis is dependent on study design as well as the nature of the data. The statistical methodology should be clearly documented for clinical studies according to Dr. R. O'Neill of the FDA [3]. He notes, for example, that averaging data may obscure both individual results and time trends, often very relevant to experimental conclusions. He also emphasizes that the statistical model, assumptions, and calculations be clearly presented as part of the statistical documentation of clinical studies. Statistical contributions to protocol design and data analysis will be presented in the discussion of clinical trials in this book.

The above recommendations by FDA statisticians are noted here, not only because such procedures represent good scientific practice (generally accepted by scientists everywhere, including those in the pharmaceutical industry), but to highlight the increased awareness of statistical input into scientific experimentation, particularly where considerable variability exists.

Statistical applications have always been recognized as crucial to quality control procedures, tests, specifications, and definitions. Also in recent years, the application and need for statistical procedures in pre-clinical experiments have been much publicized and researched. Some more far-seeing pharmaceutical companies have been applying statistical methods in these areas for many years. More recent regulatory stimulation as well as increased exposure of the drug development process to the scrutiny of outside public and government interest groups have stimulated the growth of statistical applications in these areas. Statistics often substantiate, in a quantitative way, the "gut" feeling of the scientist, lending objective documentation to sometimes intuitive insight of experimental results.

Pharmaceutical development and technology is another area which is receiving more attention for statistical applications. In addition to being useful as aids to the decision-making process, statistically derived optimization designs are now being used to find the "best" combination of ingredients with respect to some formulation attribute. Hence, statistics now pervade almost all areas of drug development.

One concept which deserves mention can be thought of, in a sense, as the ethical aspect of statistics. Most of us, especially statisticians, are tired of the cliché concerning the three kinds of lies: "lies, damn lies, and statistics." However, one cannot deny that there are many ways of looking at data. It is not uncommon to find experts disagreeing on the best way to analyze or interpret a set of experimental data. Often, there is no one correct method. Judgment and experience are essential ingredients of the analysis. It would be disturbing, however, if disagreement on the approach or interpretation resulted in disparate and conflicting conclusions. Fortunately, when alternate methods are sound, this is rarely the case. The misuse of statistics, which consists in part of (a) coming to a firm conclusion with poor data due to design or observational flaws, or (b) *selecting* only the data which proves a pre-determined hypothesis, is to be condemned. The statistician is a scientist, and as is the case with all scientists, integrity is key to success, both inward and outward. Data maneuvering or falsification will satisfy only very immediate and temporary objectives.

This book is an attempt to acquaint the student and pharmaceutical scientist—from clinical monitor, to the analytical chemist, to all members of the pharmaceutical research community—with some basic concepts and analyses. The approach is strictly heuristic and is by no means a systematic theoretical approach. Most examples of problems and data analysis which arise in practice are not simple, often having unexpected wrinkles which invalidate the hoped-for simple analysis and interpretation promised by the elegant experimental design. Most of the time, professional statisticians should be consulted before proceeding with an analysis or publishing the results and conclusion of a study.

To summarize, the aim of this book is to educate the medical and pharmaceutically oriented scientist in statistical usage. If those who read and learn from this book are able to understand and intelligently incorporate some of these statistical ideas into their experimental toolbags, this objective will have been achieved.

REFERENCES

1. Dubey, S. D., *Statistical Documentation: Why and What*, Bureau of Drugs, FDA, Rockville, Md., Nov. 19, 1975.
2. Litt, B. D., *The How Aspect of Statistical Documentation*, Bureau of Drugs, FDA, Rockville, Md., Nov. 19, 1975.
3. O'Neill, R. T., *Statistical Documentation—Analysis*, Bureau of Drugs, FDA, Rockville, Md., Nov. 19, 1975.

Contents

Pharmaceutical Statistics

1

Basic Definitions and Concepts

Statistics has its own vocabulary. Many of the terms that comprise statistical nomenclature are familiar: some commonly used in everyday language, with perhaps, somewhat different connotations. Precise definitions are given in this chapter so that no ambiguity will exist when the words are used in subsequent chapters. Specifically, such terms as *discrete* and *continuous variables, frequency distribution, population, sample, mean, median, standard deviation, variance, range, accuracy, and precision* are introduced and defined. The methods of calculation of the mean, median, standard deviation, and range are also presented. When studying any discipline, the initial efforts are most important. The first chapters of this book are important in this regard. Although most of the early concepts are relatively simple, a firm grasp of this material is essential for understanding the more difficult material to follow.

1.1 VARIABLES AND VARIATION

Variables are the measurements, the values, which are characteristic of the data collected in experiments. These are the data that will usually be displayed, analyzed, and interpreted in a research report or publication. In statistical terms, these observations are more correctly known as *random variables*. Random variables take on values, or numbers, according to some corresponding probability function. Although we will wait until Chap. 3 to discuss the concept of probability, for the present we can think of a random variable as the typical experimental observation that we, as scientists, deal with on a daily basis. Because these measurements may take on different values, repeat measurements observed under apparently identical conditions do not, in general, give the identical results (i.e., they are usually not exactly reproducible). Duplicate determinations of serum concentration of a drug 1 hr after an injection will not be identical no matter if the duplicates come from (a) the same blood sample or (b) from separate samples from two different persons or (c) from the same person on two different occasions. Variation is an inherent part of experimental observations. To isolate and to identify particular causes of variability require special experimental designs and analysis. Variation in observations is due to a number of causes. For example, an assay will vary depending on:

1. The instrument used for the analysis
2. The analyst performing the assay
3. The particular sample chosen
4. Unidentified, uncontrollable background error, commonly known as "noise"

This inherent variability in observation and measurement is a principal reason for the need of statistical methodology in experimental design and data analysis. In the absence of variability, scientific experiments would be short and simple: interpretation of experimental results from well-designed experiments would be

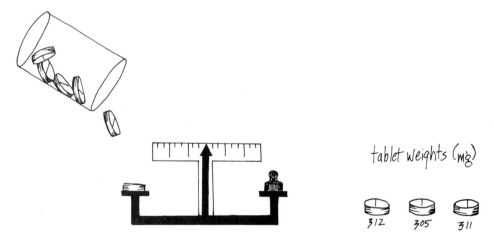

tablet weights (mg)

312   305   311

Tablet weights: an example of a variable measurement (a random variable).

unambiguous. In fact, without variability, single observations would often be sufficient to define the properties of an object or a system. Since few, if any, processes can be considered absolutely invariant, statistical treatment is often essential for summarizing and defining the nature of data, and for making decisions or inferences based on these variable experimental observations.

1.1.1 Continuous Variables

Experimental data come in many forms.* Probably the most commonly encountered variables are known as *continuous variables*. A continuous variable is one that can take on *any* value within some range or interval (i.e., within a specified lower and upper limit). The limiting factor for the total number of possible observations or results is the sensitivity of the measuring instrument. When weighing tablets or making blood pressure measurements, there are an infinite number of possible values that can be observed if the measurement could be made to an unlimited number of decimal places. However, if the balance, for example, is sensitive only to the nearest milligram, the data will appear as discrete values. For tablets targeted at 1 g and weighed to the nearest milligram, the tablet weights might range from 900 to 1100 mg, a total of 201 possible integral values (900, 901, 902, 903, . . . , 1098, 1099, 1100). For the same tablets weighed on a more sensitive balance, to the nearest 0.1 mg, values from 899.5 to 1100.4 might be possible, a total of 2010 possible values, and so on.

Often, continuous variables cannot be easily measured but can be ranked in order of magnitude. In the assessment of pain in a clinical study of analgesics, a patient can have a continuum of pain. To measure pain on a continuous numerical scale would be difficult. On the other hand, a patient may be able to differentiate slight pain from moderate pain, moderate pain from severe pain, and so on. In analgesic studies, scores are commonly assigned to pain severity, such as no pain = 0, slight pain = 1, moderate pain = 2, and severe pain = 3. Although the scores cannot be thought of as an exact characterization of pain, the value 3 does represent more intense pain than the values 0, 1, or 2. The scoring system above is a representation of a continuous variable by discrete "scores" which can be rationally ordered or ranked from low to high. This is commonly known as a *rating scale*.

---

*For a further discussion of different kinds of variables, see Sec. 15.1 in Chap. 15, Nonparametric Methods.

1.2.2   Discrete Variables

In contrast to continuous variables, *discrete variables* can take on a
countable number of values. These kinds of variables are commonly
observed in biological and pharmaceutical experiments and are exemplified by measurements such as the number of anginal episodes in
1 week or the number of side effects of different kinds after drug
treatment. Although not continuous, discrete data often have values
associated with them which can be numerically ordered according to
their magnitude, as in the examples given earlier of a rating scale
for pain and the number of anginal episodes per week.

Discrete data that can be named (nominal), categorized into two
or more classes, and counted are called categorical variables, or
attributes; for example, the attributes may be different side effects
resulting from different drug treatments or the presence or absence
of a defect in a finished product. These kinds of data are frequently observed in clinical and pharmaceutical experiments and processes.
Finished tablets classified in quality control as "defective" or "not
defective" are an example of a categorical or attribute type of variable. In clinical studies, the categorization of a patient by sex
(male or female) or race is a classification according to attributes.
When calculating ED_{50} or LD_{50}, animals are categorized as "respond-
ers" or "nonresponders" to various levels of a therapeutic agent, a
categorical response. These examples describe variables that cannot be ordered. A male is not associated with a higher or lower
numerical value than a female.

Classification by attributes: patients categorized by weight.

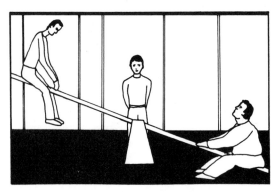

Underweight   Normal weight   Overweight

Continuous variables can always be classified into discrete classes where the classes are ordered. For example, patients can be categorized as "underweight," "normal weight," or "overweight" based on criteria such as those listed in Metropolitan Life Insurance tables of "Desirable Weights for Men and Women" [1]. In this example, "overweight" represents a condition that is greater than "underweight."

Thus we can roughly classify data as:

1. *Continuous* (blood pressure, weight)
2. *Discrete, associated with numbers and ordered* (number of anginal episodes per week)
3. *Attributes: categorical, ordered* (degree of overweight)
4. *Attributes: categorical, not ordered* (male or female)

1.2 FREQUENCY DISTRIBUTIONS AND CUMULATIVE FREQUENCY DISTRIBUTIONS

1.2.1 Frequency Distributions

An important function of statistics is to facilitate the comprehension and meaning of large quantities of data by constructing simple data summaries. The *frequency distribution* is an example of such a data summary, a table or categorization of the frequency* of occurrence of variables in various class intervals. Sometimes a frequency distribution of a set of data is simply called a "distribution." For continuous data, in general, a frequency distribution is constructed by classifying the observations (variables) into a number of discrete intervals. For categorical data, a frequency distribution is simply a listing of the number of observations in each class or category, such as 20 males and 30 females entered in a clinical study. This procedure results in a more manageable presentation of the data.

Table 1.1 is a tabulation of serum cholesterol changes resulting from the administration of a cholesterol-lowering agent to a group of 156 patients. The data are presented in the order in which results were reported from the clinic.

A frequency distribution derived from the 156 cholesterol values is shown in Table 1.2. This table shows a tabulation of the frequency, or number, of occurrences of values that fall into the various class intervals of "serum cholesterol changes." Clearly, the condensation of the data as shown in the frequency distribution in

---

*The frequency is the number of observations in a specified interval or class: for example, tablets weighing between 300 and 310 mg, or the number of patients who are female.

Table 1.1 Serum Cholesterol Changes (mg %) for 156 Patients After Administration of a Drug Tested for Cholesterol-Lowering Effect[a]

17	-12	25	-37	-29	-39
-22	0	-22	-63	34	-31
-64	-12	-49	5	-8	33
-50	-7	16	-11	-38	-17
0	-9	-21	1	2	-30
-32	-34	-14	-18	5	6
24	-6	-49	-8	-49	-37
-25	-12	14	10	-41	-66
-31	35	21	-19	-27	17
-6	-17	-6	1	-28	40
-31	17	-54	-27	-16	16
-44	10	-3	-3	5	6
-19	9	-10	-20	-9	-8
-10	-11	11	-39	19	-32
4	-15	-18	35	6	20
46	24	-27	-19	5	-60
27	23	-22	-1	12	-27
-13	-39	39	-34	-97	-26
38	14	-47	8	16	-15
-62	12	-53	11	21	-47
-54	-11	-5	0	55	34
-69	-11	-44	20	-50	19
0	-25	-24	-4	14	2
-34	16	-23	-71	-58	9
9	2	-2	-58	13	14
17	-13	-22	-3	-17	1

[a]A negative number means a decrease and a positive number means an increase.

Table 1.2 Frequency Distribution of Serum Cholesterol Changes (Data Taken from Table 1.1)

Class interval	Frequency
-100 to -81 (-100.5 to -80.5)	1
-80 to -61 (-80.5 to -60.5)	6
-60 to -41 (-60.5 to -40.5)	16
-40 to -21 (-40.5 to -20.5)	31
-20 to -1 (-20.5 to -0.5)	40
+0 to +19 (-0.5 to +19.5)	43
+20 to +39 (+19.5 to +39.5)	16
+40 to +59 (+39.5 to + 59.5)	3

Table 1.3 Frequency Distribution of Serum Cholesterol Changes Using 16 Class Intervals

Class interval	Frequency	Class interval	Frequency
-100 to -91	1	-20 to -11	22
-90 to -81	0	-10 to -1	18
-80 to -71	1	0 to +9	22
-70 to -61	5	+10 to +19	21
-60 to -51	6	+20 to +29	9
-50 to -41	10	+30 to +39	7
-40 to -31	14	+40 to +49	2
-30 to -21	17	+50 to +59	1

Table 1.2 allows for a better "feeling" of the experimental results than do the raw data represented by the individual 156 results. For example, one can readily see that most of the patients had a lower cholesterol value in response to the drug (a negative change) and that most of the data lie between -50 and +19 mg %.

When constructing a frequency distribution, two problems must be addressed. The first problem is how many classes or intervals should be constructed, and the second problem is the specification of the width of each interval (i.e., specifying the upper and lower limit of each interval). There are no definitive answers to these questions. The choices depend on the nature of the data and good judgment. The number of intervals chosen should result in a table that considerably improves the readability of the data. The following rules of thumb are useful to help select the intervals for a frequency table:

1. Choose intervals that have significance in relation to the nature of the data. For example, for the cholesterol data, intervals such as 18 to 32 would be cumbersome and confusing. Intervals of width 10 or 20, such as those in Tables 1.2 and 1.3, are more easily comprehended and manipulated arithmetically.
2. Try not to have too many empty intervals (i.e., intervals with no observations). The half of the total number of intervals that contain the least number of observations should contain at least 10% of the data. The intervals with the least number of observations in Table 1.2 are the first two intervals (-100 to -81 and -80 to -61) and the last two intervals (+20 to +39 and +40 to +59) (one-half of the eight intervals), which contain 26 or 17% of the 156 observations.
3. Eight to twenty intervals are usually adequate.

Table 1.3 shows the same 156 serum cholesterol changes in a
frequency table with 16 intervals. Which table gives you a better
feeling for the results of this study, Table 1.2 or Table 1.3? (See
also Exercise Problem 3.)

The width of all of the intervals, in general, should be the
same. This makes the table easy to read and allows for simple computations of statistics such as the mean and standard deviation.
The intervals should be mutually exclusive so that no ambiguity
exists when classifying values. In Tables 1.2 and 1.3 we have defined the intervals so that a value can only be categorized in one
class interval. In this way, we avoid problems that can arise when
observations are exactly equal to the boundaries of the class intervals. If the class intervals were defined so as to be continguous,
such as -100 to -90, -90 to -80, -80 to -70, and so on, one must
define the class to which a borderline value belongs, either the
class below or the class above, a priori. For example, a value of
-80 might be defined to be in the interval -80 to -70.

Another way to construct the intervals is to have the boundary
values have one more "significant figure" than the actual measurements so that none of the values can fall on the boundaries. The
extra figure is conveniently chosen as 5. In the cholesterol example, measurements were made to the nearest mg %; all values are
whole numbers. Therefore, two adjacent values can be no less different than 1 mg %, +10 and +11, for example. The class intervals
could then have a decimal of 0.5 at the boundaries, which means
that no value can fall exactly on a boundary value. The intervals
in parentheses in Table 1.2 were constructed in this manner. This
categorization, using an extra figure that is halfway between the
two closest possible values, makes sense from another point of view.
After rounding off, a value of +20 can be considered to be between
19.5 and 20.5, and would naturally be placed in the interval 19.5
to 39.5, as shown in Table 1.2.

1.2.2 Stem-and-Leaf Plot

An expeditious and compact way of summarizing and tabulating large
amounts of data, by hand, known as the *stem-and-leaf method* [2],
is best illustrated with an example. We will use the data from Table
1.1 to demonstrate the procedure.

An ordered series of integers is conveniently chosen (see below)
to cover the range of values. The integers consist of the first
digit(s) of the data, as appropriate, and are arranged in a vertical
column, the "stem." By adding another digit(s) to one of the integers in the stem column (the "leaves"), we can tabulate the data
in class intervals as in a frequency table. For the data of Table

1.1, the numbers range from approximately -100 to +60. The stem is conveniently set up as follows:

-10	-1
-9	-0
-8	+0
-7	+1
-6	+2
-5	+3
-4	+4
-3	+5
-2	+6

In this example, the stem is the first digit(s) of the number and the leaf is the last digit. The first value in Table 1.1 is 17. Therefore, we place a 7 (leaf) next to the +1 in the stem column. The next value in Table 1.1 is -22. We place a 2 (leaf) next to -2 in the stem column; and so on. Continuing this process for each value in Table 1.1 results in the following stem-and-leaf diagram.

```
-10
 -9  7
 -8
 -7  1
 -6  4 2 9 3 6 0
 -5  0 4 4 3 8 0 8
 -4  4 9 9 7 4 1 9 7
 -3  2 1 1 4 4 9 7 9 4 8 9 1 0 7 2
 -2  2 5 5 2 1 7 2 4 3 2 7 0 9 7 8 6 7
 -1  9 0 3 2 2 2 7 1 5 1 1 3 4 0 8 1 8 9 9 6 7 7 5
 -0  6 7 9 6 6 3 5 2 8 3 1 4 3 8 9 8
 +0  0 4 0 9 0 9 2 5 1 1 8 0 2 5 5 6 5 6 6 2 9 1
 +1  7 7 0 7 4 2 6 6 4 1 0 1 9 2 6 4 3 7 6 9 4
 +2  4 7 4 3 5 1 0 1 0
 +3  8 9 9 5 4 3 4
 +4  6 0
 +5  5
 +6
```

This is a list of all of the values in Table 1.1. The distribution of this data set is easily visualized with no further manipulation. However, if necessary, one can easily construct a frequency distribution from the configuration of data resulting from the stem-and-leaf tabulation. (Note that all categories in this particular example can contain as many as 10 different numbers except for the -0 category, which can contain only nine numbers, -1 to -9 inclusive. This "anomaly" occurs because of the presence of both positive and negative values and the value 0. In this example, 0 is arbitrarily assigned a positive value.) In addition to the advantages of this tabulation noted above, the data is in the form of a histogram, which is a common way of graphically displaying data distributions (see Chap. 2).

1.2.3   Cumulative Frequency Distributions

A large set of data can be conveniently displayed using a cumulative frequency table or plot. The data are first ordered and, with a large data set, may be arranged in a frequency table with n class intervals. The frequency, often expressed as a proportion (or percentage), of values equal to or less than a given value, X_i, is calculated for each specified value of X_i, where X_i is the upper point of the class interval (i = 1 to n). A plot of the cumulative proportion versus X can be used to determine the proportion of values that lie in some interval, i.e., between some specified limits. The cumulative distribution for the tablet potencies in Table 1.4 is shown in Table 1.5 and plotted in Fig. 1.1. The cumulative proportion represents the proportion of values less than or equal to X_i (e.g., 29% of the values are less than or equal to 98.5). Also, for

Table 1.4   Frequency Distribution of Tablet Potencies

Potency (mg)	Frequency, W_i[a]	X_i[b]	Potency (mg)	Frequency, W_i	X_i
89.5– 90.5	1	90	100.5–101.5	17	101
90.5– 91.5	0	91	101.5–102.5	13	102
91.5– 92.5	2	92	102.5–103.5	9	103
92.5– 93.5	1	93	103.5–104.5	0	104
93.5– 94.5	5	94	104.5–105.5	0	105
94.5– 95.5	1	95	105.5–106.5	5	106
95.5– 96.5	2	96	106.5–107.5	4	107
96.5– 97.5	7	97	107.5–108.5	0	108
97.5– 98.5	10	98	108.5–109.5	0	109
98.5– 99.5	8	99	109.5–110.5	2	110
99.5–100.5	13	100		$\Sigma/W_i = 100$	

[a] W_i is the frequency.
[b] X_i is the midpoint of the interval.

Table 1.5   Cumulative Frequency Distribution of
Tablet Potencies (Taken from Table 1.4)

Potency, X_i (mg)[a]	Cumulative frequency ($\leqslant$ X)	Cumulative proportion
90.5	1	0.01
92.5	3	0.03
93.5	4	0.04
94.5	9	0.09
95.5	10	0.10
96.5	12	0.12
97.5	19	0.19
98.5	29	0.29
99.5	37	0.37
100.5	50	0.50
101.5	67	0.67
102.5	80	0.80
103.5	89	0.89
106.5	94	0.94
107.5	98	0.98
110.5	100	1.00

[a]X_i is the upper point of the class interval in
Table 1.4, excluding null intervals.

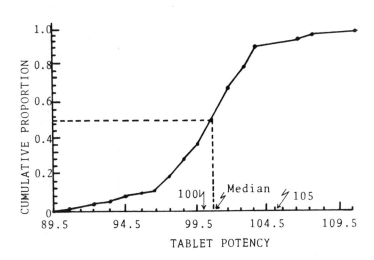

Figure 1.1   Cumulative proportion plot for data in Table 1.5
(tablet potencies).

example, from an inspection of Fig. 1.1, one can estimate the proportion of tablets with potencies between 100 and 105 mg inclusive,
equal to approximately 0.48 (0.91 at 105 mg minus 0.43 at 100 mg).
(See also Exercise Problem 5.)

The cumulative distribution is a very important concept in
statistics. In particular, the application of the cumulative normal
distribution, which is concerned with continuous data, will be discussed in Chap. 3. A more detailed account of the construction and
interpretation of frequency distribution is given in Refs. 3−5.

1.3 SAMPLE AND POPULATION

Understanding the concepts of samples and populations is important
when discussing statistical procedures. *Samples* are usually a relatively small number of observations taken from a relatively large
population or universe. The sample values are the observations,
the data, obtained from the population. The population consists of
data with some clearly defined characteristic(s). For example, a
population may consist of all patients with a particular disease, or
tablets from a production batch. The sample in these cases could
consist of a selection of patients to participate in a clinical study,
or tablets chosen for a weight determination. The sample is only
part of the available data. In the usual experimental situation, we
make observations on a relatively small sample in order to make
inferences about the characteristics of the whole, the population.
The totality of available data is the population or universe. When
designing an experiment, the population should be clearly defined
so that samples chosen are representative of the population. This
is important in clinical trials, for example, where inferences to the
treatment of disease states are crucial. The exact nature or character of the population is rarely known, and often impossible to as-
certain, although we can make assumptions about its properties.
Theoretically, a population can be finite or infinite in the number of
its elements. For example, a finished package contains a finite number of tablets; all possible tablets made by a particular process,
past, present, and future, can be considered infinite in concept.
In most of our examples, the population will be considered to be
infinite, or at least very large compared to the sample size. Table
1.6 shows some populations and samples, examples which should be
familiar to the pharmaceutical scientist.

1.3.1 Population Parameters and Sample Statistics

"Any measurable characteristic of the universe is called a *parameter*"
[6]. For example, the average weight of a batch of tablets or the

Table 1.6 Examples of Samples and Populations

Population	Sample
Tablet batch	Twenty tablets taken for content uniformity
Normal males between ages 18 and 65 years available to hospital	Twenty-four subjects selected for a phase I clinical study
Sprague-Dawley Weaning rats	100 rats selected to test possible toxic effects of a new drug candidate
Analysts working for company X	Three analysts from a company to test a new assay method
Persons with diastolic blood pressure between 105 and 120 mmHg in the United States	120 patients with diastolic pressure between 105 and 120 mmHg to enter clinical study to compare two antihypertensive agents
Serum cholesterol levels of one patient	Blood samples drawn once a week for 3 months from a single patient

average blood pressure of hypertensive persons in the United States are parameters of the respective populations. Parameters are generally denoted by Greek letters; for example, the mean of the population is denoted as μ. Note that parameters are characteristic of the population, and are values that are usually unknown to us.

Quantities derived from the sample are called *sample statistics*. Corresponding to the true average weight of a batch of tablets is the average weight for the small sample taken from the population of tablets. We should be very clear about the nature of samples. Emphasis is placed here (and throughout this book) on the variable nature of such sample statistics. A parameter, for example, the mean weight of a batch of tablets, is a fixed value; it does not vary. Sample statistics are variable. Their values depend on the particular sample chosen and the variability of the measurement. The average weight of 10 tablets will differ from sample to sample because:

1. We choose 10 different tablets at each sampling.
2. The balance (and our ability to read it) is not exactly reproducible from one weighing to another.

   An important part of the statistical process is the characterization of a population by estimating its parameters. The parameters
can be estimated by evaluating suitable sample statistics. The reader will probably have little trouble in understanding that the average
weight of a sample of tablets (a sample statistic) estimates the true
mean weight (a parameter) of the batch. This concept is elucidated
and expanded in the remaining sections of this chapter.

1.4   MEASURES DESCRIBING THE CENTER
OF DATA DISTRIBUTIONS

1.4.1   The Average

Probably the most familiar statistical term in popular use is the
average, denoted by $\overline{X}$ (X bar). The average is also commonly
known as the *mean* or *arithmetic average*. The average is a summarizing statistic and is a measure of the center of a distribution,
particularly meaningful if the data are symmetrically distributed
below and above the average. Symbolically, the mean is equal to

$$\frac{\sum_{i=1}^{N} X_i}{N} \tag{1.1}$$

the sum of the observations divided by the number of observations.
$\sum_{i=1}^{N} X_i$ is the sum of the N values, each denoted by X_i (X_1, X_2,
. . . , X_n), where i can take on the values 1, 2, 3, 4, . . . , N.*
The average of the values 7, 11, 6, 5, and 4 is

$$\frac{7 + 11 + 6 + 5 + 4}{5} = 6.6$$

This is an unweighted average, each value contributing equally to
the average. A *weighted average* is one in which the contribution,
or weights, of the different data points that comprise the mean are
not the same. A weighted mean is calculated as

$$\frac{\sum W_i X_i}{\sum W_i} \tag{1.2}$$

---

*For the most part, when using summation notation in this book, we
will not use the full notation, such as $\sum_{i=1}^{N} X_i$, but rather $\sum X$, the
i notation being implied, unless otherwise stated.

where W_i is the weight associated with X_i. The weights for the calculation of a weighted average are often the number of observations associated with the values X_i. This concept is illustrated for the calculation of the average for data categorized in the form of a frequency distribution. Table 1.4 shows a frequency distribution of 100 tablet potencies. The frequency is the number of observations of tablets in a given class interval, as defined previously. The frequency or number of tablets in a "potency" interval is the *weight* used in the computation of the weighted average. The value X associated with the weight is taken as the midpoint of the interval; for example, for the first interval, 89.5 to 90.5, $X_1 = 90$. Applying Eq. (1.2), the weighted average is $\Sigma\ W_i X_i / \Sigma\ W_i$:

$$\frac{1 \times 90 + 0 \times 91 + 2 \times 92 + 1 \times 93 + 5 \times 94 + \cdots + 4 \times 107 + 2 \times 110}{1 + 0 + 2 + 1 + 5 \cdots + 4 + 2}$$

which equals $10,023/100 = 100.23$ mg.

Two other kinds of averages that are sometimes found in statistical procedures are the geometric and harmonic means. The *geometric mean* is defined as

$$\sqrt[n]{X_1 \cdot X_2 \cdot X_3 \cdots X_n}$$

or the nth root of the product of n observations.

The geometric mean of the numbers 50, 100, and 200 is

$$\sqrt[3]{50 \cdot 100 \cdot 200} = \sqrt[3]{1,000,000} = 100$$

If a measurement of population growth shows 50 at time 0, 100 after one day, and 200 after 2 days, the geometric mean (100) is more meaningful than the arithmetic mean (116.7). The geometric mean is always less than or equal to the arithmetic mean, and is meaningful for data with logarithmic relationships. Note that the logarithm of $\sqrt[3]{50 \cdot 100 \cdot 200}$ is equal to $[\log 50 + \log 100 + \log 200]/3$, which is the average of the logarithms of the observations. The geometric mean is the antilog of this average (the antilog of the average is 100).

The harmonic mean is the appropriate average following a reciprocal transformation (Chap. 10). The harmonic mean is defined as

$$\frac{N}{\Sigma\ 1/X_i}$$

For the 3 observations 2, 4, and 8 (N = 3), the harmonic mean is

$$\frac{3}{1/2 + 1/4 + 1/8} = 3.429$$

1.4.2   The Median

Although the average is the most often used measure of centrality, the *median* is also a common measure of the center of a data set. When computing the average, very large or very small values can have a significant effect on the magnitude of the average. For example, the average of the numbers 0, 1, 2, 3, and 34 is 8. The arithmetic average acts as the fulcrum of a balanced beam, with weights placed at points corresponding to the individual values, as shown in Fig. 1.2. The single value 34 needs four values, 0, 1, 2, and 3, as a counterbalance.

The *median* represents the center of a data set, without regard for the distance of each point from the center. The median is that value which divides the data in half, half the values being less than and half the values greater than the median value. The median is easily obtained when the data are ranked in order of magnitude. The median of an odd number of *different** observations is the middle value. For $2N + 1$ values, the median is the $(N + 1)$th ordered value. The median of the data 0, 1, 2, 3, and 34 is the third (middle) value, 2 ($N = 2$, $2N + 1 = 5$ values). By convention, the median for an even number of data points is considered to be the average of the two center points. For example, the median of the numbers 0, 1, 2, and 3 is the average of the center points, 1 and 2, equal to $(1 + 2)/2 = 1.5$. The median is often used as a description of the center of a data set when the data have an asymmetrical distribution. In the presence of either extremely high or extremely low outlying values, the median appears to describe the distribution better than does the average. The median is more stable than the average in the presence of extreme observations. A very large or very small value has the same effect on the calculation of the median as any other value, larger or smaller than the median, respectively. On the other hand, as noted previously, very large and very small values have a significant effect on the magnitude of the mean.

The distribution of individual yearly incomes, which have relatively few very large values (the multimillionaires), serves as a good example of the use of the median as a descriptive statistic. Because of the large influence of these extreme values, the average income is higher than one might expect on an intuitive basis. The

---

*If the median value is not unique, that is, two or more values are equal to the median, the median is calculated by interpolation [3].

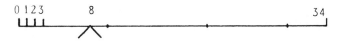

0 1 2 3   8   3 4

Figure 1.2 Average illustrated as balancing forces.

median income, which is less than the average income, represents a
figure that is readily interpreted; that is, one-half of the population earns more (or less) than the median income.

The distribution of particle sizes for bulk powders used in
pharmaceutical products is often skewed. In these cases, the
median is a better descriptor of the centrality of the distribution
than is the mean [7]. The median is less efficient than the mean
as an estimate of the center of a distribution; that is, the median
is more variable [8]. For most of the problems discussed in this
book, we will be concerned with the mean rather than the median
as a measure of centrality.

The median is also known as the *50th percentile* of a distribution. To compute percentiles, the data are ranked in order of
magnitude, from smallest to largest. The nth percentile denotes a
value below which n percent of the data are found, and above which
(100 - n) percent of the data are found. The 10th, 25th, and 75th
percentiles represent values below which 10%, 25%, and 75%, respectively, of the data occur. For the tablet potencies shown in
Table 1.5, the 10th percentile is 95.5 mg; 10% of the tablets contain less than 95.5 mg and 90% of the tablets contain more than
95.5 mg of drug. The 25th, 50th, and 75th percentiles are also
known as the first, second, and third quartiles, respectively.

The *mode* is less often used as the central, or typical, value of
a distribution. The mode is that value which occurs with the
greatest frequency. For a symmetrical distribution that peaks in
the center, such as the normal distribution (see Chap. 3) the mode,
median, and mean are identical. For data skewed to the right
(e.g., incomes), which contain a relatively few very large values,
the mean is larger than the median, which is larger than the mode
(see Fig. 10.1, Ch. 10).

1.5 MEASUREMENT OF THE SPREAD
OF DATA

The mean (or median) alone gives no insight or information about
the spread or range of values that comprise a data set. For example, a mean of five values equal to 10 may be comprised of the
numbers

0, 5, 10, 15, and 20   or   5, 10, 10, 10, and 15

The mean, coupled with the *standard deviation* or *range*, is a suc-
cinct and minimal description of a group of experimental observations or a data distribution. The standard deviation and the range
are measures of the spread of the data; the larger the magnitude of
the standard deviation or range, the more spread out the data are.
A standard deviation of 10 implies a wider range of values than a
standard deviation of 3, for example.

1.5.1   Range

The *range*, denoted as R, is the difference between the smallest
and the largest values in the data set. For the data in Table 1.1,
the range is 152, from -97 to +55 mg %. The range is based on
only two values, the smallest and largest, and is more variable than
the standard deviation (i.e., it is less stable).

1.5.2   Standard Deviation and Variance

The *standard deviation*, denoted as s.d. or S, is calculated as

$$\sqrt{\frac{\Sigma \ (X \ - \ \overline{X})^2}{N \ - \ 1}} \tag{1.3}$$

where N is the number of data points (or sample size) and $\Sigma \ (X \ - \ \overline{X})^2$
is the *sum of squares* of the differences of each value from the
mean, $\overline{X}$. The standard deviation is more difficult to calculate than
is the range.

Consider a group of data points: 101.8, 103.2, 104.0, 102.5,
and 103.5. The mean is 103.0. Details of the calculation of the
standard deviation are shown in Table 1.7. Each value is sub-
tracted from the mean: $X - \overline{X}$. These differences are squared,
$(X - \overline{X})^2$, and summed. The sum of the squared differences
divided by N - 1 is calculated, and the square root of this result
is the standard deviation.

With the accessibility of electronic calculators and computers, it
is rare, nowadays, to hand-compute a mean and standard deviation
(or any other calculation, for that matter). Nevertheless, when
computing the standard deviation by hand (or with the help of a
calculator), a well-known shortcut computing formula is recommended. The short-cut is based on the identity

$$\Sigma \ (X \ - \ \overline{X})^2 = \Sigma \ X^2 - \frac{(\Sigma \ X)^2}{N}$$

Table 1.7 Calculation of the Standard Deviation

X	$\overline{X}$	$X - \overline{X}$	$(X - \overline{X})^2$
101.8	103	-1.2	1.44
103.2	103	0.2	0.04
104.0	103	1.0	1.00
102.5	103	-0.5	0.25
103.5	103	0.5	0.25

$\Sigma X = 515$ $\qquad\qquad\qquad\qquad \Sigma (X - \overline{X})^2 = 2.98$

$$\text{s.d.} = \sqrt{\frac{\Sigma (X - \overline{X})^2}{N - 1}} = \sqrt{\frac{2.98}{4}} = 0.86$$

Therefore,

$$\text{s.d.} = \sqrt{\frac{\Sigma X^2 - (\Sigma X)^2/N}{N - 1}} \qquad (1.4)$$

where ΣX^2 is the sum of each value squared and $(\Sigma X)^2$ is the square of the sum of all the values $[(\Sigma X)^2/N$ is also known as the *correction term*]. We will apply this important formula, Eq. (1.4), to the data above to illustrate the calculation of the standard deviation. This result will be compared to that obtained by the more time-consuming method of squaring each deviation from the mean (Table 1.7).

$$\Sigma (X - \overline{X})^2 = 101.8^2 + 103.2^2 + 104.0^2 + 102.5^2 + 103.5^2 - \frac{515^2}{5}$$

$$= 2.98$$

The standard deviation is $\sqrt{2.98/4} = 0.86$, as before.

The *variance* is the square of the standard deviation, often represented as S^2. The variance is calculated as

$$S^2 = \frac{\Sigma (X - \overline{X})^2}{N - 1} \qquad (1.5)$$

In the example of the data in Table 1.7, the variance, S^2, is

$$\frac{2.98}{4} = 0.745$$

A question that often puzzles new students of statistics is: Why use N - 1 rather than N in the denominator in the expression for the standard deviation or variance [Eqs. (1.3) and (1.5)]?

The *variance of the population*, a parameter traditionally denoted as σ^2 (sigma squared), is calculated as*

$$\sigma^2 = \frac{\Sigma \ (X - \overline{X})^2}{N} \tag{1.6}$$

where N is the number of all possible values in the population. The use of N - 1 rather than N in the calculation of the variance of a *sample* (a sample statistic) makes the sample variance an *unbiased estimate* of the population variance. Because the sample variance is variable (a random variable), in any given experiment, S^2 will not be exactly equal to the true population variance, σ^2. However, in the long run, S^2 (calculated with N - 1 in the denominator) will equal σ^2, on the average. "On the average" means that if samples of size N were repeatedly randomly selected from the population, and the variance calculated for each sample, the averages of these calculated variance estimates would equal σ^2. Note that the sample variance is an *estimate* of the true population variance σ^2.

If S^2 estimates σ^2 on the average, the sample variance is an unbiased estimate of the population variance. It can be proven that the sample variance calculated with N - 1 in the denominator is an unbiased estimate of σ^2. To try to verify this fact by repeating exactly the same laboratory or clinical experiment (if the population variance were known) would be impractical. However, for explanatory purposes, it is often useful to illustrate certain theorems by showing what would happen upon repeated sampling from the same population. The concept of the unbiased nature of the sample variance can be demonstrated using a population that consists of three values: 0, 1, and 2. The population variance, $\Sigma \ (X - \overline{X})^2/3$, is equal to 2/3 [see Eq. (1.6)]. Using the repeated sampling approach noted above, samples of size 2 are repeatedly selected at random from this population. The first choice is replaced before selection of the second choice so that each of the three values has an equal chance of being selected on both the first and second selection. (This is known as *sampling with replacement*.) The following possibilities of samples of size 2 are equally likely to be chosen:

---

*Strictly speaking, this formula is for a population with a finite number of data points.

0, 1; 1, 0; 0, 2; 2, 0; 1, 2; 2, 1; 1, 1; 2, 2; 0, 0

The *sample variance** of these nine pairs are [$\Sigma (X - \overline{X})^2/(N - 1)$]
0.5, 0.5, 2, 2, 0.5, 0.5, 0, 0, and 0, respectively. The average
of the nine equally likely possible variances is

$$\frac{0.5 + 0.5 + 2 + 2 + 0.5 + 0.5 + 0 + 0 + 0}{9} = \frac{6}{9} = \frac{2}{3}$$

exactly equal to the population variance. This demonstrates the unbiased character of the sample variance. The sample standard deviation [Eq. (1.3)] is not an unbiased estimate of the *population
standard deviation*, σ, which for a finite population is calculated as

$$\sqrt{\frac{\Sigma (X - \overline{X})^2}{N}} \tag{1.7}$$

The unbiased nature of a *sample estimate* of a *population parameter*,
such as the variance or the mean, is a desirable characteristic. $\overline{X}$,
the sample estimate of the true population mean, is also an unbiased
estimate of the true mean. (The true mean is designated by the
Greek letter μ. In general, population parameters are denoted by
Greek letters, as noted previously.)

One should be aware that some calculators which have a built-in
function for calculating the standard deviation use N in the denominator of the formula for the standard deviation. As we have emphasized above, this is correct for the calculation of the population
standard deviation (or variance), and will be close to the calculation
of the unbiased sample standard deviation when N is large.

The value of N - 1 is also known as the *degrees of freedom* for
the sample (later we will come across situations where degrees of
freedom are less than N - 1). The concept of degrees of freedom
(denoted as d.f.) is very important in statistics, and we will have
to know the degrees of freedom for the variance estimates used in
statistical tests to be described in subsequent chapters.

1.5.3 Coefficient of Variation

The variability of data may often be better described as a relative
variation rather than as an absolute variation, such as that represented by the standard deviation or range. One common way of

---

*For samples of size 2, the variance is simply calculated as the
square of the difference of the values divided by 2, $d^2/2$. For
example, the variance of 0 and 1 is $(1 - 0)^2/2 = 0.5$.

expressing the variability, which takes into account its relative magnitude, is the ratio of the standard deviation to the mean, s.d./ $\bar{X}$. This ratio, often expressed as a percentage, is called the *coefficient of variation*, abbreviated as C.V. A coefficient of variation of 0.1 or 10% means that the s.d. is one-tenth of the mean. This way of expressing variability is useful in many situations. It puts the variability in perspective relative to the magnitude of the measurements and allows a comparison of the variability of different kinds of measurements. For example, a group of rats of average weight 100 g and s.d. of 10 g has the same relative variation (C.V.) as a group of animals with average weight 70 g and standard deviation of 7 g. Many measurements have an almost constant C.V., the magnitude of the s.d. being proportional to the mean. In biological data, the coefficient of variation is often between 20 and 50%, and one would not be surprised to see an occasional C.V. as high as 100% or more. The relatively large C.V. observed in biological experiments is due mostly to "biological variation," the lack of reproducibility in living material. On the other hand, the variability in chemical and instrumental analyses of drugs is usually relatively small. Thus it is not unusual to find a C.V. of less than 1% for some analytical procedures.

1.5.4   Standard Deviation of the Mean
(Standard Error of the Mean)

The standard deviation is a measure of the spread of a group of individual observations, a measure of their variability. In statistical procedures to be discussed in this book, we are more concerned with making inferences about the mean of a distribution rather than with individual values. In these cases, the variability of the mean rather than the variability of individual values is of interest. The sample mean is a random variable, just as the individual values that comprise the mean are variable. Thus repeated sampling of means from the same population will result in a distribution of means which has its own mean and standard deviation.

The *standard deviation of the mean*, commonly known as the *standard error of the mean*, is a measure of the variability of the mean. For example, the average potency of the 100 tablets shown in Table 1.4 may have been determined to estimate the average potency of the population, in this case, a production batch. An estimate of the variability of the mean value would be useful. The mean tablet potency is 100.23 mg and the standard deviation is 3.687. To compute the standard deviation of the mean (also designated as $S_{\bar{X}}$), we might assay several more sets of 100 tablets and calculate the mean potency of each sample. This repeated sampling would result in a group of means, each composed of 100 tablets,

Table 1.8   Means of Potencies of Five
Sets of 100 Tablets Selected from a
Production Batch

Sample	Mean potency
1	99.84
2	100.23
3	100.50
4	100.96
5	100.07

with different values, such as the five means shown in Table 1.8.
The standard deviation of this group of means can be calculated in
the same manner as the individual values are calculated [Eq. (1.3)].
The standard deviation of these five means is 0.431. We can anticipate that the s.d. of the means will be considerably smaller
than the s.d. calculated from the 100 individual potencies. This
fact is easily comprehended if one conceives of the mean as
"averaging out" the extreme individual values that may occur among
the individual data. The means of very large samples taken from
the same population are very stable, tending to cluster closer together than the individual data, as illustrated in Table 1.8.

Fortunately, we do not have to perform real or simulated
sampling experiments, such as weighing five sets of 100 tablets each,
to obtain replicate data in order to estimate the s.d. of means.
Statistical theory shows that the standard deviation of mean values
is equal to the standard deviation calculated from the individual
data divided by $\sqrt{N}$, where N is the sample size:*

$$S_{\overline{X}} = \frac{S}{\sqrt{N}} \tag{1.8}$$

The standard deviation of the numbers shown in Table 1.4 is 3.687.
Therefore, the standard deviation of the mean for the potencies of
100 tablets shown in Table 1.4 is estimated as $S/\sqrt{N} = 3.687/\sqrt{100} =$
0.3687. This theory verifies our intuition; the s.d. of means is
smaller than the s.d. of the individual data points. The student
should not be confused by the two estimates of the standard deviation of the mean illustrated above. In the usual circumstance, the

---

*The variance of a mean, $S_{\overline{X}}^2$, is S^2/N.

estimate is derived as $S/\sqrt{N}$ (0.3687 in this example). The data in Table 1.8 were used only to illustrate the concept of a standard deviation of a mean. In any event, the two estimates are not expected to agree exactly; after all, the s.d. *is* also a random variable and *only* estimates the true value, $\sigma/\sqrt{N}$.

As the sample size increases, the standard deviation of the mean becomes smaller and smaller. We can reduce the s.d. of the mean, $S_{\overline{X}}$, to a very small value by increasing N. Thus means of very large samples hardly vary at all. The concept of the standard deviation of the mean is important, and the student will find it well worth the extra effort made to understand the meaning and implications of $S_{\overline{X}}$.

1.6   CODING

From both a practical and a theoretical point of view, it is useful to understand how the mean and standard deviation of a group of numbers are affected by certain arithmetic manipulations, particularly adding a constant to, or subtracting a constant from each value; and multiplying or dividing each value by a constant.

Consider the following data to exemplify the results described below:

$$\boxed{2,\ 3,\ 5,\ 10}$$

Mean = $\overline{X}$ = 5

Variance = S^2 = 12.67

Standard deviation = S = 3.56

1. Addition or subtraction of a constant will cause the mean to be increased or decreased by the constant, but will not change the variance or standard deviation. For example, adding +3 to each value results in the following data:

$$\boxed{5,\ 6,\ 8,\ 13}$$

$\overline{X}$ = 8

S = 3.56

Subtracting 2 from each value results in

$$\boxed{0,\ 1,\ 3,\ 8}$$

$\overline{X} = 3$

$S = 3.56$

This property may be used to advantage when hand calculating the mean and standard deviation of very large or cumbersome numbers. Consider the following data:

$$1251, \ 1257, \ 1253, \ 1255$$

Subtracting 1250 from each value we obtain

$$1, \ 7, \ 3, \ 5$$

$\overline{X} = 4$

$S = 2.58$

To obtain the mean of the original values, add 1250 to the mean obtained above, 4. The standard deviation is unchanged. For the original data

$\overline{X} = 1250 + 4 = 1254$

$S = 2.58$

This manipulation is expressed in Eq. (1.9) where X_i represents one of n observations from a population with variance σ^2. C is a constant and $\overline{X}$ is the average of the X_i's.

$$\text{Average } (X_i + C) = \Sigma(X_i + C)/n = \overline{X} + C \tag{1.9}$$

$$\text{Variance } (X_i + C) = \sigma^2$$

2. If the mean of a set of data is $\overline{X}$ and the standard deviation is S, multiplying or dividing each value by a constant k results in a new mean of $k\overline{X}$ or $\overline{X}/k$, respectively, and a new standard deviation of kS or S/k, respectively. Multiplying each of the original values above by 3 results in

$$6, \ 9, \ 15, \ 30$$

$\overline{X} = 15$ (3 × 5)

$S = 10.68$ (3 × 3.56)

Dividing each value by 2 results in

| 1, 1.5, 2.5, 5 |

$\overline{X} = 2.5$ $(5/2)$

$S = 1.78$ $(3.56/2)$

In general,

Average $(C \cdot X_i) = C \ \overline{X}$ (1.10)

Variance $(C \cdot X_i) = C^2 \ \sigma^2$

These results can be used to show that a set of data with mean $\overline{X}$ and standard deviation equal to S can be converted to data with a mean of 0 and a standard deviation of 1 (as in the "standardization" of normal curves, discussed in Sec. 3.4.1). If the mean is sub-tracted from each value, and this result is divided by S, the re-sultant data have a mean of 0 and a standard deviation of 1. The transformation is

$$\frac{X - \overline{X}}{S}$$ (1.11)

Standard scores are values that have been transformed according to Eq. (1.11) [9]. For the original data, the first value 2 is changed to $(2 - 5)/3.56$ equal to -0.84. The interested reader may verify that transforming the values in this way results in a mean of 0 and a s.d. of 1.

1.7   PRECISION, ACCURACY, AND BIAS

When dealing with variable measurements, the definitions of *precision* and *accuracy*, often obscure and not distinguished in ordinary usage, should be clearly defined from a statistical point of view.

1.7.1   Precision

In the vocabulary of statistics, *precision* refers to the extent of variability of a group of measurements observed under similar ex-perimental conditions. A precise set of measurements is compact. Observations, relatively close in magnitude, are considered to be precise as reflected by a small standard deviation. (Note that means are more precisely measured than individual observations according to this definition.) An important, sometimes elusive concept is that a precise set of measurements may have the same mean as an imprecise set. In most experiments with which we will be concerned, the mean and standard deviation of the data are independent (i.e., they are unrelated). Fig. 1.3 shows the results of two assay methods, each performed in triplicate. Both methods have an average result of 100%, but method II is more precise.

1.7.2 Accuracy

Accuracy refers to the closeness of an individual observation or mean to the true value. The "true" value is that result which would be observed in the absence of error (e.g., the true mean tablet potency or the true drug content of a preparation being assayed). In the example of the assay results shown in Fig. 1.3, both methods are apparently equally accurate (or inaccurate).

Figure 1.4 shows the results of two dissolution methods for two formulations of the same drug, each formulation replicated four times by each method. The objective of the in vitro dissolution test is to simulate the in vivo oral absorption of the drug from the two dosage-form modifications. The first dissolution method, A, is very precise but does not give an accurate prediction of the in vivo results. According to the dissolution data for method A, we would expect that formulation I would be more rapidly and extensively absorbed in vivo. The actual in vivo results depicted in Fig. 1.4 show the contrary result. The less precise method, method B in this example, is a more *accurate* predictor of the true in vivo results. This example is meant to show that a precise measurement need not be accurate, nor an accurate measurement precise.

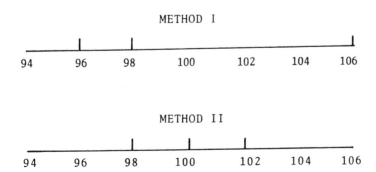

Figure 1.3 Representation of two analytical methods with the same accuracy but different precisions.

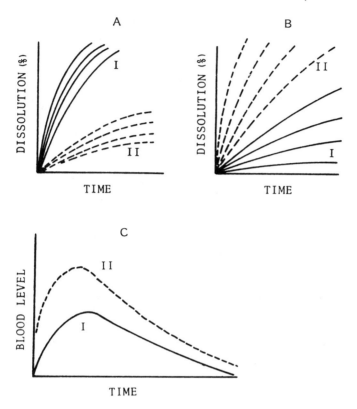

Figure 1.4 In vitro dissolution results for two formu̶a̶t̶i̶o̶ns using two different methods and in vivo blood level versus time results. Methods A and B, in vitro; C, in vivo.

Of course, the best circumstance is to have data that are both precise and accurate. If possible, we should make efforts to improve both the accuracy and precision of experimental observations. For example, in drug analysis, advanced electronic instrumentation can greatly increase the accuracy and precision of assay results.

1.7.3   Bias

Accuracy can also be associated with the term *bias*. The notion of bias has been discussed in Sec. 1.4 in relation to the concept of unbiased estimates (e.g., the mean and variance). The meaning of bias in statistics is similar to the everyday definition in terms of "fairness." An accurate measurement, no matter what the precision,

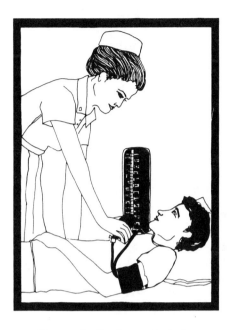 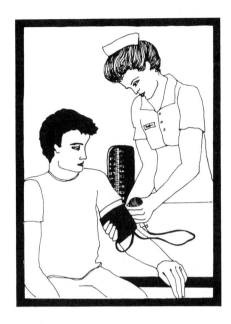

Nurse 1 (before study)   Nurse 2 (during study)

Figure 1.5 Bias in determining the effect of an antihypertensive drug.

can be thought of as unbiased, because an accurate measurement is
a "fair" estimate of the true result. A biased estimate is systematically either higher or lower than the true value. A biased estimate can be thought of as giving an "unfair" notion of the true
value. For example, when estimating the average result of experimental data, the mean, $\overline{X}$, represents an estimate of the true population parameter, μ, and in this sense is considered accurate and
unbiased. An average blood pressure reduction of 10 mmHg due to
an antihypertensive agent, derived from data from a clinical study
of 200 patients, can be thought of as an unbiased estimate of the
true blood pressure reduction due to the drug, provided that the
patients are appropriately selected at "random." The true reduction in this case is the average reduction that would be observed
if the antihypertensive effect of the drug were known for all members of the population (e.g., all hypertensive patients). The

outcome of a single experiment, such as the 10 mmHg reduction observed in the 200 patients above, will in all probability not be
identical to the true mean reduction. But the mean reduction as
observed in the 200 patients is an accurate and unbiased assessment
of the population average. A biased estimate is one which, on the
average, does not equal the population parameter. In the example
cited above for hypertensives, a biased estimate would result if for
all patients one nurse took all the measurements before therapy and
another nurse took all measurements during therapy, and each nurse
had a different criterion or method for determining blood pressure.
See Fig. 1.5 for a clarification as to why this procedure leads to a
biased estimate of the drug's effectiveness in reducing blood pressure. If the supine position results in higher blood pressure than
the sitting position, the results of the study will tend to show a
bias in the direction of too large a blood pressure reduction.

The statistical estimates that we usually use, such as the mean
and variance, are unbiased estimates. Bias often results from (a)
the improper use of experimental design; (b) improper choice of
samples; (c) unconscious bias, due to lack of blinding, for example;
or (d) improper observation and recording of data, such as that
illustrated in Fig. 1.5.

1.8   THE QUESTION OF SIGNIFICANT FIGURES

The question of *significant figures* is an important consideration in
statistical calculations and presentations. In general, the ordinary
rules for retaining significant figures are *not* applicable to statistical
computations. Contrary to the usual rules for retaining significant
figures, one should retain as many figures as possible when performing statistical calculations, not rounding off until all computations
are complete.

The reason for not rounding off during statistical computations
is that untenable answers may result when using computational procedures which involve taking differences between values very close
in magnitude if values are rounded off prior to taking differences.
This may occur when calculating "sums of squares" (the sum of
squared differences from the mean) using the shortcut formula,
Eq. (1.4), for the calculation of the variance or standard deviation.
The shortcut formula for $\Sigma (X - \bar{X})^2$ is $\Sigma X^2 - (\Sigma X)^2/N$, which cannot be negative, and will be equal to zero only if all the data have
the same value. If the two terms, ΣX^2 and $(\Sigma X)^2/N$, are very
similar in magnitude, rounding off before taking their difference
may result in a zero or negative difference. This problem is illustrated by calculating the standard deviation of the three numbers,
1.19, 1.20, and 1.21. If the squares of these numbers are first

rounded off to two decimal places, the following calculation of the standard deviation results:

$$S = \sqrt{\frac{\Sigma\ X^2 - (\Sigma\ X)^2/N}{N - 1}} = \sqrt{\frac{1.42 + 1.44 + 1.46 - 3.6^2/3}{2}}$$

$$= \sqrt{\frac{4.32 - 4.32}{2}} = 0$$

The correct standard deviation calculated without rounding off is 0.01.

Computers and calculators carry many digits when performing calculations and do not round off further unless instructed to do so. These instruments retain as many digits as their capacity permits through all arithmetic computations. The possibility of rounding off, even considering the large capacity of modern computers, can cause unexpected problems in sophisticated statistical calculations, and must be taken into account in preparing statistical software programs. These problems can usually be overcome by using special programming techniques.

At the completion of the calculations, as many figures as are appropriate to the situation can be presented. Common sense and the usual rules for reporting significant figures should be applied (see Ref. 7 for a detailed discussion of significant figures). Sokal and Rohlf [7] recommend that, if possible, observations should be measured with enough significant figures so that the range of data is between 30 and 300 possible values. This flexible rule results in a relative error of less than 3%. For example, when measuring diastolic blood pressure, the range of values for a particular group of patients might be limited to 60 to 130 mmHg. Therefore, measurements to the nearest mmHg would result in approximately 70 possible values, and would be measured with sufficient accuracy according to this rule. If the investigator can make the measurement only in intervals of 2 mmHg (e.g., 70 and 72 mmHg can be measured, but not 71 mmHg), we would have 35 possible data points, which is still within the 30 to 300 suggested by this rule of thumb. Of course, rules should not be taken as "written in stone." All rules should be applied with judgment.

Common sense should be applied when reporting average results. For example, reporting an average blood pressure reduction of 7.42857 for 14 patients treated with an antihypertensive agent would not be appropriate. As noted above, most physicians would say that blood pressure is rarely measured to within 2 mmHg. Why should one bother to report any decimals at all for the average result? When reporting average results, it is generally good practice to report the average with a precision that is "reasonable" according

to the nature of the data. An average of 7.4 mmHg would probably suffice for this example. If the average were reported as
7 mmHg, for example, it would appear that too much information is
suppressed.

KEY TERMS

Accuracy   Precision
Attributes   Random variable
Average ($\overline{X}$)   Range
Bias   Ranking
Coding   Rating scale
Coefficient of variation (C.V.)   Sample
Continuous variables   Significant figures
Correction term (C.T.)   Standard deviation (s.d.)
Cumulative distribution   Standard error of the mean ($S_{\overline{X}}$)
Degrees of freedom (d.f.)   Standard score
Discrete variables   Treatment
Frequency distribution   Unbiased sample
Geometric mean   Universe
Harmonic mean   Variability
Mean ($\overline{X}$)   Variable
Median   Weighted average
Population

EXERCISES

1. List three experiments whose outcomes will result in each of the
    following kinds of variables.
    (a) Continuous variables
    (b) Discrete variables
    (c) Ordered variables
    (d) Categorical (attribute) variables
2. What difference in experimental conclusions, if any, would re-
    sult if the pain scale discussed in Sec. 1.1 were revised as:
    no pain = 6, slight pain = 4, moderate pain = 2, and severe
    pain = 0? (Hint: See Sec. 1.6.)
3. (a) Construct a frequency distribution containing 10 class inter-
         vals from the data in Table 1.1.
    (b) Construct a cumulative frequency plot based on the fre-
         quency distribution from part (a).
4. What is the average result based on the frequency distribution
    in part (a) of problem 3? Use a weighted-average procedure.

5. From Fig. 1.1, what proportion of tablets have potencies be-
    tween 95 and 105 mg? What proportion of tablets have a
    potency greater than 105 mg?

6. Calculate the average and standard deviation of (a) the first
    20 values in Table 1.1 and (b) the last 20 values in Table
    1.1. If these data came from two different clinical investi-
    gators, would you think that the differences in these two
    sets of data can be attributed to differences in clinical sites?
    Which set, the first or last, is more precise? Explain your
    answer.

7. What are the median and range of the first 20 values in
    Table 1.1?

8. (a) If the first value in Table 1.1 were +100 instead of +17,
        what would be the values of the median and range for
        the first 20 values?

    (b) Using the first value as 100, calculate the mean, stand-
        ard deviation, and variance. Compre the results for
        these first 20 values to the answers obtained in Prob-
        lem 6.

**9. Given the following sample characteristics, describe the pop-
    ulation from which the sample may have been derived. The
    mean is 100, the standard deviation is 50, the median is 75,
    and the range is 125.

**10. If the population average for the cholesterol reductions shown
    in Table 1.1 were somehow known to be 0 (the drug does not
    affect cholesterol levels on the average), would you believe
    that this sample of 156 patients gives an unbiased estimate of
    the true average? Describe possible situations in which
    these data might yield (a) biased results; (b) unbiased
    results.

**11. Calculate the average standard deviation using the sampling
    experiment shown in Sec. 1.5.2 for samples of size 2 taken
    from a population with values of 0, 1, and 2 (with replace-
    ment). Compare this result with the population standard
    deviation. Is the sample standard deviation an unbiased
    estimate of the population standard deviation?

12. Describe another situation that would result in a biased esti-
    mate of blood pressure reduction as discussed in Sec. 1.7.3
    (see Fig. 1.5).

13. Verify that the standard deviation of the values 1.19, 1.20,
    and 1.21 is 0.01 (see Sec. 1.8). What is the standard

**The double asterisk indicates optional, more difficult problems.

deviation of the numbers 2.19, 2.20, and 2.21? Explain the result of the two calculations above.

14. For the following blood pressure measurements: 100, 98, 101, 94, 104, 102, 108, 108, calculate (a) the mean, (b) the standard deviation, (c) the variance, (d) the coefficient of variation, (e) the range, and (f) the median.

**15. Calculate the standard deviation of the grouped data in

Table 1.2. (Hint: $S^2 = [\Sigma N_i X_i^2 - (\Sigma N_i X_i)^2 / (\Sigma N_i)] / (\Sigma N_i - 1)$;

see Ref. 3. N_i = frequency per group with midpoint X_i.)

16. Compute the arithmetic mean, geometric mean, and harmonic mean of the following set of data:

3, 5, 7, 11, 14, 57

If these data were observations on the time needed to cure a disease, which mean would you think to be most appropriate?

REFERENCES

1. *The Merck Manual*, 11th ed., Merck Sharp & Dohme, Research Laboratories, Rahway, N.J., 1966.

2. Tukey, J., *Exploratory Data Analysis*, Addison-Wesley, Reading, Mass., 1977.

3. Yule, G. U. and Kendall, M. G., *An Introduction to the Theory of Statistics*, 14th ed., Charles Griffin, London, 1965.

4. Sokal, R. R. and Rohlf, F. J., *Biometry*, W. H. Freeman, San Francisco, 1969.

5. Colton, T., *Statistics in Medicine*, Little, Brown, Boston, 1974.

6. Dixon, W. J. and Massey, F. J., Jr., *Introduction to Statistical Analysis*, 3rd ed., McGraw-Hill, New York, 1969.

7. Lachman, L., Lieberman, H. A., and Kanig, J. L., *The Theory and Practice of Industrial Pharmacy*, 2nd ed., Lea & Febiger, Philadelphia, 1976.

8. Snedecor, G. W. and Cochran, W. G., *Statistical Methods*, 7th ed., Iowa State University Press, Ames, Iowa, 1980.

9. Rothman, E. D. and Ericson, W. A., *Statistics, Methods and Applications*, Kendall Hunt, Dubuque, Iowa, 1983.

2
Data Graphics

"The preliminary examination of most data is facilitated by the use of diagrams. Diagrams prove nothing, but bring outstanding features readily to the eye; they are therefore no substitute for such critical tests as may be applied to the data, but are valuable in suggesting such tests, and in explaining the conclusions founded upon them" This quote is from Ronald A. Fisher, the father of modern statistical methodology [1]. Tabulation of raw data can be thought of as the initial and least refined way of presenting experimental results. Summary tables, such as frequency distribution tables, are much easier to digest and can be considered a second stage of refinement of data presentation. Summary statistics such as the mean, median, variance, standard deviation, and the range are concise descriptions of the properties of data, but much information is lost in this processing of experimental results. Graphic methods of displaying data are to be encouraged and are important adjuncts to data analysis and presentation. Graphical presentations clarify and also reinforce conclusions based on formal statistical analyses. Finally, the researcher has the opportunity to design aesthetic graphical presentations that command attention. The popular cliché "A picture is worth a thousand words" is especially *apropos* to statistical presentations. We will discuss some key concepts of the various ways in which data are depicted graphically.

2.1 INTRODUCTION

The diagrams and plots that we will be concerned with in our discussion of statistical methods can be placed broadly into two categories:

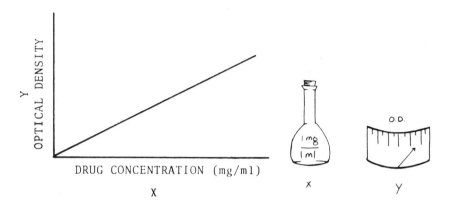

Figure 2.1   Beer's law plot illustrating a linear relationship between two variables.

1. Descriptive plots are those whose purpose is to transmit infor-
    mation. These include diagrams describing data distributions
    such as histograms and cumulative distribution plots (see Chap.
    1, Sec. 1.2.3). Bar charts and pie charts are examples of
    popular modes of communicating survey data or differences be-
    tween products.
2. Plots that describe *relationships* between variables. These plots
    usually show an underlying, but unknown analytic relationship
    between the variables that we wish to describe and understand.
    These relationships can range from relatively simple to very com-
    plex, and may involve only two variables or many variables.
    One of the simplest relationships, but probably the one with
    greatest practical application, is the straight-line relationship
    between two variables, as shown in the Beer's law plot in Fig.
    2.1. Chapter 7 is devoted to the analysis of data involving
    variables that have a linear relationship.

When analyzing and depicting data that involve relationships, we
are often presented with data in pairs (X, Y pairs). In Fig. 2.1,
the optical density Y and the concentration X are the data pairs.
When considering the relationship of two variables, X and Y, one
variable can often be considered the response variable, which is
dependent on the selection of the second or causal variable. The
response variable Y (optical density in our example), is known as
the *dependent* variable. The value of Y depends on the value of
the *independent* variable, X (drug concentration). Thus, in the
example in Fig. 2.1, we think of the value of optical density as
being dependent on the concentration of drug.

2.2 THE HISTOGRAM

The *histogram*, sometimes known as a *bar graph*, is one of the most popular ways of presenting and summarizing data. All of us have seen bar graphs, not only in scientific reports but also in advertisements and other kinds of presentations illustrating the distribution of scientific data. The histogram can be considered as a visual presentation of a frequency table. The frequency, or proportion, of observations in each class interval is plotted as a bar, or

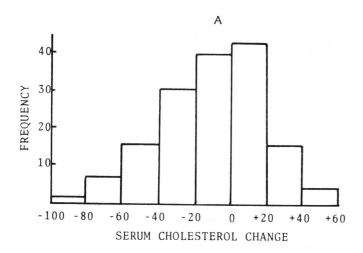

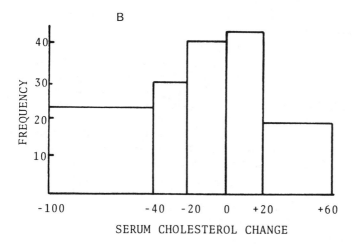

Figure 2.2   Histogram of data derived from Table 1.2.

rectangle, where the area of the bar is proportional to the frequency
(or proportion) of observations in a given interval. An example of
a histogram is shown in Fig. 2.2, where the data from the frequency
table in Table 1.2 have been used as the data source. As is the
case with frequency tables, class intervals for histograms should be
of equal width. When the intervals are of equal width, the height
of the bar is proportional to the frequency of observations in the
interval. If the intervals are not of equal width, the histogram is
not easily or obviously interpreted, as shown in Fig. 2.2B.

The choice of intervals for a histogram depends on the nature
of the data, the distribution of the data, and the purpose of the
presentation. In general, rules of thumb similar to that used for
frequency distribution tables (Sec. 1.2) can be used. Eight to
twenty equally spaced intervals usually are sufficient to give a good
picture of the data distribution.

2.3   CONSTRUCTION AND LABELING
OF GRAPHS

Proper *construction and labeling* of graphs are crucial elements in
graphic data representation. The design and actual construction of
graphs are not in themselves difficult. The preparation of a *good*
graph, however, requires careful thought and competent technical
skills. One needs not only a knowledge of statistical principles,
but also, in particular, computer and drafting competency. There
are no firm rules for preparing good graphical presentations. Mostly, we rely on experience and a few guidelines. Both books and
research papers have addressed the need for a more scientific
guide to optimal graphics which, after all, is measured by how well
the graph communicates the intended message(s) to the individuals
who are intended to read and interpret the graphs. Still, no rules
will cover all situations. One must be clear that no matter how well
a graph or chart is conceived, if the draftmanship and execution
is poor, the graph will fail to achieve its purpose.
     A "good" graph or chart should be as *simple* as possible, yet
clearly transmit its intended message. Superfluous notation, confusing lines or curves, and inappropriate draftmanship (lettering,
etc.) that can distract the reader are signs of a poorly constructed
graph. The book, *Statistical Graphics*, by C. F. Schmid [2] is
recommended for those who wish to study examples of good and
poor renderings of graphic presentations. For example, Schmid

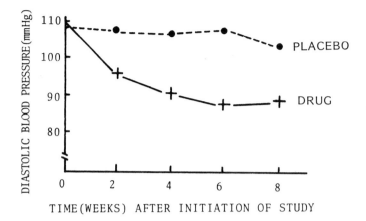

Figure 2.3 Blood pressure as a function of time in a clinical study comparing drug and placebo with a regimen of one tablet per day. ● placebo (average of 50 patients); + drug (average of 45 patients).

notes that visual contrast should be intentionally used to emphasize important characteristics of the graph. Here, we will present a few examples to illustrate the recommendations for good graphic presentation as well as examples of graphs that are not prepared well or fail to illustrate the facts fairly.

Figure 2.3 shows the results of a clinical study that was designed to compare an active drug to a placebo for the treatment of hypertension. This graph was constructed from the X, Y pairs, *time* and *blood pressure*, respectively. Each point on the graph (+, ●) is the average blood pressure for either drug or placebo at some point in time subsequent to the initiation of the study.

Proper construction and labeling of the typical rectilinear graph should include the following considerations:

1. A *title* should be given. The title should be brief and to the point, enabling the reader to understand the purpose of the graph without having to resort to reading the text. The title can be placed below or above the graph as in Fig. 2.3.

2. The *axes* should be *clearly* delineated and *labeled*. In general, the zero (0) points of both axes should be clearly indicated. The ordinate (the Y axis) is usually labeled with the descritpion parallel to the Y axis. Both the ordinate and abcissa (X axis) should be each appropriately labeled and subdivided in units of

equal width (of course, the X and Y axes almost always have different subdivisions). In the example in Fig. 2.3, note the units of mmHg and weeks for the ordinate and abcissa, respectively. Grid lines may be added (see Fig. 2.4E) but, if used, should be kept to a minimum, not be prominent and should not interfere with the interpretation of the figure.

3. The numerical *values* assigned to the axes should be *appropriately spaced* so as to nicely cover the extent of the graph. This can easily be accomplished by trial and error and a little manipulation. The scales and proportions should be constructed to present a fair picture of the results and should not be exaggerated so to prejudice the interpretation. Sometimes it may be necessary to skip or omit some of the data to achieve this objective. In these cases, the use of a "broken line" is recommended to clearly indicate the range of data not included in the graph (see Fig. 2.3).

4. If appropriate, a *key* explaining the symbols used in the graph should be used. For example, at the bottom of Fig. 2.3, the key defines ● as the symbol for placebo and + for drug. In many cases, labeling the curves directly on the graph (Fig. 2.3) results in more clarity.

5. In situations where the graph is derived from laboratory data, inclusion of the *source* of the data (name, laboratory notebook number, and page number, for example) is recommended.

Usually graphs should stand on their own, independent of the main body of the text.

Examples of various ways of plotting data, derived from a study of exercise time at various time intervals after administration of a single dose of two long-acting nitrate products to anginal patients, is shown in Fig. 2.4A–E. All of these plots are accurate representations of the experimental results, but each gives the reader a different impression. It would be wrong to expand or contract the axes of the graph, or otherwise distort the graph, in order to convey an incorrect impression to the reader. Most scientists are well aware of how data can be manipulated to give different impressions. If obvious deception is intended, the experimental results will not be taken seriously.

When examining the various plots in Fig. 2.4, one could not say which plot best represents the meaning of the experimental results without knowledge of the experimental details, in particular the objective of the experiment, the implications of the experimental outcome, and the message that is *meant* to be conveyed. For example, if an improvement of exercise time of 120 sec for one drug compared to the other is considered to be significant from a medical point of view, the graphs labeled A, C, and E in Fig. 2.4 would all seem appropriate in conveying this message. The graphs labeled B and D show this difference less clearly. On the other hand, if 120 sec

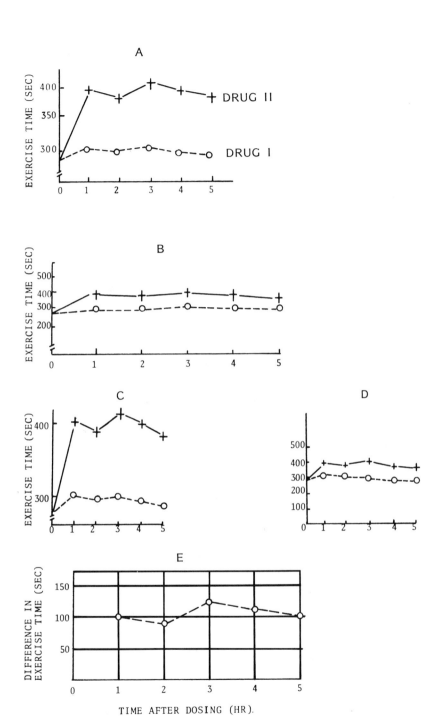

Figure 2.4 Various graphs of the same data presented in different ways. Exercise time at various times after administration of single doses of two nitrate products. ○ drug I; + drug II.

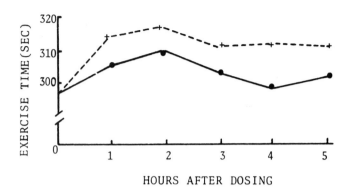

Figure 2.5   Exercise time at various times after administration of
two nitrate products. ● product I; + product II.

is considered to be of little medical significance, B and D might be
a better representation of the data.

Note that in plots A, B, and C of Fig. 2.4, the ordinate (exercise time) is broken, indicating that some values have been skipped.
This is not meant to be deceptive, but is intentionally done to show
better the differences between the two drugs.   As long as the zero
point and the break in the axis are clearly indicated, and the message is not distorted, such a procedure is entirely acceptable.

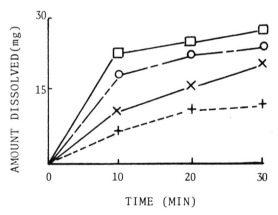

Figure 2.6   Plot of dissolution of four successive batches of a commercial tablet product.   □ batch I; ○ batch II; × batch III; +
batch IV.

Figures 2.4B and 2.5 are exaggerated examples of plots that may be considered not to reflect accurately the significance of the experimental results. In Fig. 2.4B, the clinically significant difference of approximately 120 sec is made to look very small, tending to diminish drug differences in the viewer's mind. Also, fluctuations in the hourly results appear to be less than the data truly suggest. In Fig. 2.5, a difference of 5 sec in exercise time between the two drugs appears very large. Care should be taken when constructing (as well as reading) graphs so that experimental conclusions come through clear and true.

6. If more than one curve appears on the same graph, a convenient way to differentiate the curves is to use different symbols for the experimental points (e.g., ○, ×, △, □, +) and, if necessary, connecting the points in different ways (e.g., —— · —— · —— · , ..., — · — · — · —). A key or label is used, which is helpful in distinguishing the various curves, as shown in Figs. 2.3 to 2.6. Other ways of differentiating curves include different kinds of cross-hatching and use of different colors.

7. One should take care not to place too many curves on the same graph, as this can result in confusion. There are no specific rules in this regard. The decision depends on the nature of the data, and how the data look when they are plotted. The curves graphed in Fig. 2.7 are cluttered and confusing. The curves should be presented differently or separated into two or more graphs. Figure 2.8 is a clearer depiction of the dissolution results of the five formulations shown in Fig. 2.7.

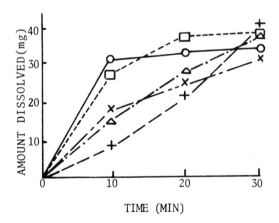

TIME (MIN)

Figure 2.7 Plot of dissolution time of five different commercial formulations of the same drug. ○ Product A; □ product B; × product C; △ product D; + product E.

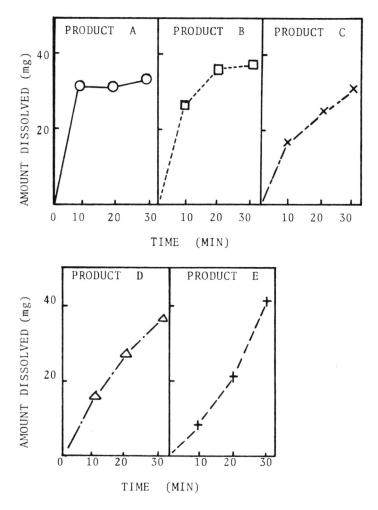

Figure 2.8   Individual plots of dissolution of the five formulations shown in Fig. 2.7.

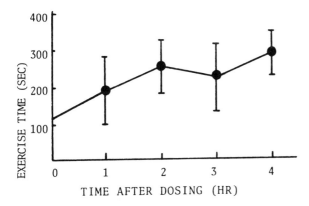

Figure 2.9 Plot of exercise time as a function of time for an anti-anginal drug showing mean values and standard error of the mean.

8. The *standard deviation* may be indicated on graphs as shown in Fig. 2.9. However, when the standard deviation is indicated on a graph (or in a table, for that matter), it should be made clear whether the variation described in the graph is an indication of the standard deviation (S) or the standard deviation of the mean ($S_{\overline{X}}$). The standard deviation of the mean, if appropriate, is often preferable to the standard deviation not only because the values on the graph are mean values, but because $S_{\overline{X}}$ is smaller than the s.d., and therefore less cluttering. *Overlapping* standard deviations, as shown in Fig. 2.10, should be avoided, as this representation of the experimental results is usually more confusing than clarifying.

9. The manner in which the points on a graph should be connected is not always obvious. Should the individual points be connected by straight lines, or should a smooth curve that approximates the points be drawn through the data? (See Fig. 2.11.) If the graphs represent flunctional relationships, the data should probably be connected by a smooth curve. For example, the blood level versus time data shown in Fig. 2.11 are described most accurately by a smooth curve. Although, theoretically, the points should not be connected by straight lines as shown in Fig. 2.11A, such graphs are often depicted this way. Connecting the individual points with straight lines may be considered acceptable if one recognizes that this representation is meant to clarify the graphical presentation, or is done for some other appropriate reason. In the blood-level example, the area under the curve is proportional to the amount of drug absorbed. The area is often computed by the trapezoidal

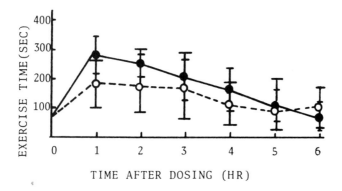

Figure 2.10   Graph comparing two antianginal drugs which is confusing and cluttered because of the overalapping standard deviations.
● drug A; ○ drug B.

rule [2], and depiction of the data as shown in Fig. 2.11A makes it
easier to visualize and perform such calculations.

Figure 2.12 shows another example in which connecting points
by straight lines is convenient but may *not* be a good representation of the experimental outcome.   The straight line connecting the
blood pressure at zero time (before drug administration) to the blood
pressure after 2 weeks of drug administration suggests a gradual
decrease (a linear decrease) in blood pressure over the 2-week
period.   In fact, no measurements were made during the initial

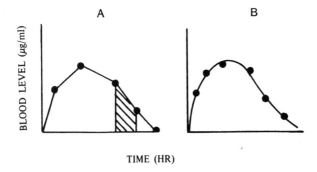

Figure 2.11   Plot of blood level versus time data illustrating two
ways of drawing the curves.

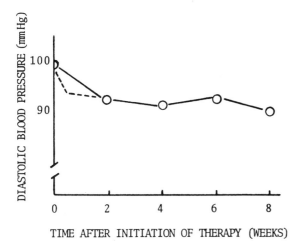

TIME AFTER INITIATION OF THERAPY (WEEKS)

Figure 2.12   Graph of blood pressure reduction with time of anti-hypertensive drug illustrating possible misinterpretation that may occur when points are connected by straight lines.

2-week interval.   The 10-mmHg decrease observed after 2 weeks of therapy may have occurred before the 2-week reading (e.g., in 1 week, as indicated by the dashed line in Fig. 2.12).   One should be careful to ensure that graphs constructed in such a manner are not misinterpreted.

2.4   SCATTER PLOTS (CORRELATION DIAGRAMS)

Although the applications of *correlation* will be presented in some detail in Chap. 7, we will introduce the notion of *scatter plots* (also called correlation diagrams or scatter diagrams) at this time.   This type of plot or diagram is commonly used when presenting results of experiments.   A typical scatter plot is illustrated in Fig. 2.13. Data are collected in pairs (X and Y) with the objective of demonstrating a trend or relationship (or lack of relationship) between the X and Y variables.   Usually, we are interested in showing a linear relationship between the variables (i.e., a straight line).   For example, one may be interested in demonstrating a relationship (or correlation) between time to 80% *dissolution* of various tablet formulations of a particular drug and the *fraction of the dose absorbed* when human subjects take the various tablets.   The data plotted in

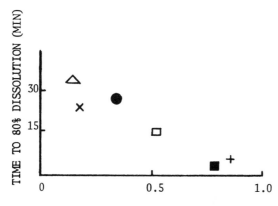

FRACTION OF DOSE ABSORBED IN VIVO

Figure 2.13   Scatter plot showing the correlation of dissolution time and in vivo absorption of six tablet formulations. △ formulation A; × formulation B; ● formulation C; □ formulation D; ■ formulation E; + formulation F.

Fig. 2.13 show pictorially that as dissolution increases (i.e., the time to 80% dissolution decreases) in vivo absorption increases. Scatter plots involve data pairs, X and Y, both of which are variable. In this example, *dissolution time* and *fraction absorbed* are both random variables.

2.5   SEMILOGARITHMIC PLOTS

Several important kinds of experiments in the pharmaceutical sciences result in data such that the *logarithm* of the response (Y) is linearly related to an independent variable, X.   The semilogarithmic plot is useful when the response (Y) is best depicted as proportional changes relative to changes in X, or when the spread of Y is very large and cannot be easily depicted on a rectilinear scale. Semilog graph paper has the usual equal interval scale on the X axis and the logarithmic scale on the Y axis.   In the logarithmic scale, equal intervals represent equal ratios.   For example, the distance between 1 and 10 will exactly equal the distance between 10 and 100 on a logarithmic scale.   In particular first-order kinetic processes, often apparent in drug degradation and pharmacokinetic systems show a linear relationship when log C is plotted versus

Table 2.1 Blood Levels After Intravenous
Injection of Drug

Time after injection, t (hr)	Blood level, C (μg/mL)	Log blood level
0	20	1.301
1	10	1.000
2	5	0.699
3	2.5	0.398
4	1.25	0.097

time. First-order processes can be expressed by the following
equation:

$$\log C = \log C_0 - \frac{kt}{2.3} \qquad (2.1)$$

where

C = concentration at time t

C_0 = concentration at time 0

k = first-order rate constant

t = time

log = logarithm to the base 10

Table 2.1 shows blood-level data obtained after an intravenous injection of a drug described by a one-compartment model [3].
    Figure 2.14 shows two ways of plotting the data in Table 2.1 to
demonstrate the linearity of the log C versus t relationship.
    1. Figure 2.14A shows a plot of log C versus time. The re-
sulting straight line is a consequence of the relationship of log concentration and time as shown in Eq. (2.1). This is an equation of
a straight line with the Y intercept equal to log C_0 and a slope
equal to $-k/2.3$. Straight-line relationships are discussed in more
detail in Chap. 8.
    2. Figure 2.14B shows a more convenient way of plotting the
data of Table 2.1, making use of *semilog graph paper*. This paper
has a logarithmic scale on the Y axis and the usual arithmetic,
linear scale on the X axis. The logarithmic scale is constructed so
that the spacing corresponds to the logarithms of the numbers on

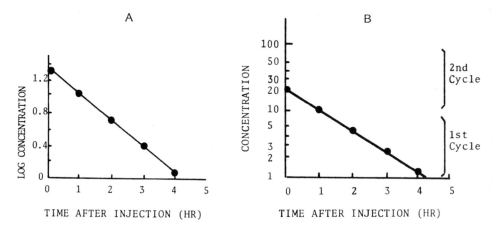

Figure 2.14   Linearizing plots of data from Table 2.1.   Plot A:
log C vs. time; plot B: semilog plot.

the Y axis. For example, the distance between 1 and 2 is the same
as that between 2 and 4. (Log 2 - log 1) is equal to (log 4 - log 2).
The semilog graph paper depicted in Fig. 2.14B is two-cycle paper.
The Y (log) axis has been repeated two times. The decimal point
for the numbers on the Y axis is accommodated to the data. In our
example, the data range from 1.25 to 20 and the Y axis is adjusted
accordingly, as shown in Fig. 2.14B. The data may be plotted directly on this paper without the need to look up the logarithms of
the concentration values.

2.6   OTHER DESCRIPTIVE FIGURES

Most of the discussion in this chapter has been concerned with
plots that show relationships between variables such as blood pressure changes following two or more treatments, or drug decomposition as a function of time. Often occasions arise in which graphical
presentations are better made using other more pictorial techniques.
These approaches include the popular bar and pie charts. Schmid
[2] differentiates bar charts into two categories, (a) *column charts*
in which there is a vertical orientation and *bar charts* in which the
bars are horizontal. In general, the bar charts are more appropriate for comparison of categorical variables, whereas the column

chart is used for data showing relationships such as comparisons of drug effect over time.

Bar charts are very simple but effective visual displays. They are usually used to compare some experimental outcome or other relevant data where the length of the bar represents the magnitude. There are many variations of the simple bar chart [2]; an example is shown in Figure 2.15. In Fig. 2.15A, patients are categorized as having a good, fair, or poor response. Forty percent of the patients had a good response, 35% had a fair response, and 25% had a poor response.

Figure 2.15B shows bars in pairs to emphasize the comparative nature of two treatments. It is clear from this diagram that Treatment X is superior to Treatment Y. Figure 2.15C is another way of displaying the results shown in Fig. 2.15B. Which chart do you think better sends the message of the results of this comparative study, Fig. 2.15B or 2.15C? One should be aware that the results correspond only to the length of the bar. If the order in which the bars are presented is not obvious, displaying bars in order of magnitude is recommended. In the example in Fig. 2.15, the order is based on the nature of the results, "Good," "Fair," and "Poor." Everything else in the design of these charts is superfluous and the

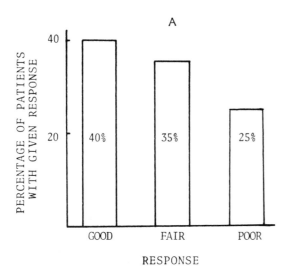

Figure 2.15   Graphical representation of patient responses to drug therapy.

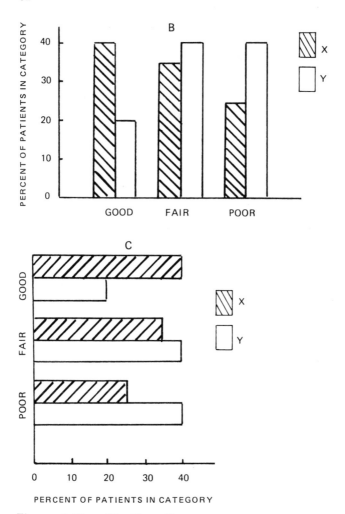

Figure 2.15 (Continued)

otherwise principal objective is to prepare an aesthetic presentation
that emphasizes but does not exaggerate the results. For example,
the use of graphic techniques such as shading, cross-hatching, and
color, tastefully executed, can enhance the presentation.

Column charts are prepared in a similar way to bar charts. As
noted above, whether or not a bar or column chart is best to dis-
play data is not always clear. Data trends over time usually are
best shown using columns. Figure 2.16 shows the comparison of
exercise time for two drugs using a column chart. This is the

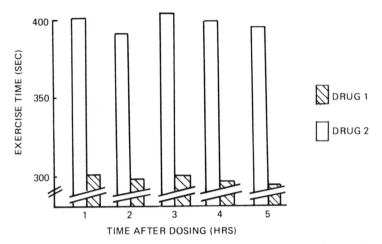

Figure 2.16 Exercise time for two drugs in the form of a column chart using data of Fig. 2.4A.

same data used to prepare Fig. 2.4A (also, see Exercise Problem 8 at the end of this chapter).

Pie charts are popular ways of presenting categorical data. Although the principles used in the construction of these charts are relatively simple, thought and care are necessary to convey the correct message. For example, dividing the circle into too many categories can be confusing and misleading. As a rule of thumb, no more than 6 sectors should be used. Another problem with pie charts is that it is not always easy to differentiate two segments that are reasonably close in size, whereas in the bar graph, values close in size are easily differentiated, since length is the critical feature.

The circle (or pie) represents 100%, or *all* of the results. Each segment (or slice of pie) has an area proportional to the area of the circle, representative of the contribution due to the particular segment. In the example shown in Fig. 2.17A, the pie represents the entire anti-inflammatory drug market. The slices are proportions of the market accounted for by major drugs in this therapeutic class. These charts are frequently used for business and economic descriptions, but can be applied to the presentation of scientific data in appropriate circumstances. Figure 2.17B shows the proportion of patients with good, fair, and poor responses to a drug in a clinical trial (see also Fig. 2.15).

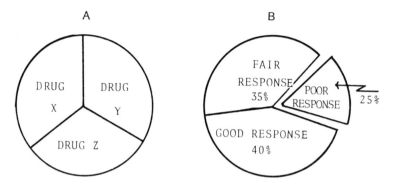

Figure 2.17   Examples of pie charts.

Of course, we have not exhausted all possible ways of presenting data graphically. We have introduced the cumulative plot in
Sec. 1.2.3. Other kinds of plots are the stick diagram (analogous
to the histogram) and frequency polygon [4]. The number of ways
in which data can be presented is limited only by our own ingenuity.
An elegant pictorial presentation of data can "make" a report or
government submission. On the other hand, poor presentation of
data can detract from an otherwise good report. The book *Statistical
Graphics* by Calvin Schmid is recommended for those who wish detailed information on the presentation of graphs and charts.

KEY TERMS

Bar charts   Independent variables
Bar graphs   Key
Column charts   Pie charts
Correlation   Scatter plots
Data pairs   Semilog plots
Dependent variables   Trapezoidal rule
Histogram

EXERCISES

1. Plot the following data, preparing and labeling the graph ac-
    cording to the guidelines outlined in this chapter. These data
    are the result of preparing various modifications of a formulation
    and observing the effect of the modifications on tablet hardness.

Formulation modification

Starch (%)	Lactose (%)	Tablet hardness (kg)
10	5	8.3
10	10	9.1
10	15	9.6
10	20	10.2
5	5	9.1
5	10	9.4
5	15	9.8
5	20	10.4

(Hint: Plot these data on a single graph where the Y axis is tablet hardness and the X axis is lactose concentration. There will be two curves, one at 10% starch and the other at 5% starch.)

2. Prepare a histogram from the data of Table 1.3. Compare this histogram to that shown in Fig. 2.2A. Which do you think is a better representation of the data distribution?

3. Plot the following data and label the graph appropriately.

Patient	X: response to product A	Y: response to product B
1	2.5	3.8
2	3.6	2.4
3	8.9	4.7
4	6.4	5.9
5	9.5	2.1
6	7.4	5.0
7	1.0	8.5
8	4.7	7.8

What conclusion(s) can you draw from this plot if the responses are pain relief scores, where a high score means more relief?

4. A batch of tables was shown to have 70% with no defects, 15% slightly chipped, 10% discolored, and 5% dirty. Construct a pie chart from these data.

5. The following data from a dose-response experiment, a measure of physical activity, is the response of five animals at each of three doses.

Dose (mg)	Responses
1	8, 12, 9, 14, 6
2	16, 20, 12, 15, 17
4	20, 17, 25, 27, 16

Plot the individual data points and the average at each dose versus (a) dose; (b) log dose.

6. The concentration of drug in solution was measured as a function of time:

Time (weeks)	Concentration
0	100
4	95
8	91
26	68
52	43

(a) Plot concentration versus time.
(b) Plot log concentration versus time.

7. Plot the following data and label the axes appropriately.

Patient	X: Cholesterol (mg %)	Y: Triglycerides (mg %)
1	180	80
2	240	180
3	200	70
4	300	200
5	360	240
6	240	200

Tablet	X: Tablet potency (mg)	Y: Tablet weight (mg)
1	5	300
2	6	300
3	4	280
4	5	295
5	6	320
6	4	290

8. Which figure do you think best represents the results of the exercise time study, Fig. 2.16 or Fig. 2.4A? If the presentation were to be used in a popular nontechnical journal read by laymen and physicians, which figure would you recommend?

REFERENCES

1. Fisher, R. A., *Statistical Methods for Research Workers*, 13th ed., Hafner, New York, 1963.
2. Schmid, C. F., *Statistical Graphics*, Wiley, New York, 1983.
3. Gibaldi, M. and Perrier, D., *Pharmacokinetics*, 2nd ed., Marcel Dekker, New York, 1982.
4. Dixon, W. J. and Massey, F. J., Jr., *Introduction to Statistical Analysis*, 3rd ed., McGraw-Hill, New York, 1969.

3
Introduction to Probability: The Binomial and Normal Probability Distributions

The theory of statistics is based on probability. Some basic definitions and theorems are introduced in this chapter. This elementary discussion leads to the concept of a probability distribution, a mathematical function that assigns probabilities for outcomes in its domain. The properties of (a) the binomial distribution, a discrete distribution, and (b) the normal distribution, a continuous distribution, are presented. The normal distribution is the basis of modern statistical theory and methodology. One of the chief reasons for the pervasion of the normal distribution in statistics is the central limit theorem, which shows that means of samples from virtually all probability distributions tend to be normal for large sample sizes. Also, many of the probability distributions used in statistical analyses are based on the normal distribution. These include the t, F, and Chi-square distributions. The binomial distribution is applicable to experimental results that have two possible outcomes, such as pass or fail in quality control, or cured or not cured in a clinical drug study. With a minimal understanding of probability, one can apply statistical methods intelligently to the simple but prevalent problems that crop up in the analysis of experimental data.

3.1   INTRODUCTION

Most of us have an intuitive idea of the meaning of probability. The meaning and use of probability in everyday life is a subconscious integration of experience and knowledge that allows us to say, for example: "If I purchase this car at my local dealer, the convenience and good service will *probably* make it worthwhile despite the greater initial cost of the car." From a statistical point of view, we will try to be more precise in the definition of probability. The *Random House Dictionary of the English Language* defines probability as "The likelihood of an occurrence expressed by the ratio of the actual occurrences to that of all possible occurrences; the relative frequency with which an event occurs, or is likely to occur." Therefore, the probability of observing an event can be defined as the proportion of such events which will occur in a large number of observations or experimental trials.

The approach to probability is often associated with odds in gambling or games of chance, and picturing probability in this context will help its understanding. When placing a bet on the outcome of a coin toss, the game of "heads and tails," one could reasonably *guess* that the probability of a head or tail is one-half (1/2) or 50%. One-half of the outcomes will be heads and one-half will be tails. Do you think that the probability of observing a head (or tail) on a single toss of the coin is exactly 0.5 (50%)? Probably not; a probability of 50% would result only if the coin is absolutely balanced. The only way to verify the probability is to carry out an extensive experiment, tossing a coin a million times or more and counting the proportion of heads or tails that result.

The gambler who knows that the odds in a game of craps favor the "house" will lose in the long run. Why should a knowledgable person play a losing game? Other than for psychological reasons, the gambler may feel that a reasonably good chance of winning on any single bet is worth the chance, and maybe "Lady Luck" will be on his side. Probability is a measure of uncertainty. We may be able to predict accurately some average result in the long run, but the outcome of a single experiment cannot be anticipated with certainty.

3.2 SOME BASIC PROBABILITY

The concept of probability is "probably" best understood when discussing discontinuous or *discrete* variables. These variables have a countable number of outcomes. Consider an experiment in which only one of two possible outcomes can occur. For example, the result of treatment with an antibiotic is that an infection is either *cured* or *not cured* within 5 days. Although this situation is conceptually analogous to the coin-tossing example, it differs in the following respect. For the coin-tossing example, the probability can be determined by a rational examination of the nature of the experiment. If the coin is balanced, heads and tails are equally likely; the probability of a head is equal to the probability of a tail = 0.5. In the case of the antibiotic cure, however, the probability of a cure is not easily ascertained a priori, i.e., prior to performing an experiment. If the antibiotic were widely used, based on his or her own experience, a physician prescriber of the product might be able

to give a good estimate of the probability of a cure for patients
treated with the drug. For example, in the physician's practice, he
or she may have observed that approximately three of four patients
treated with the antibiotic are cured. For this physician, the probability that a patient will be cured when treated with the antibiotic
is 75%.

A large multicenter clinical trial would give a better estimate of
the probability of success after treatment. A study of 1000 patients
might show 786 patients cured; the *probability of a cure* is estimated
as 0.786 or 78.6%. This does not mean that the exact probability is
0.786. The exact probability can be determined only by treating
the total population and observing the proportion cured, a practical
impossibility in this case. In this context, it would be fair to say
that exact probabilities are nearly always unknown.

3.2.1   Some Elementary Definitions and Theorems

1. $0 \leq P(A) \leq 1$ (3.1)

where $P(A)$ is the probability of observing event A. The probability of any event or experimental outcome, $P(A)$, cannot be less
than 0 or greater than 1. An impossible event has a probability of
0. A certain event has a probability of 1.

2. If events A, B, C, . . . are *mutually exclusive*, the probability of observing A or B or C . . . is the sum of the probabilities
of each event, A, B, C, ... If two or more events are
"Mutually exclusive," the events cannot occur simultaneously, i.e.,
if one event is observed, the other event(s) cannot occur. For example, we cannot observe both a head and and a tail on a single
toss of a coin.

$P(A \text{ or } B \text{ or } C \text{ . . .}) = P(A) + P(B) + P(B) + \text{ . . .}$ (3.2)

An example frequently encountered in quality control illustrates
this theorem. Among 1,000,000 tablets in a batch, 50,000 are known
to be flawed, perhaps containing *specks* of grease. The probability
of finding a *randomly* chosen tablet with specks is 50,000/1,000,000 =
0.05 or 5%. The process of *randomly* choosing a tablet is akin to a
lottery. The tablets are well mixed, ensuring that each tablet has
an equal chance of being chosen. While blindfolded, one figuratively
chooses a single tablet from a container containing the 1,000,000
tablets (see Chap. 4 for a detailed discussion of random sampling).
A gambler making an equitable bet would give odds of 19 to 1

against a specked tablet being chosen (1 of 20 tablets is specked). Odds are defined as

$$\frac{P(A)}{1 - P(A)}$$

There are other defects among the 1,000,000 tablets. Thirty thousand, or 3%, have *chipped* edges and 40,000 (4%) are *discolored*. If these defects are mutually exclusive, the probability of observing any one of these events for a single tablet is 0.03 and 0.04, respectively (see Fig. 3.1A). According to Eq. (3.2), the probability of choosing an unacceptable tablet (specked, chipped, or discolored) at random is 0.05 + 0.03 + 0.04 = 0.12, or 12%. (The probability of choosing an acceptable tablet is 1 - 0.12 = 0.88.)

3.   P(A) + P(B) + P(C) + . . . = 1   (3.3)

where A, B, C, . . . are mutually exclusive and exhaust all possible outcomes.

If the set of all possible experimental outcomes are mutually exclusive, the sum of the probabilities of all possible outcomes is equal to 1. This is equivalent to saying that we are certain that one of the mutually exclusive outcomes will occur.

The four events in Fig. 3.1 do not all have to be mutually exclusive. In general:

4.   *If two events are not mutually exclusive,*

P(A or B) = P(A) + P(B) - P(A and B)   (3.4)

Note that if A and B are mutually exclusive, P(A and B) = 0, and for two events, A and B. Eqs. (3.2) and (3.4) are identical. (A and B) means the simultaneous occurrence of A and B. (A or B) means that A or B or both A and B occur. For example, some tablets with chips may also be specked. If 20,000 tablets are both chipped *and* specked in the example above, one can verify that 60,000 tablets are specked *or* chipped.

P(specked or chipped) = P(specked) + P(chipped)

                         - P(specked and chipped)

                      = 0.05 + 0.03 - 0.02 = 0.06

The probability of finding a specked or chipped tablet is 0.06. Thirty thousand tablets are *only* specked, 10,000 tablets are *only* chipped, and 20,000 tablets are both specked and chipped; a total

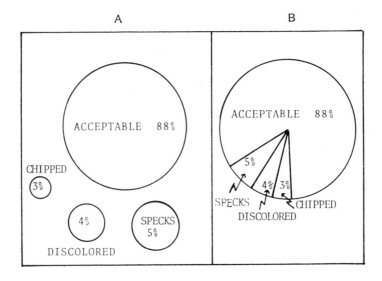

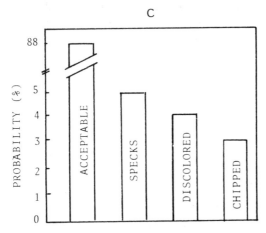

Figure 3.1   Probability distribution for tablet attributes.

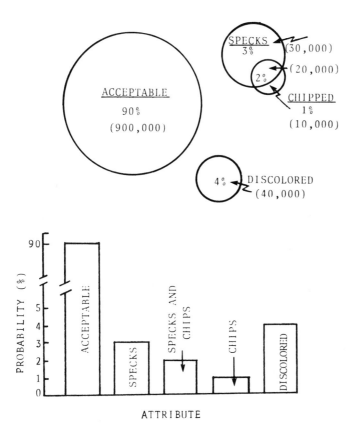

Figure 3.2 Distribution of tablet attributes where attributes are not all mutually exclusive.

of 60,000 tablets specked or chipped. The distribution of tablet attributes under these conditions is shown in Fig. 3.2.

With reference to this example of tablet attributes, we can enumerate all possible mutually exclusive events. In the former case, where each tablet was acceptable or had only a single defect, there are four possible outcomes (specked, chipped edges, discolored, and acceptable tablets). These four outcomes and their associated probabilities make up a *probability distribution*, which can be represented in several ways, as shown in Fig. 3.1. The distribution of attributes where some tablets may be both specked and chipped is shown in Fig. 3.2. The notion of a probability distribution is discussed further later in this chapter (Sec. 3.3).

5. *The multiplicative law of probability states that*

$$P(A \text{ and } B) = P(A|B)P(B) \tag{3.5}$$

where $P(A|B)$ is known as the conditional probability of A given that B occurs. In the present example, the probability that a tablet will be specked given that the tablet is chipped is [from Eq. (3.5)]

$$P(\text{specked}|\text{chipped}) = \frac{P(\text{specked and chipped})}{P(\text{chipped})}$$

$$= \frac{0.02}{0.03} = \frac{2}{3}$$

Referring to Fig. 3.2, it is clear that 2/3 of the chipped tablets are also specked. Thus the probability of a tablet being specked given that it is also chipped is 2/3.

3.2.2   Independent Events

In games of chance, such as roulette, the probability of winning (or losing) is theoretically the same on each turn of the wheel, irrespective of prior outcomes. Each turn of the wheel results in an independent outcome. The events, A and B, are said to be independent if a knowledge of B does not affect the probability of A. Mathematically, two events are independent if

$$P(A|B) = P(A) \tag{3.6}$$

Substituting Eq. (3.6) into Eq. (3.5), we can say that if

$$P(A \text{ and } B) = P(A)P(B) \tag{3.7}$$

then A and B are independent. When sampling tablets for defects, if each tablet is selected at random and the batch size is very large, the sample observations may be considered independent. Thus, in the example of tablet attributes shown in Fig. 3.4, the probability of selecting an acceptable tablet (A) followed by a defective tablet (B) is

$$(0.88)(0.12) = 0.106$$

The probability of selecting two tablets, both of which are acceptable, is $0.88 \times 0.88 = 0.7744$.

3.3   PROBABILITY DISTRIBUTIONS —
THE BINOMIAL DISTRIBUTION

To understand probability further, one should have a notion of the
concept of a probability distribution, introduced in Sec. 3.2.   A
probability distribution is a mathematical representation (function)
of the probabilities associated with the values of a random variable.

For discrete data, the concept can be illustrated using the
simple example of the outcome of antibiotic therapy introduced earlier
in this chapter.   In this example, the outcome of a patient following
treatment can take on one of two possibilities: a cure with a probability of 0.75 or a failure with a probability of 0.25.   Assigning
the value 1 for a cure and 0 for a failure, the probability distribution is simply:

$f(1) = 0.75$

$f(0) = 0.25$

Figure 3.3 shows the probability distribution for this example,
the random variable being the outcome of a patient treated with
the antibiotic.   This is an example of a binomial distribution.
Another example of a binomial distribution is the coin tossing game,
heads or tails where the two outcomes have equal probability, 0.5.
This binomial distribution ($p = 0.5$) has application in statistical
methods, preference tests (Chap. 14, Sec. 14.2.1) and the sign test
(Chap. 15, Sec. 15.2), for example.

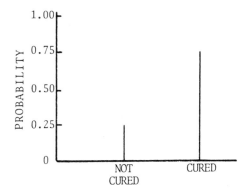

Figure 3.3   Probability distribution of a binomial outcome based on
a single observation.

When a single observation can be dichotomized, that is, the observation can be placed into one of two possible categories, the binomial distribution can be used to define the probability characteristics of one or more such observations. The binomial distribution is a very important probability distribution in applications in pharmaceutical research. The few examples noted in Table 3.1 reveal its pervading presence in pharmaceutical processes.

3.3.1 Some Definitions

A *binomial trial* is a single binomial experiment or observation. The treatment of a single patient with the antibiotic is a binomial trial. The trial must result in only one of two outcomes, where the two outcomes are *mutually exclusive*. In the antibiotic example, the only possible outcomes are that a patient is either cured or not cured. In addition, only one of these outcomes is possible after treatment. A patient cannot be both cured and not cured after treatment. Each binomial trial must be *independent*. The result of a patient's treatment does not influence the outcome of the treatment for a different patient. In another example, when randomly sampling tablets for a binomial attribute, chipped or not chipped, the observation of a chipped tablet does not depend upon or influence the outcome observed for any other tablet.

Table 3.1   Some Examples of Binomial Data in Pharmaceutical Research

Experiment or process	Dichotomous data
LD_{50} determination	Animals *live* or *die* after dosing. Determine dose that kills 50% of animals.
ED_{50} determination	Drug is *effective* or *not effective*. Determine dose that is effective in 50% of animals.
Sampling for defects	In quality control, product is sampled for defects. Tablets are *acceptable* or *unacceptable*.
Clinical trials	Treatment is *successful* or *not successful*.
Formulation modification	A. Palatability preference for *old* and *new* formulation. B. New formulation is *more* or *less available* in crossover design.

The binomial distribution is completely defined by two parameters: (a) the probability of one or the other outcome, and (b) the number of trials or observations, N. Given these two parameters, we can calculate the probability of any specified number of successes in N trials. For the antibiotic example, the probability of success is 0.75. With this information, we can calculate the probability that 3 of 4 patients will be cured (N = 4). We could also calculate this result, given the probability of failure (0.25). The probability of 3 of 4 patients being cured is exactly the same as the probability of 1 of 4 patients not being cured.

The probability of success (or failure) lies between 0 and 1. The probability of failure (the complement of a success) is 1 minus the probability of success [1 - P(success)]. Since the outcome of a binomial trial must be either success or failure, P(success) + P(failure) = 1 [see Eq. (3.3)].

The standard deviation of a binomial distribution with probability of success, p, and N trials is $\sqrt{pq/N}$, where q = 1 - p. The s.d. of

NUMBER OF OBSERVATIONS (N)   AND   PROBABILITY OF SUCCESS

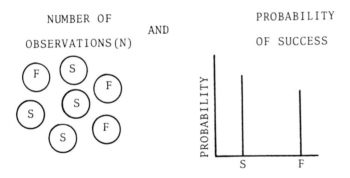

PROVIDE COMPLETE KNOWLEDGE OF DISTRIBUTION

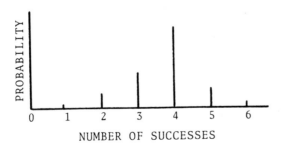

NUMBER OF SUCCESSES

the proportion of successes of antibiotic treatment in 16 trials is
$\sqrt{0.75 \times 0.25/16} = 0.108$. (Also see Sec. 3.3.2 in Chap. 3.)

The probability of the outcome of a binomial experiment consisting of N trials can be computed from the expansion of the expression

$$(p + q)^N \qquad\qquad (3.8)$$

where p is defined as the probability of success and q is the probability of failure. For example, consider the outcomes that are possible after three tosses of a coin. There are four (N + 1) possible results

1. Three heads
2. Two heads and one tail
3. Two tails and one head
4. Three tails

For the outcome of the treatment of three patients in the antibiotic example, the four possible results are

1. Three cures
2. Two cures and one failure
2. Two failures and one cure
4. Three failures

The probabilities of these events can be calculated from the individual terms from the expansion of $(p + q)^N$, where N = 3, the number of binomial trials.

$$(p + q)^3 = p^3 + 3p^2q + 3pq^2 + q^3$$

If p = q = 1/2, as is the case in coin-tossing, then

$$p^3 = (1/2)^3 = 1/8 = P(\text{three heads})$$

$$3p^2q = 3/8 = P(\text{two heads and one tail})$$

$$3pq^2 = 3/8 = P(\text{two tails and one head})$$

$$q^3 = 1/8 = P(\text{three tails})$$

If p = 0.75 and q = 0.25, as is the case for the antibiotic example, then

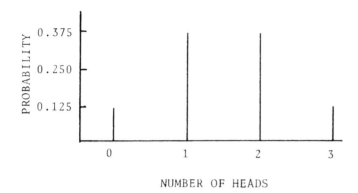

NUMBER OF HEADS

Figure 3.4 Probability distribution of binomial with p = 0.5 and N = 3.

$$p^3 = (0.75)^3 = 0.422 = P(3 \text{ cures})$$

$$3\,p^2q = 3\,(0.75)^2\,(0.25) = 0.422 \ P(2 \text{ cures and 1 failure})$$

$$3\,pq^2 = 3\,(0.75)\,(0.25)^2 = 0.141 \ P(1 \text{ cure and 2 failures})$$

$$q^3 = (0.25)^3 = 0.016 = P(3 \text{ failures})$$

The sum of the probabilities of all possible outcomes of three patients being treated or 3 sequential coin tosses is equal to 1 (e.g., 1/8 + 3/8 + 3/8 + 1/8 = 1).

This is true of any binomial experiment because $(p + q)^N$ must equal 1 by definition (i.e., p + q = 1). The probability distribuion of the coin-tossing experiment with N = 3 is shown in Fig. 3.4. Note that this is a *discrete* distribution. The particular binomial distribution shown in the figure is comprised of only *four* possible outcomes (the four sticks).

A gambler looking for a fair game, one with equitable odds, would give odds of 7 to 1 on a bet that three heads would be observed in three tosses of a coin. The payoff would be eight dollars (including the dollar bet) for a one-dollar bet. A bet that either three heads or three tails would be observed would have odds of 3 to 1. (The probability of either *three heads* or *three tails* is 1/4 = 1/8 + 1/8.)

To calculate exact probabilities in the binomial case, the expansion of the binomial, $(p + q)^N$ can be generalized by a single formula:

Probability of X successes in N trials $= \binom{N}{X} p^X q^{N-X}$ (3.9)

$\binom{N}{X}$ is defined as $\dfrac{N!}{X!(N-X)!}$

(Remember that 0! is equal to 1.)

Consider the binomial distribution with $p = 0.75$ and $N = 4$ for the antibiotic example. This represents the distribution of outcomes after treating four patients. There are five possible outcomes:

No patients are cured
One patient is cured
Two patients are cured
Three patients are cured
Four patients are cured

The probability that three of four patients are cured can be calculated from Eq. (3.9)

$\binom{4}{3} (0.75)^3 (0.25)^1$

$= \dfrac{4 \cdot 3 \cdot 2 \cdot 1}{1 \cdot 3 \cdot 2 \cdot 1} (0.42188) (0.25) = 0.42188$

The meaning of this particular calculation will be explained in detail in order to gain some insight into solving probability problems. There are four ways in which three patients can be cured and one patient not cured (see Table 3.2). Denoting the 4 patients as A, B, C, and D, the probability that patients A, B, and C are cured and patient D is not cured is equal to

$(0.75) (0.75) (0.75) (0.25) = 0.1055$ (3.10)

where 0.25 is the probability that patient D will *not* be cured. There is no reason why any of the four possibilities shown in Table 3.2 should occur more or less frequently than any other (i.e., each possibility is equally likely). Therefore, the probability that the antibiotic will successfully cure exactly three patients is four times the probability calculated in Eq. (3.10):

$4 (0.1055) = 0.422$

Table 3.2   Four Ways in Which 3 of 4 Patients are Cured

	1	2	3	4
Patients cured	A, B, C	A, B, D	A, C, D	B, C. D
Patients not cured	D	C	B	A

The expression $\binom{4}{3}$ represents a combination, a selection of three objects, disregarding order, from four distinct objects. The combination, $\binom{4}{3}$, is equal to 4, and, as we have just demonstrated, there are four ways in which three cures can be obtained from 4 patients. Each one of these possible outcomes has a probability of $(0.75)^3$ $(0.25)^1$. Thus, the probability of three cures in four patients is

$$4 \ (0.75)^3 \ (0.25)^1$$

as before.

The probability distribution based on the possible outcomes of an experiment in which four patients are treated with the antibiotic (the probability of a cure is 0.75) is shown in Table 3.3 and Fig. 3.5. Note that the sum of the probabilities of the possible outcomes equals 1, as is also shown in the cumulative probability function plotted in Fig. 3.5B. The cumulative distribution is a nondecreasing function starting at a probability of zero and ending at a probability of 1. Figures 3.1 and 3.2, describing the distribution of tablet attributes in a batch of tablets, are examples of other discrete probability distributions.

Table 3.3   Probability Distribution for Outcomes
of Treating Four Patients with an Antibiotic

Outcome	Probability
No cures	0.00391
One cure	0.04688
Two cures	0.21094
Three cures	0.42188
Four cures	0.31641

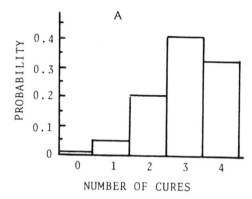

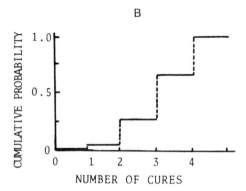

Figure 3.5   Probability distribution graph for outcomes of treating four patients with an antibiotic.

Statistical hypothesis testing, a procedure for making decisions based on variable data is based on probability theory. In the following example, we use data observed in a coin tossing game to decide whether or not we believe the coin to be loaded (biased).

You are an observer of a coin-tossing game and you are debating whether or not you should become an active participant. You note that only one head occurred among 10 tosses of the coin. You calculate the probability of such an event because it occurs to you that one head in 10 tosses of a coin is very unlikely; something is amiss (a "loaded" coin!). Thus, if the probability of a head is 0.5, the chances of observing one head in 10 tosses of a coin is less than 1 in 100 (Exercise Problem 18). This low probability suggests a coin that is not balanced. However, you properly note that the probability of any *single event* or outcome (such as one head in 10 trials) is apt to be small if N is sufficiently large. You decide to calculate the probability of this perhaps, unusual result *plus* all other possible outcomes which are equally or less probable. In our example, this includes possibilities of no heads in 10 tosses, in addition to one or no tails in 10 tosses. These four probabilities (no heads, one head, no tails, and one tail) total approximately 2.2%. This is strong evidence in favor of a biased coin. Such a decision is based on the fact that the chance of obtaining an event as unlikely or less likely than one head in 10 tosses is about 1 in 50 (2.2%) if the coin is *balanced*. You might wisely bet on tails on the next toss. You have made a decision: "The coin has a probability of less than 0.5 of showing heads on a single toss."

The probability distribution for the number of heads (or tails) in 10 tosses of a coin (p = 0.5 and N = 10) is shown in Fig. 3.6. Note the symmetry of the distribution. Although this is a discrete distribution, the "sticks" assume a symmetric shape similar to the

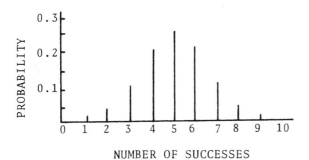

NUMBER OF SUCCESSES

Figure 3.6   Probability distribution for p = 0.5 and N = 10.

normal curve. The two unlikely events in each "tail" (i.e., no heads or tails or one head or one tail) have a total probability of 0.022. The center and peak of the distribution is observed to be at X = 5, equal to Np, the number of trials times the probability of success. (See also Table IV.3, p = 0.5, N = 10.)

The application of binomial probabilities can be extended to more practical problems than gambling odds for the pharmaceutical scientist. When tablets are inspected for attributes or patients treated with a new antibiotic, we can apply a knowledge of the properties of the binomial distribution to estimate the true proportion or probability of success, and make appropriate decisions based on these estimates.

3.3.2 Summary of Properties of the Binomial Distribution

1. The binomial distribution is defined by N and p. With a knowledge of these parameters, the probability of any outcome of N binomial trials can be calculated from Eq. (3.9). We have noted that the sum of all possible outcomes of a binomial experiment with N trials is 1, which conforms to the notion of a probability distribution.

2. The results of a binomial experiment can be expressed either as the *number of successes* or as a *proportion*. Thus, if six heads are observed in 10 tosses of a coin, we can also say that 60% of the tosses are heads. If 16 defective tablets are observed in a random sample of 1000 tablets, we can say that 1.6% of the tablets sampled are defective. In terms of proportions, the *true mean* of the binomial population is equal to the probability of success, p. The sample proportion (0.6 in the coin-tossing example and 0.016 in the example of sampling for defective tablets) is an estimate of the true proportion.

3. The variability of the results of a binomial experiment is expressed as a standard deviation. For example, when inspecting tablets for the number of defectives, a different number of defective tablets will be observed depending on which 1000 tablets happen to be chosen. This variation, dependent on the particular sample inspected, is also known as *sampling error*. The standard deviation of a binomial distribution can be expressed in two ways, depending on the manner in which the mean is presented (i.e., as a proportion or as the number of successes). The standard deviation in terms of proportion of successes is

$$\sqrt{\frac{pq}{N}}$$

(3.11)

In terms of number of successes, the standard deviation is

$$\sqrt{Npq} \qquad\qquad (3.12)$$

where N is the sample size, the number of binomial trials. As shown in Eqs. (3.11) and (3.12), the standard deviation is dependent on the value of p for binomial variables. The maximum s.d. occurs when $p = q = 0.5$, because pq is maximized. The value of pq does not change very much with varying p and q until p or q reach low or high values, close to or more extreme than 0.2 and 0.8.

p	q	pq
0.5	0.5	0.25
0.4	0.6	0.24
0.3	0.7	0.21
0.2	0.8	0.16
0.1	0.9	0.09

4. When dealing with proportions, the variability of the observed proportion can be made as small as we wish by increasing the sample size [similar to the s.d. of the mean of samples of size N, Eq. (1.8)]. This means that we can estimate the proportion of "successes" in a population with very little error if we choose a sufficiently large sample. In the case of the tablet inspection example above, the variability (s.d.) of the proportion for samples of size 100 is

$$\sqrt{\frac{(0.016)(0.984)}{100}} = 0.0125$$

By sampling 1000 tablets, we can reduce the variability by a factor of 3.16 ($\sqrt{100/1000} = 1/3.16$). The variability of the estimate of the true proportion (i.e., the sample estimate) is not dependent on the population size (the size of the entire batch of tablets in this example), but is dependent only on the size of the sample selected for observation. This interesting fact is true if the sample size is considerably smaller than the size of the population. Otherwise, a correction must be made in the calculation of the standard deviation [4]. If the sample size is no more than 5% of the population size, the correction is negligible. In virtually all of the examples that concern us in pharmaceutical experimentation, the sample size is considerably less than the population size. Since binomial data are often easy to obtain, large sample sizes can often be accommodated to obtain very precise estimates of population parameters. An oft-quoted example is that a sample size of 6000 to 7000 randomly selected voters will be sufficient to estimate the outcome of a national election within 1% of the total popular vote. Similarly, when sampling tablets for defects, 6000 to 7000 tablets will estimate the proportion of a property of the tablets (e.g., defects) within at most 1% of the true value. (The least precise estimate occurs when p = 0.5.)

3.4 CONTINUOUS DATA DISTRIBUTIONS

Another view of probability concerns continuous data such as tablet dissolution time. The probability that any single tablet will have a particular specified dissolution result is 0, because the number of possible outcomes for continuous data is infinite. Probability can be conceived as the ratio of the number of times that an event occurs to the total number of possible outcomes. If the total number of outcomes is infinite, the probability of any single event is zero. This concept can be confusing. If one observes a large number of dissolution results, such as time to 90% dissolution, any particular observation might appear to have a finite probability of occurring. Analogous to the discussion for discrete data, could we not make an equitable bet that a result for dissolution of exactly 5 min 13 sec, for example, would be observed? The apparent contradiction is due to the fact that data which are *continuous, in theory*, appears as *discrete* data *in practice* because of the limitations of measuring instruments, as discussed in Chap. 1. For example, a sensitive clock could measure time to virtually any given precision (i.e., to small fractions of a second). It would be difficult to conceive of winning a bet that a 90% dissolution time would occur at a very specific time, where time can be measured to any specified degree of precision (e.g., 30 min 8.21683475 . . . sec).

With *continuous* variables, we cannot express probabilities in as simple or intuitive a fashion as was done with discrete variables. Applications of calculus are necessary to describe concepts of probability with continuous distributions. Continuous cumulative probability distributions are represented by smooth curves (Fig. 3.7B) rather than the steplike function shown in Fig. 3.5B. The area under the probability distribution curve (also known as the probability density) is equal to 1 for all probability functions. Thus the area under the normal distribution curve in Fig. 3.7A is equal to 1.

3.4.1 The Normal Distribution

The normal distribution is an example of a continuous probability density function. The normal distribution is most familiar as the

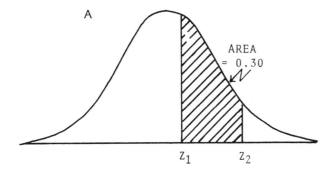

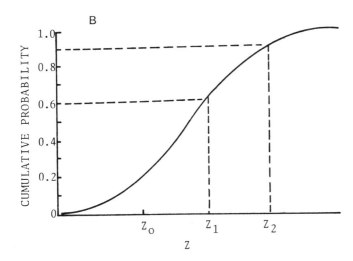

Figure 3.7   A normal distribution.

symmetrical, bell-shaped curve shown in Fig. 3.8.   A theoretical
normal distribution is a continuous probability distribution and consists of an infinite number of values.   In the theoretical normal distribution, the data points extend from positive infinity to negative
infinity.   It is clear that scientific data from pharmaceutical experiments cannot possibly fit this definition.   Neverthless, if real data
conform reasonably well with the theoretical definition of the normal
curve, adequate approximations, if not very accurate estimates of
probability, can be computed based on normal curve theory.

The equation for the normal distribution (normal probability
density) is

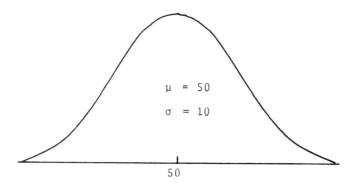

Figure 3.8   A typical normal curve.

$$Y = \frac{1}{\sigma\sqrt{2\pi}}\, e^{-(1/2)(X - \mu)^2/\sigma^2}$$ (3.13)

where

σ = standard deviation

μ = mean

X = value of the observation

e = base of natural logarithms, 2.718 . . .

Y = ordinate of normal curve, a function of X

The normal distribution is defined by its mean, μ, and its standard deviation, σ [see Eq. (3.13)]. This means that if these two parameters of the normal distribution are known, all the properties of the distribution are known. There are any number of different normal distributions. They all have the typical symmetrical, bell-shaped appearance. They are differentiated only by their means, a measure of location, and their standard deviation, a measure of spread. The normal curve shown in Fig. 3.8 can be considered to define the distribution of the potencies of tablets in a batch of tablets. Most of the tablets have a potency close to the mean potency of 50 mg. The farther the assay values are from the mean, the fewer the number of tablets there will be with these more extreme values. As noted above, the spread or shape of the normal distribution is dependent on the standard deviation. A large standard deviation means that the spread is large. In this example,

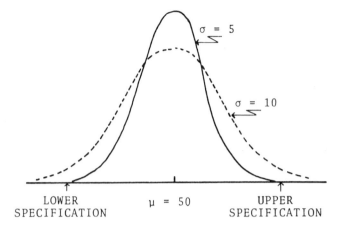

Figure 3.9 Two normal curves with different standard deviations.

a larger s.d. means that there are more tablets far removed from the mean, perhaps far enough to be out of specifications (see Fig. 3.9).

In real-life situations, the distribution of a finite number of values often closely approximates a normal distribution. Weights of tablets taken from a single batch may be approximately normally distributed. For practical purposes, any continuous distribution can be visualized as being constructed by categorizing a large amount of data in small equilength intervals and constructing a histogram. Such a histogram can similarly be constructed for normally distributed variables.

Suppose that all the tablets from a large batch are weighed and categorized in small intervals or boxes (see Fig. 3.10). The number of tablets in each box is counted and a histogram plotted as in

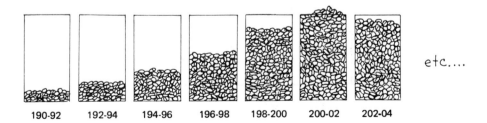

Figure 3.10 Categorization of tablets from a tablet batch by weight.

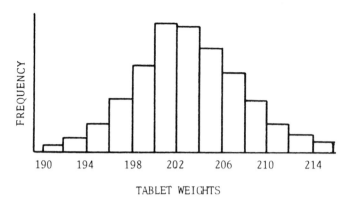

TABLET WEIGHTS

Figure 3.11   Histogram of tablet weights.

Fig. 3.11. As more boxes are added and the intervals made shorter,
the intervals will eventually be so small that the distinction between
the bars in the histogram is lost and a smooth curve results, as
shown in Fig. 3.12. In this example, the histogram of tablet weights
looks like a normal curve.

Areas under the normal curve represent probabilities and are
obtained by appropriate integration of Eq. (3.13). In Fig. 3.7, the
probability of observing a value between Z_1 and Z_2 is calculated by
integrating the normal density function between Z_1 and Z_2.

This function is not easily integrated. However, tables are
available that can be used to obtain the area between any two values

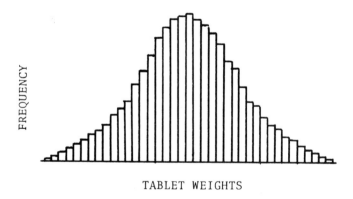

TABLET WEIGHTS

Figure 3.12   Histogram of tablet weights with small class intervals.

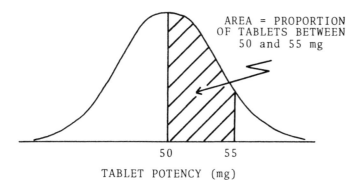

AREA = PROPORTION
OF TABLETS BETWEEN
50 and 55 mg

50   55

TABLET POTENCY (mg)

Figure 3.13   Area under normal curve as a representation of proportion of tablets in an interval.

of the variable, Z.   Such an area is illustrated in Fig. 3.7A.   If
the area between Z_1 and Z_2 in Fig. 3.7 is 0.3, the probability of
observing a value between Z_1 and Z_2 is 3 in 10 or 0.3.   In the
case of the tablet potencies, the area in a specified interval can be
thought of as the proportion of tablets in the batch contained in
the interval.   This concept is illustrated in Fig. 3.13
    Probabilities can be determined directly from the cumulative
distribution plot as shown in Fig. 3.7B (see Exercise Problem 9).
The probability of observing a value below Z_1 is 0.6.   The probability of observing a value below Z_2 is 0.9.   Therefore, the probability of observing a value between Z_1 and Z_2 is 0.9 - 0.6 = 0.3.
    There are an infinite number of normal curves depending on
μ and σ.   However, the area in any interval can be calculated from
tables of cumulative areas under the *standard normal curve*.   The
standard normal curve has a mean of 0 and a standard deviation of
1.   Table IV.2 in App. IV is a table of cumulative areas under the
standard normal curve, giving the area below Z (i.e., the area
between -∞ and Z).   For example, for Z = 1.96, the area in Table
IV.2 is 0.975.   This means that 97.5% of the values comprising the
standard normal curve are less than 1.96, lying between -∞ and
1.96.   The normal curve is symmetrical about its mean.   Therefore,
the area below -1.96 is 0.025 as depicted in Fig. 3.14.   The area
between Z equal to -1.96 and +1.96 is 0.95.   Referring to Table
IV.2, the area below Z equal to +2.58 is 0.995, and the area below
Z = 2.58 is 0.005.   Thus the area between Z equal to -2.58 and
+2.58 is 0.99.   It would be very useful for the reader to memorize
the Z values and the corresponding areas between ±Z as shown in

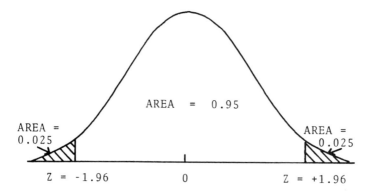

AREA = 0.95

AREA =
0.025

AREA =
0.025

Z = -1.96   0   Z = +1.96

Figure 3.14   Symmetry of the normal curve.

Table 3.4. These values of Z are commonly used in statistical analyses and tests.

The area in any interval of a normal curve with a mean and standard deviation different from 0 and 1, respectively, can be computed from the standard normal curve table by using a transformation. The transformation changes a value from the normal curve with mean μ and standard deviation σ, to the corresponding value, Z, in the standard normal curve. The transformation is

$$Z = \frac{X - \mu}{\sigma} \tag{3.14}$$

Table 3.4   Area Between ±Z for Some
Commonly Used Values of Z

Z	Area between ±Z
0.84	0.60
1.00	0.68
1.28	0.80
1.65	0.90
1.96	0.95
2.32	0.98
2.58	0.99

The area (probability) between -∞ and X (i.e., the area below X)
corresponds to the value of the area below Z from the cumulative
standard normal curve table. Note that if the normal curve which
we are considering is the standard normal curve itself, the transformation results in the identity

$$Z = \frac{X - 0}{1} = X$$

Z is exactly equal to X, as expected. Effectively the transformation
changes variables with a mean of μ and a standard deviation of σ to
variables with a mean of 0 and a standard deviation of 1.

Suppose in the example of tablet potencies that the mean is 50
and the standard deviation is 5 mg. Given these two parameters,
what proportion of tablets in the batch would be expected to have
more than 58.25 mg of drug? First we calculate the transformed
value, Z. Then the desired proportion (equivalent to probability)
can be obtained from Table IV.2. In this example, X = 58.25, μ =
50, and σ = 5. Referring to Eq. (3.14), we have

$$Z = \frac{X - \mu}{\sigma}$$

$$= \frac{58.25 - 50}{5} = 1.65$$

According to Table IV.2, the area between -∞ and 1.65 is 0.95.
This represents the probability of a tablet having 58.25 mg or less
of drug. Since the question was, "What proportion of tablets in
the batch have a potency greater than 58.25 mg?", the area above
58.25 mg is the correct answer. The area under the entire curve
is 1; the area above 58.25 mg is 1 - 0.95, equal to 0.05. This is
equivalent to saying that 5% of the tablets have at least 58.25 mg
(58.25 mg or more) of drug in this particular batch or distribution
of tablets. This transformation is illustrated in Fig. 3.15.

One should appreciate that since the normal distribution is a
perfectly symmetrical continuous distribution which extends from -∞
to +∞, real data never exactly fit this model. However, data from
distributions reasonably similar to the normal can be treated as being
normal, with the understanding that probabilities will be approximately correct. As the data are closer to normal, the probabilities
will be more exact. Methods exist to test if data can reasonably be
expected to be derived from a normally distributed population [1].
In this book, when applying the normal distribution to data we will
either (a) assume that the data are close to normal according to
previous experience or from an inspection of the data, or (b) that

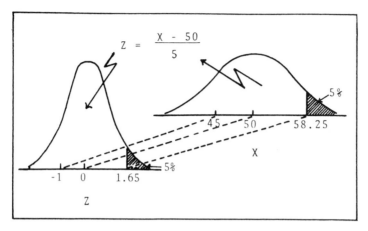

Figure 3.15   Z transformation for tablets with mean of 50 mg and s.d. of 5 mg.

normality will not greatly distort the probabilities based on the normal distribution.

Several examples are presented below which further illustrate applications of the normal distribution.

Example 1:   The U.S. Pharmacopia (USP) weight test for tablets states that for tablets weighing up to 100 mg, not more than 2 of 20 tablets may differ from the average weight by more than 10%, and no tablet may differ from the average weight by more than 20% [2]. To ensure that batches of a 100-mg tablet (labeled as 100 mg) will pass this test consistently, a statistician recommended that 98% of the tablets in the batch should weigh within 10% of the mean. One thousand tablets from a batch of 3,000,000 were weighed and the mean and standard deviation were calculated as 101.2 ± 3.92 mg. Before performing the official USP test, the quality control supervisor wishes to know if this batch meets the statistician's recommendation.   The calculation to answer this problem can be made using areas under the standard normal curve if the tablet weights can be assumed to have a distribution that is approximately normal. For purposes of this example, the sample mean and standard deviation will be considered equal to the true batch mean and standard deviation.   Although not exactly true, the sample estimates will be close to the true values when a sample as large as 1000 is used. For this large sample size, the sample estimates are very close to the true parameters.   However, one should clearly understand that to compute probabilities based on areas under the normal curve, both the mean and standard deviation must be known.   When these

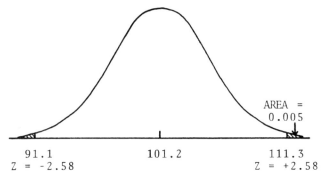

X = TABLET WEIGHT

Figure 3.16 Distribution of tablets with mean weight 101.2 mg and standard deviation equal to 3.92.

parameters are estimated from the sample statistics, other derived distributions can be used to calculate probabilities.

Figure 3.16 shows the region where tablet weights will be outside the limits, 10% from the mean ($\mu \pm 0.1 \mu$), that is, 10.12 mg or more from the mean for an average tablet weight of 101.2 mg (101.2 ± 10.12 mg). The question to be answered is: What proportion of tablets is between 91.1 and 111.3 mg? If the answer is 98% or greater, the requirements are met. The proportion of tablets between 91.1 and 111.3 mg can be estimated by computing the area under the normal curve in the interval 91.1 to 111.3, the unshaded area in Fig. 3.16. This can be accomplished by use of the Z transformation and the table of areas under the standard normal curve (Table IV.2). First we calculate the area below 111.3 using the Z transformation:

$$Z = \frac{X - \mu}{\sigma} = \frac{111.3 - 101.2}{3.92} = 2.58$$

This corresponds to an area of 0.995 (see Table IV.2). The area above 111.3 is (1 - 0.995) = 0.005 or 1/200. Referring to Fig. 3.16, this area represents the probability of finding a tablet that weighs 111.3 mg or more. The probability of a tablet weighing 91.1 mg or less is calculated in a similar manner.

$$Z = \frac{91.1 - 101.2}{3.92} = -2.58$$

Table IV.2 shows that this area is 0.005; that is, the probability of a tablet weighing between -∞ and 91.1 mg is 0.005. The probability that a tablet will weigh more than 111.3 mg or less than 91.1 mg is 0.005 + 0.005, equal to 0.01. Therefore, 99% (1.00 - 0.01) of the tablets weigh between 91.1 and 111.3 mg and the statistician's recommendation is more than satisfied. The batch should have no trouble passing the USP test.

The fact that the normal distribution is symmetric around the mean simplifies calculations of areas under the normal curve. In the example above, the probability of values exceeding Z equal to 2.58 is exactly the same as the probability of values being less than Z equal to -2.58. This is a consequence of the symmetry of the normal curve, 2.58 and -2.58 being equidistant from the mean. This is easily seen from an examination of Fig. 3.16.

Although this batch of tablets should pass the USP weight uniformity test, if *some* tablets in the batch are out of the 10 or 20% range, there is a chance that a random sample of 20 will fail the USP test. In our example, about 1% or 30,000 tablets will be more than 10% different from the mean (less than 91.1 or more than 111.3 mg). It would be of interest to know the chances, albeit small, that of 20 randomly chosen tablets, more than 2 would be "aberrant." When 1% of the tablets in a batch deviate from the batch mean by 10% or more, the chances of finding more than 2 such tablets in a sample of 20 is approximately 0.001 (1/1000). This calculation makes use of the binomial probability distribution.

Example 2: During clinical trials, serum cholesterol, among other serum components, is frequently monitored to ensure that a patient's cholesterol is within the normal range, as well as to observe possible drug effects on serum cholesterol levels. A question of concern is: What is an abnormal serum cholesterol value? One way to define "abnormal" is to tabulate cholesterol values for apparently normal healthy persons, and to consider values very remote from the average as abnormal. The distribution of measurements such as serum cholesterol often have an approximately normal distribution.

The results of the analysis of a large number of "normal" cholesterol values showed a mean of 215 mg % and a standard deviation of 35 mg %. This data can be depicted as a normal distribution as shown in Fig. 3.17. "Abnormal" can be defined in terms of the proportion of "normal" values that fall in the extremes of the distribution. This may be thought of in terms of a gamble. By choosing to say that extreme values observed in a new patient are abnormal, we are saying that persons observed to have very low or high cholesterol levels could be "normal," but the likelihood or probability that they come from the population of normal healthy persons is small. By defining an abnormal cholesterol value as one

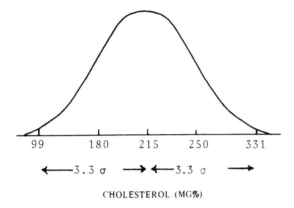

CHOLESTEROL (MG%)

Figure 3.17 Distribution of "normal" cholesterol values.

that has a 1 in 1000 chance of coming from the distribution of values from normal healthy persons, cutoff points can be defined for abnormality based on the parameters of the normal distribution. According to the cumulative standard normal curve, Table IV.2, a value of Z equal to approximately 3.3 leaves 0.05% of the area in the upper tail. Because of the symmetry of the normal curve, 0.05% of the area is below Z = -3.3. Therefore, 0.1% (1/1000) of the values will lie outside the values of Z equal to ±3.3 in the standard normal curve. The values of X (cholesterol levels) corresponding to Z = ±3.3 can be calculated from the Z transformation.

$$Z = \frac{X - \mu}{\sigma} = \frac{X - 215}{35} = \pm 3.3$$

$$X = 215 \pm (3.3)(35) = 99, 331$$

This is equivalent to saying that cholesterol levels which deviate from the average of "normal" persons by 3.3 standard deviation units or more are deemed to be abnormal. For example, the lower limit is the mean of the "normals" minus 3.3 times the standard deviation of 215 - (3.3)(35) = 99. The cutoff points are illustrated in Fig. 3.17.

Example 3: The standard normal distribution may be used to calculate the proportion of values in any interval from any normal distribution. As an example of this calculation, consider the data of cholesterol values in Example 2. We may wish to calculate the proportion of cholesterol values between 200 and 250 mg %.

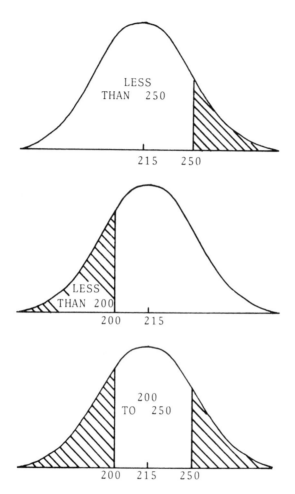

Figure 3.18 Illustration of the calculation of proportion of cholesterol values between 200 and 250 mg %.

Examination of Fig. 3.18 shows that the area (probability) under the normal curve between 200 and 250 mg % is the probability of a value being less than 250 *minus* the probability of a value being less than 200. Referring to Table IV.2, we have:
    Probability of a value less than 250:

$$\frac{250 - 215}{35} = 1 = Z \qquad \text{probability} = 0.841$$

Probability of a value less than 200:

$$\frac{200 - 215}{35} = -0.429 = Z \qquad \text{probability} = 0.334$$

Therefore, the probability of a value falling between 250 and 200 is

0.841 - 0.334 = 0.507

3.4.2 Central Limit Theorem

"Without doubt, the most important theorem in statistics is the central limit theorem" [3]. This theorem states that the distribution of sample means of size N taken from *any* distribution with a finite variance σ^2 and mean μ tends to be *normal* with variance σ^2/N and mean μ. We have previously discussed the fact that a sample mean of size N has a variance equal to σ^2/N. The new and important feature here is that if we are dealing with means of *sufficiently large sample size*, the means have a normal distribution, regardless of the form of the distribution from which the samples were selected.

How large is a "large" sample? The answer to this question depends on the form of the distribution from which the samples are taken. If the distribution is normal, any size sample results in means that are normally distributed. For distributions that deviate greatly from normality, larger samples will be needed to approximate normality than distributions which are more similar to the normal distributions (e.g., symmetrical distributions).

The power of this theorem is that the normal distribution can be used to describe most of the data with which we will be concerned, provided that the means come from samples of sufficient size. An example will be presented to illustrate how means of distributions far from normal tend to be normally distributed as the sample size increases. Later in this chapter we will see that even the discrete binomial distribution, where only a very limited number of outcomes are possible, closely approximates the normal distribution with sample sizes as small as 10 in symmetrical cases (e.g., p = q = 0.5).

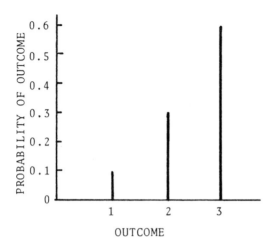

Figure 3.19   Probability distribution of outcomes 1, 2, and 3.

Consider a distribution which consists of outcomes 1, 2, and 3 with probabilities depicted in Fig. 3.19. The probabilities of observing values of 1, 2, and 3 are 0.1, 0.3, and 0.6, respectively. This an asymmetric distribution, with only three discrete outcomes. The mean is 2.5. Sampling from this population can be simulated by placing 600 tags marked with the number 3, 300 tags marked with the number 2, and 100 tags marked with the number 1 in a box. We will mix up the tags, select 10 (replacing each tag and mixing after each individual selection), and *compute the mean of the 10 samples*. A typical result might be five tags marked 3, four tags marked 2, and one tag marked 1, an average of 2.4. With a computer or programmable calculator, we can simulate this drawing of 10 tags. The distributions of 100 such means for samples of sizes 10 and 20 obtained from a computer simulation are shown in Fig. 3.20. The distribution is closer to normal as the sample size is increased from 10 to 20. This is an empirical demonstration of the central limit theorem. Of course, under ordinary circumstances, we would not draw 100 samples each of size 10 (or 20) to demonstrate a result that can be proved mathematically.

3.4.3   Normal Approximation to the Binomial

A very important result in statistical theory is that the binomial probability distribution can be approximated by the normal distribution if the sample size is sufficiently large (see Sec. 3.4.2). A

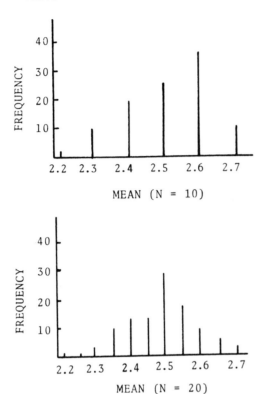

Figure 3.20 Distribution of means of sizes 10 and 20 from population shown in Fig. 3.19.

conservative rule of thumb is that if Np (the product of the number of observations and the probability of success) and Nq are both greater than or equal to 5, we can use the normal distribution to approximate binomial probabilities. With symmetric binomial distributions, when p = q = 0.5, the approximation works well for Np less than 5.

To demonstrate the application of the normal approximation to the binomial, we will examine the binomial distribution described above, where N = 10 and p = 0.5. We can superimpose a normal curve over the binomial with μ = 5 (number of successes) and standard deviation $\sqrt{Npq} = \sqrt{10(0.5)(0.5)} = 1.58$, as shown in Fig. 3.21.

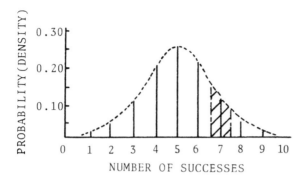

Figure 3.21   Normal approximation to binomial distribution: Np = 5 and s.d. = 1.58.

The probability of a discrete result can be calculated using the binomial probability [Eq. (3.9)] or Table IV.3.   The probability of seven successes, for example, is equal to 0.117.   In a normal distribution, the probability of a single value cannot be calculated. We can only calculate the probability of a range of values within a specified interval.   The area that approximately corresponds to the probability of observing seven successes in 10 trials is the area between 6.5 and 7.5, as illustrated in Fig. 3.21.   This area can be obtained using the Z transformation discussed earlier in this chapter [Eq. (3.14)].   The area between 6.5 and 7.5 is equal to the area below 7.5 minus the area below 6.5.

Area below 6.5:

$$Z = \frac{6.5 - 5}{1.58} = 0.948 \qquad \text{from Table IV.2, area} = 0.828$$

Area below 7.5:

$$Z = \frac{7.5 - 5}{1.58} = 1.58 \qquad \text{from Table IV.2, area} = 0.943$$

Therefore, the area (probability) between 6.5 and 7.5 is

$$0.943 - 0.828 = 0.115$$

This area is very close to the exact probability of 0.117.

The use of X ± 0.5 to help estimate the probability of a discrete value, X, using a continuous distribution (e.g., the normal distribution) is known as a continuity correction. We will see that the continuity correction is commonly used to improve the estimation of binomial probabilities by the normal approximation (Chap. 5).

Most of our applications of the binomial distribution will involve data that allow for the use of the normal approximation to binomial probabilities. This is convenient because calculations using exact binomial probabilities are tedious and much more difficult than the calculations using the standard normal cumulative distribution (Table IV.2), particularly when the sample size is large.

3.5 OTHER COMMON PROBABILITY DISTRIBUTIONS

3.5.1 The Poisson Distribution

Although we will not discuss this distribution further in this book, the Poisson distribution deserves some mention. The Poisson distribution can be considered to be an approximation to the binomial distribution when the sample size is large and the probability of observing a specific event is small. In quality control, the probability of observing a defective item is often calculated using the Poisson. The probability of observing X events of a given kind in N observations, where the probability of observing the event in a single observation is P, is

$$p(X) = \frac{\lambda^X e^{-\lambda}}{X!} \tag{3.15}$$

$\lambda = NP$

e = base of natural logarithms (2.718 . . .)

N = number of observations

We may use the Poisson distribution to compute the probability of finding one defective tablet in a sample of 100 taken from a batch with 1% defective tablets. Applying Eq. (3.15), we have

$$N = 100 \quad P = 0.01 \quad NP = \lambda = (100)(0.01) = 1$$

$$P(1) = \frac{(1)^1 (e^{-1})}{1!} = e^{-1} = 0.368$$

The exact probability calculated from the binomial distribution is 0.370. (See Exercise Problem 8.)

3.5.2   The t Distribution ("Student's t")

The t distribution is an extremely important probability distribution. This distribution can be constructed by repeatedly taking samples of size N from a normal distribution and computing the statistic

$$t = \frac{\overline{X} - \mu}{S/\sqrt{N}}$$ (3.16)

where $\overline{X}$ is the sample mean, μ the true mean of the normal distribution, and S the sample standard deviation. The distribution of the t's thus obtained forms the t distribution. The exact shape of the t distribution depends on sample size (degrees of freedom), but the t distribution is symmetrically distributed about a mean of zero, as shown in Fig. 3.22A.

To elucidate further the concept of a sampling distribution obtained by repeated sampling, as discussed for the t distribution above, a simulated sampling of 100 samples each of size 4 (N = 4) was performed. These samples were selected from a normal distribution with mean 50 and standard deviation equal to 5, for this example. The mean and standard deviation of each sample of size 4 were calculated and a t ratio [Eq. (3.16] constructed. The distribution of the 100 t values thus obtained is shown in Table 3.5. The data are plotted (histogram) together with the theoretically derived t distribution with 3 degrees of freedom (N - 1 = 4 - 1 = 3) in Fig. 3.23. Note that the distribution is symmetrically centered around a mean of 0, and that 5% of the t values are 3.18 or more units from the mean (theoretically).

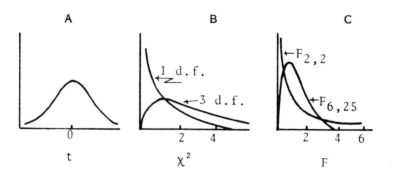

Figure 3.22   Examples of typical probability distributions.

Table 3.5 Frequency Distribution of 100 t Values Obtained by Simulated Repeat Sampling from a Normal Distribution with Mean 50 and Standard Deviation 5[a]

Class interval	Frequency
-5.5 to -4.5	1
-4.5 to -3.5	2
-3.5 to -2.5	2
-2.5 to -1.5	11
-1.5 to -0.5	18
-0.5 to +0.5	29
+0.5 to +1.5	21
+1.5 to +2.5	9
+2.5 to +3.5	4
+3.5 to +4.5	2
+4.5 to +5.5	1

[a]Sample size = 4.

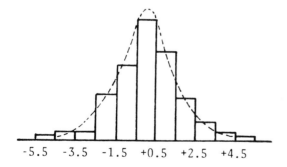

-5.5   -3.5   -1.5   +0.5   +2.5   +4.5

Figure 3.23 Simulated t distribution (d.f. = 3) compared to a theoretical t distribution.

3.5.3   The Chi-Square (χ^2) Distribution

Another important probability distribution in statistics is the chi-square distribution. The chi-square distribution may be derived from normally distributed variables, defined as the sum of squares of independent normal variables, each of which has mean 0 and standard deviation 1. Thus, if Z is normal with $\mu = 0$ and $\sigma = 1$,

$$\chi^2 = \Sigma\, Z_i^2 \qquad\qquad\qquad (3.17)$$

Applications of the chi-square distribution are presented in Chaps. 5 and 15. The chi-square distribution is often used to assess probabilities when comparing discrete values from comparative groups, where the normal distribution can be used to approximate discrete probabilities.

As with the t distribution, the distribution of chi-square depends on degrees of freedom, equal to the number of independent normal variables as defined in Eq. (3.17). Figure 3.22B shows chi-square distributions with 1 and 3 degrees of freedom.

3.5.4   The F Distribution

After the normal distribution, the F distribution is probably the most important probability distribution used in statistics. This distribution results from the sampling distribution of the ratio of two independent variance estimates obtained from the same normal distribution. Thus the first sample consists of N_1 observations and the second sample consists of N_2 observations:

$$F = \frac{S_1^2}{S_2^2} \qquad\qquad\qquad (3.18)$$

The F distribution depends on two parameters, the degrees of freedom in the numerator ($N_1 - 1$) and the degrees of freedom in the denominator ($N_2 - 1$). This distribution is used to test for differences of means (analysis of variance) as well as to test for the equality of two variances. The F distribution is discussed in more detail in Chaps. 5 and 8 as applied to the comparison of two variances and testing of equality of means in the analysis of variance, respectively.

KEY TERMS

Binominal distribution
Binominal formula
Binominal trial
Central limit theorem
Chi-square distribution
Combinations
Conditional probability
Continuous distribution
Cumulative distribution
Density function
Discontinuous variable
Discrete distribution
Distribution
Equally likely
Event
Factorial
Failure
F distribution

Independent events
Multiplicative probability
Mutually exclusive
Normal distribution
Outcome
Poisson distribution
Population
Probability
Probability distribution
Proportion
Random
Randomly chosen
Standard normal distribution
Success
t distribution
Variability
Z transformation

EXERCISES

1. Explain why you think that a controlled multicenter clinical study better estimates the probability of a patient responding to treatment than the observations of a single physician in daily practice.
2. Describe the population that represents the multicenter antibiotic clinical study described in Sec. 3.3.
3. Give three examples of probability distributions that describe the probability of outcomes in terms of attributes.
4. Explain why 30,000 tablets are only specked if 20,000 tablets are both chipped and specked as described in Sec. 3.2. What is the probability, in the example described in Sec. 3.2, of finding a specked tablet *or* a chipped tablet? (Hint: Count all the tablets that have either a speck or a chip.) See Eq. (3.4).
5. In a survey of hospital patients, it was shown that the probability that a patient has high blood pressure given that he or she is diabetic was 0.85. If 10% of the patients are diabetic and 25% have high blood pressure:
    (a) What is the probability that a patient has both diabetes and high blood pressure?
    (b) Are the conditions of diabetes and high blood pressure independent?
    [Hint: See Eqs. (3.5), (3.6), and (3.7).]

6. Show how the result 0.21094 is obtained for the probability of
    two of four patients being cured if the probability of a cure is
    0.75 for each patient and the outcomes are independent (see
    Table 3.2). (Enumerate all ways in which two of four patients
    can be cured, and compute the probability associated with each
    of these ways.)

7. What is the probability that three of six patients will be cured
    if the probability of a cure is 60%?

8. Calculate the probability of one success in 100 trials if p = 0.01.

9. From the cumulative plot in Fig. 3.7B, estimate the probability
    that a value, selected at random, will be (a) greater than Z_0;
    (b) less than Z_0.

10. What is the probability that a normal patient has a cholesterol
    value below 170 (μ = 215, σ = 35)?

11. If the mean and standard deviation of the potency of a batch of
    tablets are 50 mg and 5 mg, respectively, what proportion of
    the tablets have a potency between 40 and 60 mg?

12. If a patient has a serum cholesterol value outside normal limits,
    does this mean that the patient is abnormal in the sense of
    having a disease or illness?

13. Serum sodium values for normal persons have a mean of 140
    mEq/L and a s.d. of 2.5. What is the probability that a per-
    son's serum sodium will be between 137 and 142 mEq/L?

14. Data were collected over many years on cholesterol levels of
    normal persons in a New York hospital with the following results
    based on 100,000 readings. The mean is 205 mg %; the standard
    deviation is 45. Assuming that the data have a normal distribu-
    tion, what is the probability that a normal patient has a value
    greater than 280 mg %?

15. In the game of craps, two dice are thrown, each die having an
    equal probability of showing one of the numbers 1 to 6 inclusive.
    Explain why the probability of observing a point of 2 (the sum
    of the numbers on the two dice) is 1/36.

16. Is the probability of observing two heads and one tail the same
    under the two following conditions: (a) simultaneously throwing
    three coins; (b) tossing one coin three consecutive times? Ex-
    plain your answer.

17. What odds would you give of finding either none *or* one defec-
    tive tablet in a sample of size 20 if the batch of tablets has 1%
    defective? Answer the same question if the sample size is 100.

18. What is the probability of observing exactly one head in 10
    tosses of a coin?

**19. The chance of obtaining a cure using a conventional treat-
    ment for a particular form of cancer is 1%. A new treatment
    being tested cures two of the first four patients tested.

Would you announce to the world that a major breakthrough in the treatment of this cancer is imminent? Explain your answer.

20. What is the standard deviation for the binomial experiments described in Problems 17 and 19? (Answer in terms of Npq and pq/N.)

**21. In screening new compounds for pharmacological activity, the compound is administered to 20 animals. For a standard drug, 50% of the animals show a response on the average. Fifteen of the twenty animals show the response after administration of a new drug. Is the new drug a promising candidate? Why? [Hint: Compute the s.d. of the response based on p = 0.5. See if the observed response is more than 2 s.d.'s greater than 0.5.]

22. Using the binomial formula, calculate the probability that a sample of 30 tablets will show 0 or 1 defect if there are 1% defects in the batch. (What is the probability that there will be more than one defect in the sample of 30?)

REFERENCES

1. Hald, A., *Statistical Theory and Engineering Applications*, Wiley, New York, 1965.
2. *United States Pharmacopeia*, 20th Rev., and *National Formulary*, 15th ed., USP Pharmacopeial Convention, Inc., Rockville, Md., 1980.
3. Ostle, B., *Statistics in Research*, 3rd ed., Iowa State University Press, Ames, Iowa, 1981.
4. Dixon, W. J. and Massey, F. J., Jr., *Introduction to Statistical Analysis*, 3rd ed., McGraw-Hill, New York, 1969.

4
Choosing Samples

The samples are the units that provide the experimental observations, such as tablets sampled for potency, patients sampled for plasma cholesterol levels, or tablets inspected for defects. The sampling procedure is an essential ingredient of a good experiment. An otherwise excellent experiment or investigation can be invalidated if proper attention is not given to choosing samples in a manner consistent with the experimental design or objectives. Statistical treatment of data and the inference based on experimental results depend on the sampling procedure. The way in which samples should be selected is not always obvious, and requires careful thought.

The implementation of the sampling procedure may be more or less difficult depending on the experimental situation, such as that which we may confront when choosing patients for a clinical trial or choosing tablets for quality control tests. In this chapter we discuss various ways of choosing samples and assigning treatments to experimental units (e.g., assigning different drug treatments to patients). We will briefly discuss various types of sampling schemes, such as simple random sampling, stratified sampling, systematic sampling, and cluster sampling. In addition, the use of random number tables to assign experimental units to treatments in designed experiments will be described.

4.1   INTRODUCTION

There are many different ways of selecting samples. We all take samples daily, although we usually do not think of this in a statistical sense. Cooks are always sampling their wares, tasting the soup to see if it needs a little more spice, or sampling a gravy or sauce to see if it needs more mixing. When buying a car, we take a test ride in a "sample" to determine if it meets our needs and desires.

The usual purpose of observing or measuring a property of a sample is to make some inference about the population from which the sample is drawn. In order to have reasonable assurance that we will not be deceived by the sample observations, we should take care that the samples are not biased. We would clearly be misled if the test car was not representative of the line, but had somehow been modified to entice us into a sale. We can never be sure that the sample we observe mirrors the entire population. If we could observe the entire population, we would then know its exact nature. However, 100% sampling is virtually never done. (One well-known exception is the U.S. census.) It is costly, time consuming, and may result in erroneous observations. For example, to inspect each and every one of 2 million tablets for specks, a tedious and time consuming task, would probably result in many errors due to fatigue of the inspectors.

Destructive testing precludes 100% sampling. To assay each tablet in a batch does not make sense. Under ordinary circumstances, no one would assay every last bit of bulk powder to ensure that it is not adulterated.

The sampling procedure used will probably depend on the experiemental situation. Factors to be considered when devising a sampling scheme include:

1. The nature of the population. For example, can we enumerate the individual units, such as packaged bottles of a product, or is the population less easily defined, as in the case of hypertensive patients?
2. The cost of sampling in terms of both time and money.
3. Convenience. Sometimes it may be virtually impossible to carry out a particular sampling procedure.
4. Desired precision. The accuracy and precision desired will be a function of the sampling procedure and sample size.

Sampling schemes may be roughly divided into *probability sampling* and *nonprobability sampling* (sometimes called authoritative sampling). Nonprobability sampling methods often are conceptually convenient and simple. These methods are considered as methods of *convenience* in many cases. Samples are chosen in a particular manner because alternatives are difficult. For example, when sampling powder from 10 drums of a shipment of 100 drums, those drums that are most easily accessible might be the ones chosen. Or, when sampling tablets from a large container, we may conveniently choose from those at the top. A "judgment" sample is chosen with possible knowledge that some samples are more "representative" than others, perhaps based on experience. A quality control inspector may decide to inspect a product during the middle of a run, feeling that the middle is more representative of the "average" product than samples obtained at the beginning or end of the run. The inspector may also choose particular containers for inspection based on knowledge of the manufacturing and bottling procedures. A "haphazard" sample is one taken without any predetermined plan, but one in which the sampler tries to avoid bias during the sampling procedure. Nonprobability samples often have a hidden bias, and it is not possible to apply typical statistical methods to estimate the population parameters (e.g., μ and σ) and the precision of the estimates. Nonprobability sampling methods should not be used unless probability sampling methods are too difficult or too expensive to implement.

We will discuss procedures and some properties of common *probability sampling methods*. Objects chosen to be included in probability samples have a known probability of being included in the sample and are chosen by some random device.

4.2   RANDOM SAMPLING

Simple *random sampling* is a common way of choosing samples. A random sample is one in which each individual (object) in the

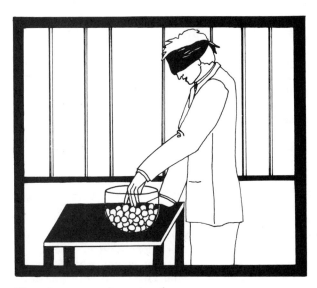

Choosing a random sample.

population to be sampled has an *equal chance of being selected.*
The procedure of choosing a random sample can be likened to a
bingo game or a lottery where the individuals (tags, balls, tablets,
etc.) are thoroughly mixed, and the sample chosen at "random."
This ensures that there is no bias; that is, on the average, the
estimates of the population parameters (e.g., the mean) will be accurate. Note that a parameter estimate, such as the mean, computed from a particular sample will, in all probability, not equal the
true parameter. Many statistical procedures are based on an assumption that samples are chosen at random. Simple random sampling is most effective when the variability is relatively small and
uniform over the population [1].

In most situations, it is not possible to mix the objects that
constitute the population and pick the samples out of a "box." But
if all members of the population can be identified, a unique identification, such as a number, can be assigned to each individual unit.
We can then choose the sample by picking numbers, randomly, from
a box using a lottery-like technique. Usually, this procedure is
more easily accomplished through the use of a table of random numbers. Random numbers have been tabulated extensively [2]. In
addition to available tables, computer-generated random numbers
may be used to select random samples or to assign experimental
units randomly to treatments as described below.

4.2.1   Table of Random Numbers

Random numbers are frequently used as a device to choose samples
to be included in a survey, a quality control inspection sample, or
to assign experimental units to treatments such as assigning patients
to drug treatments. The first step that is often necessary in the
application of a table of random numbers is to assign a number to
each of the experimental units in the population or to the units potentially available for inclusion in the sample. The numbers are
assigned consecutively from 1 to N, where N is the number of units
under consideration. The experimental units may be patients to be
assigned to one of two treatments or bottles of tablets to be inspected for defects. We then choose a "starting point" in the table
of random numbers, in some "random" manner. For example, we
can close our eyes and point a finger on a page of the random number table, and this can be the starting point. Alternatively, the
numbers thus chosen can be thought of as the page, column, and
row number of a new starting point. Using this random procedure,
having observed the numbers 3674826, we would proceed to page 367,
column 48, and row 26 in a book such as *A Million Random Digits*
[2]. This would be the starting point for the random section. If
the numbers designating the starting point do not correspond to an

available page, row, or column, the next numbers in sequence (going down or across the page as is convenient) can be used, and so on.

Table IV.1 is a typical page from a table of random numbers. The exact use of the table will depend on the specific situation. Some examples should clarify applications of the random number table table to randomization procedures.

1. A sample of 10 bottles is to be selected from a universe of 800 bottles. The bottles are numbered from 1 to 800 inclusive. A starting point is selected from the random number table and three-digit numbers are used to accommodate the 800 bottles. Suppose that the starting point is row 6 and column 21 in Table IV.1. (The first three-digit number is 177.) If a number greater than 800 appears or a number is chosen a second time (i.e., the same number appears twice or more in the table), skip the number and proceed to the next one. The first 10 numbers found in Table IV.1 with the starting point above and subject to the foregoing restraints are (reading down) 177, 703, 44, 127, 528, 43, 135, 104, 342, and 604 (see Table 4.1). Note that we did not include 964 because there is no bottle with this number; only 800 bottles are available. These numbers correspond to the 10 bottles that will be chosen for inspection.

2. Random numbers may be used to assign patients randomly to treatments in clinical trials. Initially, the characteristics and source of the patients to be included in the trial should be carefully considered. If a drug for the treatment of asthma were to be compared to a placebo treatment, the source (or population) of the samples to be chosen could be all asthmatics in this country. Clearly, even if

Table 4.1   Excerpt from Table IV.1

	Column 21
Row 6	17 7
	70 3
	04 4
	12 7
	52 8
	04 3
	13 5
	96 4
	10 4
	34 2
	60 4

we could identify all such persons, for obvious practical reasons it would not be possible to choose those to be included in the study using the simple random sampling procedure described previously. In fact, in clinical studies of this kind, patients are usually recruited by an investigator (physician), and *all* patients who meet the protocol requirements and are willing to participate are included. Most of the time, patients in the study are randomly assigned to the two or more treatments by means of a table of random numbers or a similar "random" device. Consider a study with 20 patients designed to compare an active drug substance to an identically appearing placebo. As patients enter the study, they are assigned randomly to one of the treatment groups, 10 patients to be assigned to each group. One way to accomplish this is to "flip" a coin, assigning, for example, heads to the active drug product and tails to the placebo. After 10 patients have been assigned to one group, the remaining patients are assigned to the incomplete group.

A problem with a simple random assignment of this kind is that an undesirable allocation may result by chance. For example, although improbable, the first 10 patients could be assigned to the active treatment and the last 10 to the placebo, an assignment that the randomization procedure is intended to avoid. (Note that if the treatment outcome is associated with a time trend due to seasonal effects, physician learning, personnel changes, etc., such an assignment would bias the results.) In order to avoid this possibility, the randomization can be applied to subgroups of the sample. For 20 patients, one possibility is to randomize in groups of 4, 2 actives and 2 placebos to be assigned to each group of 4. This procedure also ensures that if the study should be aborted at any time, approximately equal numbers of placebo and active treated patients will be included in the results.

If the randomization is performed in groups of 4 as recommended, the following patient allocation would result. (Use Table 4.1 for the random numbers as before, odd for placebo, even for active.)

Patient	Random no.	Drug	Comment
1	1	P	
2	7	P	
3	–	D	Assign D to patients 3 and 4 to
4	–	D	ensure equal allocation of D and P in the subgroup
5	0	D	
6	1	P	
7	5	P	
8	–	D	Assign D to patient 8 to ensure equal allocation of D and P in the subgroup.

Patient	Random no.	Drug	Comment
9	0	D	
10	1	P	
11	9	P	
12	–	D	Assign D to patient 12 to ensure equal allocation of D and P in the subgroup
13	1	P	
14	3	P	
15	–	D	Assign D to patients 15 and 16
16	–	D	to ensure equal allocation of D and P in the subgroup
17	6	D	
18	7	P	
19	0	D	
20	–	P	Assign P to patient 20 to ensure equal allocation of D and P in the subgroup

The source and methods of randomization schemes for experiments or clinical studies should be documented for U.S. Food and Drug Administration (FDA) submissions or for legal purposes. Therefore, it is a good idea to use a table of random numbers or a computer-generated randomization scheme for documentation rather than the coin-flipping technique. One should recognize, however that the latter procedure is perfectly fair, the choice of treatment being due to chance alone. Using a table of random numbers, a patient may be assigned to one treatment if an odd number appears and to the other treatment if an even number appears. We use single numbers for this allocation. If even numbers are assigned to drug treatment, the numbers in Table 4.1 would result in the following assignment to drug and placebo (read numbers down each column, one number at a time; the first number is 1, the second number is 7, the third number is 0, etc.):

Patient			Patient			Patient			Patient		
1	1	P	6	0	D	11	6	D	16	2	D
2	7	P	7	1	P	12	7	P	17	4	D
3	0	D	8	9	P	13	0	D	18	3	P
4	1	P	9	1	P	14	4	D			
5	5	P	10	3	P	15	2	D			

Table 4.2   Excerpt from Table IV.1:   Assignment of first 10 Numbers Between 1 and 20 to Placebo

					Column 11									
Row 11 —	—	—	—	—	44	22	78	84	26	04	33	46	09	52
59	29	97	68	60	71	91	38	67	54	13	58	18	24	76
48	55	90	65	72	96	57	69	36	10	96	46	92	42	45
66	37	32	20	30	77	84	57	03	29	10	45	65	04	26
68	49	69	10	82	53	75	91	93	30	34	25	20	57	27
83	62	64	11	12	67	19	—	—	—	—	—	—	—	—

Since 10 patients have been assigned to placebo (P), the remaining 2 patients are assigned to drug (D). Again, the randomization can be performed in subgroups as described in the previous paragraph. If the randomization is performed in subgroups of size 4, for example, the first 4 patients would be assigned as follows: patients 1 and 2 to placebo (random numbers 1 and 7), and patients 3 and 4 to drug to attain equal allocation of treatments in this sample of 4.

Another approach is to number the patients from 1 to 20 inclusive as they enter the study. The patients corresponding to the first 10 numbers from the random number table are assigned to one of the two treatment groups. The remaining patients are assigned to the second treatment. In our example, the first 10 numbers will be assigned to placebo and the remaining numbers to drug. In this case, two-digit numbers are used from the random number table. (The numbers 1 to 20 have at most two digits.) Starting at row 11, column 11 in Table IV.1 and reading across, the numbers in Table 4.2 represent patients to be assigned to the first treatment group, placebo. Reading across, the first 10 numbers to appear that are between 1 and 20 (disregarding repeats), underlined in Table 4.2, are 4, 9, 13, 18, 10, 20, 3, 11, 12, and 19. These patients are assigned to placebo. The remaining patients, 1, 2, 5, 6, 7, 8, 14, 15, 16, and 17, are assigned to drug.

4.3   OTHER SAMPLING PROCEDURES: STRATIFIED, SYSTEMATIC, AND CLUSTER SAMPLING

4.3.1   Stratified Sampling

Stratified sampling is a procedure in which the population is divided into subsets or strata, and random samples are selected from each strata. Stratified sampling is a recommended way of sampling when the strata are very different from each other, but objects within each stratum are alike. The precision of the estimated population mean from this sampling procedure is based on the variability within the strata. Stratified sampling will be particularly advantageous when this within-object variability is small compared to the variability between objects in different strata. In quality control procedures, items are frequently selected for inspection at random within specified time intervals (strata) rather than in a completely random fashion (simple random sampling). Thus we might sample 10 tablets during each hour of a tablet run. Often, the sample size chosen from each stratum is proportional to the size of the stratum, but in some circumstances, disproportionate sampling may be optimal. The computation of the mean and variance based on stratified sampling can be complicated, and the analysis of the data should take stratification into account [1]. In the example of the clinical study on asthmatics (Sec. 4.2.1), the stratification could be accomplished by dividing the asthmatic patients into subsets (strata) depending on age, duration of illness, or severity of illness, for example. The patients are assigned to treatments randomly within each subset. Note in this example that patients within each stratum are more alike than patients from different strata.

Consider an example of sampling tablets for drug content (assay) during a tablet run. If we believe that samples taken close in time are more alike than those taken at widely differing times, stratification would be desirable. If the tableting run takes 10 hours to complete, and a sample of 100 tablets is desired, we could take 10 tablets randomly during each hour, a stratified sample. This procedure would result in a more precise estimate of the average tablet potency than a sample of 100 tablets taken randomly over the entire 10-hour run.

Although stratified sampling often results in better precision of the estimate of the population mean, in some instances the details of its implementation may be more difficult than those of simple random sampling.

4.3.2 Systematic Sampling

Systematic sampling is often used in quality control. In this kind of sampling, every nth item is selected (e.g., every 100th item). The initial sample is selected in a random manner. Thus a quality control procedure may specify that 10 samples be taken at a particular time each hour during a production run. The time during the hour for each sampling may be chosen in a random manner. Systematic sampling is usually much more convenient, and much easier to accomplish than simple random sampling and stratified sampling. It also results in a uniform sampling over the production run, which may result in a more precise estimate of the mean. Care should be taken that the process does not show a cycle or periodic behavior, because systematic sampling will then not be representative of the

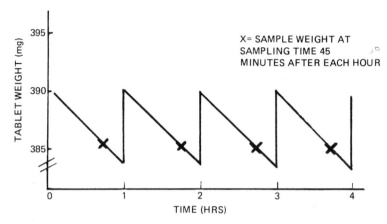

Figure 4.1 Illustration of problem with systematic sampling when process shows periodic behavior.

process. The correct variance for the mean of a systematic sample is less than that of a simple random sample if the variability of the systematic sample is greater than the variability of the entire set of data.

To illustrate the properties of a systematic sample, consider a tableting process in which tablet weights tend to decrease during the run, perhaps due to a gradual decrease in tableting pressure. The press operator adjusts the tablet pressure every hour to maintain the desired weight. The tablet weights during the run are illustrated in Fig. 4.1. If tablets are sampled 45 min after each hour, the average result will be approximately 385 mg, a biased result.

If the data appear in a random manner, systematic sampling may be desirable because it is simple and convenient to implement. As noted above, "systematic sampling is more precise than random sampling if the variance within the systematic samples is larger than the population variance as a whole. Another way of saying this is that systematic sampling is precise when units within the same sample are heterogeneous, and imprecise when they are homogeneous" [3]. In the tableting example noted in the previous paragraph, the units in the sample tend to be similar (precise) and systematic sampling is a poor choice. (See Exercise Problem 11 for an example of construction of a systematic sample.)

4.3.3   Cluster Sampling

In cluster sampling, the population is divided into groups or clusters
each of which contain "subunits." In single-stage cluster sampling,
clusters are selected at random and all elements of the clusters
chosen are included in the sample.

Two-stage cluster sampling may be used when there are many
"primary" units, each of which can be "subsampled." For example, suppose that we wish to inspect tablets visually, packaged
in the final labeled container. The batch consists of 10,000 bottles
of 100 tablets each. The primary units are the bottles and the subsample units are the tablets within each bottle. Cluster sampling,
in this example, might consist of randomly selecting a sample of 100
bottles, and then inspecting a random sample of 10 tablets from each
of these bottles, thus the nomenclature, "two-stage" sampling.
Often, cluster sampling is the most convenient way of choosing a
sample. In the example above, it would be impractical to select
1000 tablets at random from the 1,000,000 packaged tablets (10,000
bottles × 100 tablets per bottle).

For a continuous variable such as tablet weights or potency,
the estimate of the variance of the mean in two-stage cluster sampling is:

$$(1 - f_1)S_1^2/n + [S_2^2/(nm)]f_1(1 - f_2) \qquad\qquad (4.1)$$

where S_1^2 is the estimate of the variance among the primary unit
means (the means of bottles).

S_2^2 is the estimate of the variance of the subsample units, i.e.,
units within the primary units (between tablets within bottles).

f_1 and f_2 are the sampling fractions of the primary and subsample units, respectively. These are the ratios of units sampled
to the total units available. In the present example of bottled
tablets,

f_1 = 100 bottles/10,000 bottles = 0.01 (100 bottles are randomly
    selected from 10,000)

f_2 = 10 tablets/100 tablets = 0.1 (10 tablets are randomly
    selected from 100 for each of the 100 bottles)

n = number of primary unit samples (100 in this example)

m = number of units sampled from each primary unit (10 in
    this example)

If, in this example, S_1^2 and S_2^2 are 2 and 20, respectively, from Eq. (4.1), the estimated variance of the mean of 1000 tablets sampled from 100 bottles (10 tablets per bottle) is

$$(1 - 0.01)(2)/100 + [20/(100 \times 10)](0.01)(0.9) = 0.01998$$

If 1000 tablets are sampled by taking 2 tablets from each of 500 bottles, the estimated variance of the mean is

$$(1 - 0.05)(2)/500 + [20/(500 \times 2)](0.05)(0.98) = 0.00478$$

This example illustrates the increase in efficiency of sampling more primary units. The variance obtained by sampling 200 bottles is approximately one-half that of sampling 100 bottles. If f_1 is small, the variance of the mean is related to the number of primary units sampled (n) equal to approximately S_1^2/n. Cost and time factors being equal, it is more efficient to sample more primary units and fewer subsample units given a fixed sample size. However, in many situations it is not practical or economical to sample a

Tablet Sampling

large number of primary units. The inspection of tablets in finished
bottles is an example where inspection of many primary units
(bottles) would be costly and inconvenient. See Exercise Problems
9 and 10 for further illustrations.

4.4   SAMPLING IN QUALITY CONTROL

Sampling of items for inspection, chemical, or physical analysis is a
very important aspect of quality control procedures. For the mo-
ment, we will not discuss the important question: "What size sample
should we take?" This will be discussed in Chap. 6. What concerns us here is how to choose the samples. In this respect, the
important points to keep in mind from a statistical point of view are:

1.   The sample should be "representative."
2.   The sample should be chosen in a way that will be compatible
     with the objectives of the eventual data analysis.

For example, when sampling tablets, we may be interested in
estimating the mean and standard deviation of the weight or potency
of the tablet batch. If 20 tablets are chosen for a weight check
during each hour for 10 hours from a tablet press (a stratified or
systematic sample), the mean and standard deviation are computed
in the usual manner if the production run is uniform resulting in
random data. However, if warranted, the analysis should take into
account the number of tablets produced each hour and the uniformity of production during the sampling scheme. For example, in a
uniform process, an estimate of the average weight would be the
average of the 200 tablets, or equivalently, the average of the
averages of the 10 sets of 20 tablets sampled. However, if the rate
of tablet production is doubled during the 9th and 10 hours, the
averages obtained during these 2 hours should contribute twice the
weight to the overall average as the average results obtained during
the first 8 hours. For further details of the statistical analysis of
various sampling procedures, the reader is referred to Refs. 1
and 3.
      Choosing a representative sample from a bulk powder, as an ex-
ample, is often based on judgment and experience more than on scientific criteria (a "judgment" sample). Rules for sampling from
containers and for preparing powdered material or granulations for
assay are, strictly speaking, not "statistical" in nature. Bulk powder sampling schemes have been devised in an attempt to obtain a
representative sample without having to sample an inordinately large
amount of material. A common rule of thumb, taking samples from
$\sqrt{N}$ + 1 containers (N is the total number of containers), is a way

to be reasonably sure that the material inspected is representative of the entire lot, based on tradition rather than on objective grounds. Using this rule, given a batch of 50 containers, we would sample $\sqrt{50} + 1 = 8$ containers. The eight containers can be chosen using a random number table (see Exercise Problem 3).

Sampling plans for bulk powders and solid mixes such as granulations usually include the manner of sampling, the number of samples, and preparation for assay with an aim of obtaining a representative sample. One should bear in mind that a single assay will not yield information on variability. No matter what precautions we take to ensure that a single sample of a mix is representative of a batch, we can only estimate the degree of homogeneity by repeating the procedure one or more times on different portions of the mix. Repeat assays on the same sample gives an estimate of analytical error, not homogeneity of the mix.

An example of a procedure for sampling from large drums of a solid mixture is to insert a thief (a device for sampling bulk powders) and obtain a sample from the center of the container. A grain thief may be used to take samples from more than one part of the container. This procedure is repeated for an appropriate number of containers and the samples thoroughly mixed. The sample to be submitted for analysis is mixed further and quartered, rejecting two

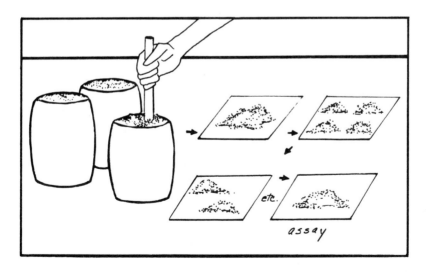

Sampling and Assaying Bulk Powders.

diagonal portions. The mixing and quartering is repeated until sufficient sample for analysis remains.

KEY TERMS

Cluster sample   Sample
Haphazard sample   Sampling with replacement
Judgment sample   Simple random sample
Multistage sample   Stratified sample
Nonprobability sample   Systematic sample
Probability sample   Table of random numbers
Representative sample   Two-stage cluster sample

EXERCISES

Use the table of random numbers (Table IV.1) to answer the following questions.

1. Twenty-four patients are recruited for a clinical study, 12 patients to be randomly assigned to each of two groups, A and B.
   The patients come to the clinic and are entered into the study
   chronologically, randomly assigned to treatment A or B. Devise
   a schedule showing to which treatment each of the 24 patients
   is assigned.
2. Devise a randomization scheme similar to that done in Problem 1
   if 24 patients are to be assigned to three treatments.
3. Thirty drums of bulk material are to be sampled for analysis.
   How many drums would you sample? If the drums are numbered
   1 to 30, explain how you chose drums and take the samples.
4. A batch of tablets is to be packaged in 5000 bottles each containing 1000 tablets. It takes 4 hours to complete the packaging
   operation. Ten bottles are to be chosen for quality control
   tests. Explain in detail how you would choose the 10 bottles.
5. Devise a randomization scheme to assign 20 patients to drug and
   placebo groups (10 patients in each group) using the numbers
   shown in Table 4.1 by using even numbers for assignment to
   drug and odd numbers for assignment to placebo.
6. Describe two different ways in which 20 tablets can be chosen
   during each hour of a tablet run.
7. One hundred bottles of a product, labeled 0 to 99 inclusive,
   are available to be analyzed. Analyze five bottles selected at
   random. Which five bottles would you choose to analyze?
8. A batch of tablets is produced over an 8-hr period. Each hour
   is divided into four 15-min intervals for purposes of sampling.

(Sampling can be done during 32 intervals, four per hour for 8 hr.) Eight samples are to be taken during the run. Devise (a) a simple random sampling scheme, (b) a stratified sampling scheme, and (c) a systematic sampling scheme. Which sample would you expect to have the smallest variance? Explain.

9. The average potencies of tablets in 20 bottles labeled 1 to 20 are

Bottle number	Potency	Bottle number	Potency
1	312	2	311
3	309	4	309
5	310	6	308
7	307	8	305
9	306	10	307
11	305	12	301
13	303	14	300
15	299	16	300
17	300	18	297
19	296	20	294

(a) Choose a random sample of 5 bottles. Calculate the mean and standard deviation.

(b) Choose a systematic sample, choosing every 4th sample, starting randomly with one of the first 4 bottles. Calculate the mean and standard deviation of the sample.

(c) Compare the averages and standard deviations of the 2 samples and explain your results. Compare your results to those obtained by other class members.

10. Ten containers each contain 4 tablets. To estimate the mean potency, 2 tablets are to be randomly selected from 3 randomly chosen containers. Perform this sampling from the data shown below. Estimate the mean and variance of the mean. Repeat the sampling, taking 3 tablets from 2 containers. Explain your results. Compute the mean potency of all 40 tablets.

Container	Tablet potencies (mg)	Container	Tablet potencies (mg)
1	290 289 305 313	2	317 300 285 327
3	288 322 306 299	4	281 305 309 289
5	292 295 327 283	6	286 327 297 314
7	311 286 281 288	8	306 282 282 285
9	313 301 315 285	10	283 327 315 322

11. Twenty-four containers of a product are produced during
     8 minutes, 3 containers each minute. The drug content of
     each container is shown below:

Minute	Container assay		
1	80	81	77
2	78	76	76
3	84	83	86
4	77	77	79
5	83	81	82
6	81	79	80
7	82	79	81
8	79	79	80

Eight containers are to be sampled and analyzed for quality
control. Take a sample of 8 as follows:

(a) Simple random sample
(b) Stratified sample; take one sample at random each minute
(c) Systematic sample; start with the first, second, or third
     container and then take every third sample thereafter.

Compute the mean and the variance of each of your 3 samples
(a, b, and c). Discuss the results. Which sample gave the
best estimate of the mean? Compare your results to those obtained from the other students in the class.

REFERENCES

1. Snedecor, G. W. and Cochran, W. G., *Statistical Methods*, 7th
    ed., Iowa State University Press, Ames, Iowa, 1980.
2. The Rand Corporation, *A Million Random Digits with 100,000
    Normal Deviates*, The Free Press, New York, 1966.
3. Cochran, W. G., *Sampling Techniques*, 3rd ed., Wiley, New
    York, 1967.
4. Stuart, A., *Basic Ideas of Scientific Sampling*, Charles Griffith
    & Co., Ltd., London, 1976.

5

Statistical Inference: Estimation and Hypothesis Testing

Parameter estimates obtained from samples are usually meant to be used to estimate the true population parameters. The sample mean and variance are typical estimators or predictors of the true mean and variance, and are often called "point" estimates. In addition, an interval that is apt to contain the true parameter often accompanies and complements the point estimate. These intervals, known as *confidence intervals*, can be constructed with a known a priori probability of bracketing the true parameter.

The question of *statistical significance* pervades much of the statistics commonly used in pharmaceutical and clinical studies. Advertising, competitive claims, and submissions of supporting data for drug efficacy to the FDA usually require evidence of superiority, effectiveness, and/or safety based on the traditional use of statistical hypothesis testing. This is the technique that leads to the familiar statement, "The difference is statistically significant" (at the 5% level or less, for example), words that open many regulatory doors. Many scientists and statisticians feel that too much is made of testing for statistical significance, and that decisions based on such statistical tests are often not appropriate. However, testing for statistical significance is one of the backbones of standard statistical methodology and the properties and applications of such tests are well understood and familiar in many experimental situations. This aspect of statistics is not only important to the pharmaceutical scientist in terms of applications to data analysis and interpretation, but is critical to an understanding of the statistical process. Since much of the material following this chapter is based largely on a comprehension of the principles of hypothesis testing, the reader is urged to make special efforts to understand the material presented in this chapter.

5.1   STATISTICAL ESTIMATION
(CONFIDENCE INTERVALS)

We will introduce the concept of statistical estimation and confidence intervals before beginning the discussion of hypothesis testing. Scientific experimentation may be divided into two classes: (a) experiments designed to estimate some parameter or property of a system, and (b) comparative experiments, where two or more treatments or experimental conditions are to be compared. The former type of experiment is concerned with estimation and the latter is concerned with hypothesis testing.

The term *estimation* in statistics has a meaning much like its meaning in ordinary usage. A population parameter is estimated based on the properties of a sample from the population. We have discussed the unbiased nature of the sample estimates of the true mean and variance, designated as $\bar{X}$ and S^2 (Secs. 1.4 and 1.5). These sample statistics estimate the population parameters and are considered to be the best estimates of these parameters from several points of view.* However, the reader should understand that statistical conclusions are couched in terms of probability. Statistical conclusions are not invariant as may be the case with results of mathematical proofs. Without having observed the entire population, one can never be sure that the sample closely reflects the population. In fact, as we have previously emphasized, sample statistics such as the mean and variance are rarely equal to the population parameters.

Nevertheless, the sample statistics (e.g., the mean and variance) are the best estimates we have of the true parameters. Thus, having calculated $\bar{X}$ and S^2 for potencies of 20 tablets from a batch, one may very well inquire about the true average potency of the batch. If the mean potency of the *20 tablets is 49.8 mg*, the *best estimate* of the true batch mean is *49.8 mg*. Although we may be almost certain that the true batch mean is not exactly 49.8 mg, there is no reason, unless other information is available, to estimate the mean to be a value different from 49.8 mg.

The discussion above raises the question of the reliability of the sample statistic as an estimate of the true parameter. Perhaps one should hesitate in reporting that the true batch mean is 49.8 mg based on data from only 20 tablets. One might question the

---

*"Point" estimates are unbiased, consistent, minimum variance estimates. Among unbiased estimators, these have minimum variance, and approach the true value with high probability as the sample size gets very large.

reliability of such an estimate. The director of quality control might inquire: "How close do you think the true mean is to 49.8 mg?" Thus it is a good policy when reporting an estimate such as a mean, to include some statement as to the reliability of the estimate. Does the 49.8-mg estimate mean that the true mean potency could be as high as 60 mg, or is there a high probability that the true mean is not more than 52 mg? This question can be answered by use of a *confidence interval*. A confidence interval is an interval within which we believe the true mean lies. We can say, for example, that the true batch mean potency is between 47.8 and 51.8 mg with 95% probability. The width of the interval depends on the properties of the population, the sample estimates of the parameters, and the degree of certainty desired (the probability statement).

Since most of the problems that we will encounter are concerned with the normal distribution, particularly sampling of means, we are most interested in confidence intervals for means. If the distribution of means is normal and σ is known, an interval with confidence coefficient, P (probability), can be computed using a table of the cumulative standard normal distribution, Table IV.2. A two-sided confidence interval, symmetric about the observed mean, is calculated as follows:

$$P\% \text{ confidence interval} = \overline{X} \pm \frac{Z_P \sigma}{\sqrt{N}} \tag{5.1}$$

where

$\overline{X}$ = observed sample mean

N = sample size

σ = population standard deviation

Z_P = normal deviate corresponding to the $(P + 1)/2$ percentile of the cumulative standard normal distribution (Table IV.2)

For the most commonly used *95%* confidence interval, *Z = 1.96*, corresponding to $(0.95 + 1)/2 = 0.975$ of the area in the cumulative standard normal distribution. Other common confidence coefficients are *90%* and *99%*, having values of Z equal to *1.65* and *2.58*, respectively. Inspection of Table IV.2 shows that the area in the tails of a normal curve beyond ±1.65, ±1.96, and ±2.58 standard deviations from the mean is 90, 95, and 99%, respectively. This is illustrated in Fig. 5.1 (see also Table 3.4).

Before presenting examples of the computation and use of confidence intervals, the reader should take time to understand the concept of a confidence interval. The confidence interval changes

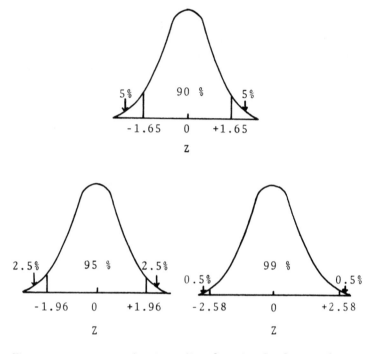

Figure 5.1   Areas in the tails of a standard normal curve.

depending on the sample chosen because, although σ* and N remain the same, $\overline{X}$ varies from sample to sample. A confidence interval using the mean from any given sample may or may not contain the true mean. Without a knowledge of the true mean, we cannot say whether or not any given interval contains the true mean. However, it can be proven that when intervals are constructed according to Eq. (5.1), P% (e.g., 95%) of such intervals will contain the true mean. Figure 5.2 shows how means of size N, taken from the same population, generate confidence intervals. Think of this as means of size 20, each mean generating a confidence interval [Eq. (5.1)]. For a 95% confidence interval, 19 of 20 such intervals will cover the true mean, μ, on the average. Any single interval has a 95% chance of covering the true mean, a priori. Of course, one would not usually take many means in an attempt to verify this concept, which can be proved theoretically. Under usual circumstances, only a single mean is observed and a confidence interval

---

*σ is assumed to be known in this example.

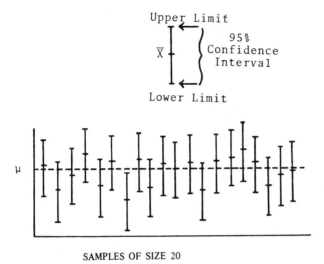

SAMPLES OF SIZE 20

Figure 5.2   Concept of the confidence interval.

computed. This interval may not cover the true mean, but we know that 19 of 20 such intervals will cover the true mean.

Looking at the confidence interval from another point of view, suppose that a mean of 49.8 mg was observed for a sample size of 20 with $\sigma/\sqrt{N}$ ($\sigma_{\overline{X}}$) equal to 2. According to Eq. (5.1), the 95% confidence interval for the true mean is $49.8 \pm 1.96(2) = 45.9$ to 53.7 mg. Figure 5.3 shows that if the true mean were outside the

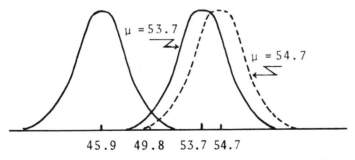

Figure 5.3   This figure shows that a mean of 49.8 is unlikely to be observed if the true mean is 54.7 (confidence interval = 45.9 to 53.7).

range 45.9 to 53.7, the observation of the sample mean, 49.8 mg, would be very unlikely. The dashed curve in the figure represents the distribution of means of size 20 with a true mean of 54.7 and $\sigma_{\overline{X}} = 2$. In this example, the true mean is outside the 95% confidence interval, and the probability of observing a mean from this distribution as small as 49.8 mg or less is less than 1% (see Exercise Problem 1). Therefore, one could conclude that the true mean is probably not as great as 54.7 mg based on the observation of a mean of 49.8 mg from a sample of 20 tablets.

5.1.1   Confidence Intervals Using the t Distribution

In most situations in which confidence intervals are computed, σ, the true standard deviation, is unknown, but is estimated from the sample data. A confidence interval can still be computed based on the sample standard deviation, S. However, the interval based on the sample standard deviation will tend to be wider than that computed with a known standard deviation. This is reasonable because if the standard deviation is not known, one has less knowledge of the true distribution and consequently less assurance of the location of the mean.

The computation of the confidence interval in cases where the standard deviation is estimated from sample data is similar to that shown in Eq. (5.1) except that a value of t is substituted for the Z value:

$$P\% \text{ confidence interval} = \overline{X} \pm \frac{tS}{\sqrt{N}} \tag{5.2}$$

Values of t are obtained from the cumulative t table, Table IV.4, corresponding to a P% confidence interval.

The appropriate value of t depends on degrees of freedom (d.f.), a concept that we encountered in Sec. 1.5.2. When constructing confidence intervals for means, the d.f. are equal to N - 1, where N is the sample size. For samples of size 20, d.f. = 19 and the appropriate values of t for *90, 95, or 99%* confidence intervals are *1.73, 2.09*, and *2.86*, respectively. Examination of the t table shows that the values of t decrease with increasing d.f., and approach the corresponding Z values (from the standard normal curve) when the d.f. are large. This is expected, because when d.f. = ∞, the standard deviation is known and the t distribution coincides with the standard normal distribution. We will talk more of the t distribution later in this chapter (see also Sec. 3.5).

5.1.2 Examples of Construction of Confidence Intervals

Example 1: Confidence interval when σ is unknown and estimated from the sample. The labeled potency of a tablet dosage form is 100 mg. Ten individual tablets are assayed according to a quality control specification. The 10 assay results shown in Table 5.1 are assumed to be sampled from a normal distribution. The sample mean is 103.0 mg and the standard deviation is 2.22. A 95% confidence interval for the true batch mean [Eq. (5.2)] is

$$103 \pm 2.26 \left(\frac{2.22}{\sqrt{10}} \right) = 101.41 \text{ to } 104.59$$

Note that the t value is 2.26. This is the value of t with 9 d.f. (N = 10) for a 95% confidence interval taken from Table IV.4.

Example 2: Confidence interval when σ is known. Suppose that the standard deviation were *known* to be equal to 2.0. The 95% confidence interval for the mean is [Eq. (5.1)]

$$\overline{X} \pm \frac{1.96\sigma}{\sqrt{N}} = 103.0 \pm \frac{1.96(2.0)}{\sqrt{10}} = 101.76 \text{ to } 104.24$$

The value 1.96 is obtained from Table IV.2 (Z = 1.96 for a two-sided symmetrical confidence interval) or from Table IV.4 for t with ∞ d.f.

Table 5.1 Assay Results for 10 Randomly Selected Tablets (mg)

101.8	104.5
102.6	100.7
99.8	106.3
104.9	100.6
103.8	105.0
$\overline{X} = 103.0$	S = 2.22

Two questions arise from this example.

1. How can we know the s.d. of a batch of tablets without assaying every tablet?
2. Why is the s.d. used in Example 2 different from that in Example 1?

Although it would be foolhardy to assay each tablet in a batch (particularly if the assay were destructive, that is, the sample is destroyed during the assay process), the variance of a "stable" process can often be precisely estimated by averaging or pooling the variance over many batches (see also Sec. 12.2 and App. I). The standard deviation obtained from this pooling is based on a large number of assays and will become very stable as long as the tableting process does not change. The pooled standard deviation can be assumed to be equal to or close to the true standard deviation (see Fig. 5.4).

The answer to the second question has actually been answered in the previous paragraph. The variance of any single sample of 10 tablets will not be identical to the true variance, 2^2 or 4 in the example above. If the average variance over many batches can be considered equal to or very close to the true variance, the pooled variance is a better estimate of the variance than that obtained from 10 tablets. This presupposes that the variance does not change from batch to batch. Under these conditions, use of the pooled variance rather than the individual sample variance will result in a narrower confidence interval, on the average.

Example 3:   Confidence Interval for a Proportion

(a) In a preclinical study, 100 untreated (control) animals were observed for the presence of liver disease. After 6 months, 25 of these animals were found to have the disease. We wish to compute a 95% confidence interval for the true proportion of animals who would have this disease if untreated (after 6 months). A confidence interval for a proportion has the same form as that for a mean. Assuming that the normal approximation to the binomial is appropriate, the confidence interval is approximately:

$$\hat{p} \pm Z \sqrt{\frac{\hat{p}\hat{q}}{N}} \tag{5.3}$$

where

$\hat{p}$ = observed proportion

Z = appropriate cutoff point from the normal distribution (Table IV.2)

N = sample size

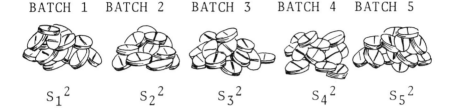

BATCH 1   BATCH 2   BATCH 3   BATCH 4   BATCH 5

S_1^2 S_2^2 S_3^2 S_4^2 S_5^2

POOLED $S^2 = \overline{S}^2 = \Sigma S^2/N$; N = NUMBER OF BATCHES

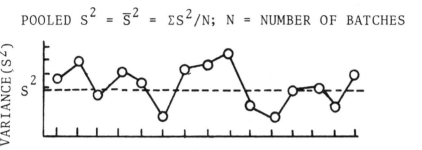

$$\overline{S} = \sqrt{\overline{S}^2}$$

Figure 5.4 Pooling variances over batches, a good estimate of the true variance of a stable process (same sample size per batch).

In the present example, a 95% confidence interval is

$$0.25 \pm 1.96 \sqrt{\frac{(0.25)(0.75)}{100}} = 0.165 \text{ to } 0.335$$

The true proportion is probably between 16.5 and 33.5%.* Notice that the mean is equal to the observed proportion and that the normal approximation to the binomial distribution makes use of the Z value of 1.96 for the 95% confidence interval from the cumulative normal distribution. The standard deviation is computed from Eq. (3.11), $\sigma = \sqrt{\hat{p}\hat{q}/N}$.

---

*Both $N\hat{p}$ and $N\hat{q}$ should be equal to or greater than 5 when using the normal approximation to the binomial (Sec. 3.4.3).

A 99% confidence interval for the true proportion is

$$0.25 \pm 2.58 \sqrt{\frac{(0.25)(0.75)}{100}} = 0.138 \text{ to } 0.362$$

Note that the 99% confidence interval is wider than the 95% interval. The greater the confidence, the wider is the interval. To be 99% "sure" that the true mean is contained in the interval, the confidence interval must be wider than that which has a 95% probability of containing the true mean.

(b) To obtain a confidence interval for the true *number of animals* with liver disease when a sample of 100 shows 25 with liver disease, we use the standard deviation according to Eq. (3.12), $\sigma = \sqrt{Np\hat{q}}$. A 95% confidence interval for the true *number* of diseased animals (where the observed number is $Np = 25$) is

$$N\hat{p} \pm 1.96 \sqrt{N\hat{p}\hat{q}} = 25 \pm 1.96 \sqrt{(0.25)(0.75)(100)}$$

$$= 16.5 \text{ to } 33.5$$

This answer is exactly equivalent to that obtained using proportions in part (a) ($16.5/100 = 0.165$ and $33.5/100 = 0.335$). Further examples of symmetric confidence intervals are presented in conjunction with various statistical tests in the remaining sections of this chapter. In particular, confidence intervals for the true difference of two means or two proportions are given in Secs. 5.22, 5.23, and 5.26.

5.1.3   Asymmetric Confidence Intervals

One-Sided Confidence Intervals

In most situations, a confidence interval symmetric about the observed mean seems most appropriate. This is the shortest interval given a fixed probability. However, there are examples where a one-sided confidence interval can be more useful. Consider the case of a clinical study in which 18 of 500 patients treated with a marketed drug report headaches as a side effect. Suppose that we are only concerned with an "upper limit" on the proportion of drug-related headaches to be expected in the population of users of the drug. In this example, when constructing a 95% interval, we use a Z (or t) value that cuts off 5% of the area in the upper tail of the distribution, rather than the 2.5% in each tail excluded in a symmetric interval. Using the normal approximation to the binomial, the upper limit is

$p + Z\sqrt{pq/N}$

$18/500 + 1.65\sqrt{(0.036)(0.964)/500}$

$0.036 + 0.014 = 0.050$

Based on the one-sided 95% confidence interval, we conclude that the true proportion of headaches among drug users is probably not greater than 5%. Note that we make no statement about the lower limit, which must be greater than 0. Another application of a one-sided confidence interval is presented in Chap. 7, Sec. 7.5, as applied to the analysis of stability data.

Other Asymmetric Confidence Intervals

In general, many P% confidence intervals can be constructed by suitably allocating $(1 - P)$% of the area to the lower and upper tails of the normal distribution. For example, a 95% confidence interval may be constructed by placing 1% of the area in the lower tail and 4% in the upper tail. This is not a common procedure and a good reason should exist before one decides to make such an allocation. Westlake [1,2] has proposed such an interval for the construction of confidence intervals in bioequivalence studies. In these studies, a ratio of some property (such as maximum serum concentration) of two products is compared. Westlake argues that an interval symmetric about the ratio 1.0 is more useful than one symmetric about the observed sample mean. The interval often has the great majority of the area in either the lower of upper tail, depending on the observed ratio. For a ratio greater than 1.0, most of the area will be in the upper tail and vice versa. Figure 5.5 illustrates this

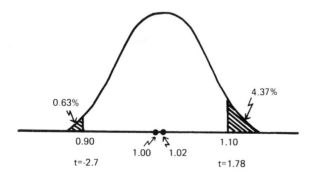

Figure 5.5 A 95% assymetric confidence interval with $\overline{X}$ = 1.02, S.D. = 0.2, and N = 20.

concept with a hypothetical example for products with an average ratio of 1.02. If the standard deviation is unknown and is estimated as 0.2 with 19 d.f. (N = 20), a 95% symmetric interval would be estimated as

$$1.02 \pm (2.1)(0.2)/\sqrt{20} = 1.02 \pm 0.094 = 0.926 \text{ to } 1.114$$

To construct the Westlake interval, a symmetric interval about 1.0, detailed tables of the t distribution are needed [1]. In this example, t values of approximately 1.78 and -2.70 will cut off 4.3% of the area in the upper tail and 0.7% in the lower tail, respectively. This results in an upper limit of 1.02 + 0.08 = 1.10 and a lower limit of 1.02 $-$ 0.12 = 0.90, symmetric about 1.0 (1.0 $\pm$ 0.1).

The remainder of this chapter will be concerned primarily with testing hypotheses, categorized as follows:

1. Comparison of the mean of a single sample (group) to some known or standard mean [single-sample (group) tests]
2. Comparison of means from two independent samples (groups) [two-independent-samples (groups) test, a form of the parallel-groups design in clinical trials]
3. Comparison of means from related samples (paired-sample tests)
4. One and two sample tests for proportions
5. Tests to compare variances

5.2   STATISTICAL HYPOTHESIS TESTING

To introduce the concept of hypothesis testing, we will use an example of the comparison of two treatment means (a two-sample test) which has many applications in pharmaceutical and clinical research. The details of the statistical test are presented in Sec. 5.2.2. A clinical study is planned to compare the efficacy of a new antihypertensive agent to a placebo. Preliminary uncontrolled studies of the drug in humans suggest antihypertensive activity of the order of a drop of 10 to 15 mmHg diastolic blood pressure. The proposed double-blind clinical trial is designed to study the effects of a once-a-day dose of tablets of the drug in a group of hypertensive patients. A second group of patients will receive an identical-appearing placebo. Blood pressure will be measured prior to the study and every 2 weeks after initiation of therapy for a total of 8 weeks. For purposes of this presentation, we will be concerned only with the blood pressure at baseline (i.e., pretreatment) and after 8 weeks of treatment. The variable that will be analyzed is the difference between the 8-week reading and the pretreatment reading. This difference, the change from baseline, will be called

Table 5.2 Average Results and Standard Deviation of a Clinical Study Comparing Drug and Placebo in the Treatment of Hypertension

	Drug	Placebo
Number of patients	11	10
Average blood pressure reduction (mmHg)	10	1
Standard deviation	11.12	7.80

δ (delta). At the completion of the experiment, the average change from baseline will be compared for the active group and the placebo group in order to come to a decision concerning the efficacy of the drug in reducing blood pressure. The design is a typical *parallel-groups* design and the implementation of the study is straightforward. The problem, and question, that is of concern is: "What statistical techniques can be used to aid us in coming to a decision regarding the treatment (placebo and active drug) difference, and ultimately to a judgment of drug efficacy?"

From a qualitative and, indeed, practical point of view, a comparison of the *average* change in blood pressure for the active and placebo groups, integrated with previous experience, can give some idea of drug efficacy. Table 5.2 shows the average results of this study. (Only 21 patients completed the study.) Based on the results, our "internal computer" might reason as follows: "The new drug reduced the blood pressure by 10 mmHg compared to a reduction of 1 mmHg for patients on placebo. That is an impressive reduction for the drug"; or "The average reduction is quite impressive, but the sample size is small, less than 12 patients per group. If the raw data were available, it would be of interest to see how many patients showed an improvement when given the drug compared to the number who showed an improvement when given placebo." Such an examination of the clinical results may give an intuitive feeling of the effectiveness of a drug product. At one time, not very long ago, presentation of such experimental results accompanied by a subjective evaluation by the clinical investigator was important evidence in the support of efficacy of drugs. If the average results showed that the drug was no better than the placebo, the drug would probably be of little, if any interest.

One obvious problem with such a subjective analysis is the potential lack of consistency in the evaluation and conclusions that may be drawn from the same results by different reviewers. Also,

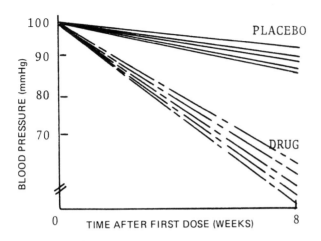

Figure 5.6   Mark of a real drug effect: A large difference between drug and placebo with small variation.

although some experimental results may appear to point unequivocally to either efficacy or lack of efficacy, the inherent variability of the experimental data may be sufficiently large to obscure the truth. In general, subjective perusal of data is not sufficient to separate drug-related effects from random variability.   Statistical hypothesis testing is an objective means of assessing whether or not observed differences between treatments can be attributed to experimental variation (error).   Good experimental design and data analysis are essential if clinical studies are to be used as evidence for drug safety and efficacy.   This is particularly critical when such evidence is part of a New Drug Application (NDA) for the FDA, or for use for advertising claims.

   The statistical evaluation or test of treatment differences is based on the *ratio* of the *observed treatment difference* (drug minus placebo in this example) to the *variability* of the difference.   A large observed difference between drug and placebo accompanied by small variability is the most impressive evidence of a real drug effect (see Fig. 5.6).

   The magnitude of the ratio can be translated into a probability or "statistical" statement relating to the true but unknown drug effect.   This is the basis of the common statement "statistically significant," implying that the difference observed between treatments is real, not merely a result of random variation.   Statistical significance addresses the question of whether or not the treatments truly differ, but does not necessarily apply to the *practical* magnitude of the drug effect. The possibility exists that a small but real drug effect has no clinical meaning. Such judgments should be made by experts who can evaluate the magnitude of the drug effect in relation to the potential use of the drug vis-à-vis other therapeutic alternatives.

The preliminary discussion above suggests the procedure used in testing statistical hypotheses. Broadly speaking, data are first collected for comparative experiments according to an appropriate plan or design. For comparative experiments similar to that considered in our example, the *ratio* of the difference of the averages of the two treatments to its experimental error (standard deviation) is referred to an appropriate tabulated probability distribution. The treatment difference is deemed "statistically significant" if the ratio is sufficiently large relative to the tabulated probability values.

The testing procedure is based on the concept of a *null hypothesis*. The null hypothesis is a hypothetical statement about a parameter (such as the mean) which will subsequently be compared to the sample estimate of the parameter, to test for treatment differences. In the present example, the null hypothesis is

$$H_0: \quad \mu_1 = \mu_2 \quad \text{or} \quad \Delta = \mu_1 - \mu_2 = 0$$

H_0 refers to the null hypothesis. μ_1 and μ_2 refer to the true blood pressure change from baseline for the two treatments. Δ is the hypothesized average difference of the change of blood pressure from baseline values for the new drug *compared* to placebo.

Δ = true average reduction in blood pressure due to drug minus true average reduction in blood pressure due to placebo

The sample estimate of Δ is designated as $\bar{\delta}$, and is assumed to have a normal distribution. The fact that H_0 is expressed as a specific difference (zero in this example), as opposed to a more general difference ($H_0: \Delta \neq 0$), is an important concept. The test of "no difference" or some specific difference (e.g., $\Delta = 2$) is usually much more easily conceptualized and implemented than a test of some nonspecific difference.

The format of the null hypothesis statement is not always immediately apparent to those unfamiliar with statistical procedures. Table 5.3 shows some examples of how null hypothesis statements can be presented. The alternative hypothesis specifies alternative values of the parameter, which we accept as true if the statistical test leads to rejection of the null hypothesis. The alternative hypothesis includes values not specified in the null hypothesis. In our example, a reasonable alternative would include all values where

Table 5.3   Examples of the Null Hypothesis for Various Experimental Situations

Study	Null hypothesis	Comments
Effect of drug therapy on cholesterol level compared to placebo	$H_0: \mu_1 = \mu_2$ or $H_0: \mu_1 - \mu_2 = 0$ or $H_0: \Delta = 0$	μ_1 refers to the true average cholesterol with drug and μ_2 refers to true average cholesterol with placebo
Effect of antibiotic on cure rate	$H_0: p_0 = 0.8$	p_0 refers to the true proportion of patients cured; H_0 states that the hypothetical cure rate is 80%
Average tablet weight for quality control	$H_0: W = 300$ mg	The target weight is a mean of 300 mg
Testing two mixing procedures with regard to homogeneity of the two mixes	$H_0: \sigma_1^2 = \sigma_2^2$	The variance of the samples from the two procedures is hypothesized to be equal
Test to see if two treatments differ	$H_0: \mu_1 \neq \mu_2$	This statement cannot be tested; H_0 must be specified as a specific difference or a limited range of differences

the true values of the two means were not equal, typically stated as follows:

$$H_a: \quad \mu_1 \neq \mu_2$$

As noted above, the magnitude of the ratio of the (observed difference minus the hypothetical difference) to its variability, the s.d. of the observed difference, determines whether or not H_0 should be accepted or rejected. A large ratio leads to rejection of H_0, and the difference is considered to be "statistically" significant. The specific details for testing simple hypotheses are presented below, beginning with the most elementary example, tests of a single mean.

5.2.1 Case I: Test of the Mean from a Single Population (One-Sample Tests), an Introduction to a Simple Example of Hypothesis Testing

The discussion above was concerned with a test to compare means from samples obtained from two groups, a drug group and a placebo group. The tests for a single mean are simpler in concept, and specific steps to construct this test are presented below. The process for other designs in which statistical hypotheses are tested is essentially the same as for the case described here. Other examples will be presented in the remainder of this chapter and, where applicable, in subsequent chapters of this book. The concept of hypothesis testing is important, and the student is well advised to make an extra effort to understand the procedures described below.

Data often come from a single population, and a comparison of the sample mean to some hypothetical or "standard" (known) value is desired. The examples shown in Table 5.4 are typical of those found in pharmaceutical research. The statistical test compares the observed value (a mean or a proportion, for example) to the hypothetical value.

To illustrate the procedure, we will consider an experiment to assess the effects of a change in manufacturing procedure on the average potency of a tablet product. A large amount of data was collected for the content of drug in the tablet formulation during a period of several years. The manufacturing process showed an average potency of 5.01 mg and a standard deviation of 0.11, both values considered to be equal to the true process parameters. A new batch was made with a modification of the usual manufacturing procedure. Twenty tablets were assayed and the results are shown in Table 5.5. The objective is to determine if the process modification results in a change of average potency from the process average of 5.01, the value of μ under the null hypothesis.

Table 5.4   Examples of Experiments Where a Single Population Mean is Observed

Sample mean	Hypothetical or standard mean
Average tablet potency of N tablets	Label potency
Preference for product A in a paired preference test	50% are hypothesized to prefer product A
Average dissolution of N tablets	Quality control specifications
Proportion of patients cured by a new drug	Cure rate of P% based on previous therapy with a similar drug
Average cholesterol level of N patients under therapy	Hypothetical or standard value based on large amount of data collected by clinical laboratory
Average blood pressure reduction in N rats in pre-clinical study	Hypothetical average reduction considered to be of biological and clinical interest
Average difference of pain relief for two drugs taken by the same patients	Average difference (Δ) is hypothesized to be 0 if the drugs are identical

Table 5.5   Results of 20 Single-Tablet Assays from a Modification of a Process with a Historical Mean of 5.01 mg

5.13	5.04	5.09	5.00
4.98	5.03	5.01	4.99
5.20	5.08	4.96	5.18
5.08	5.06	5.02	5.24
4.99	5.17	5.06	5.00

$\overline{X}$ = 5.0655 mg   S = 0.0806

σ (historical) = 0.11

The steps for designing and analyzing this experiment are as follows:

1. *Careful planning* of the experiment ensures that the objectives of the experiment are addressed by an appropriate experimental design. The testing of a hypothesis where data are derived from a poorly implemented experiment can result in invalid conclusions. Proper design includes the choice and number of experimental units (patients, animals, tablets, etc.). Other considerations of experimental design and the manner in which observations are made are addressed in Chaps. 6, 8, and 11. Sample size may be determined on a scientific, statistical basis, but the choice is often limited by cost or time considerations, or the availability of experimental units. In the present example, the routine quality control content uniformity assay of 20 tablets was the determinant of sample size, a matter of convenience. The 20 tablets were chosen at random from the newly manufactured batch.

2. The *null hypothesis* and *alternative hypothesis* are defined prior to the implementation of the experiment or study.

$$H_0: \quad \mu = \mu_0 \qquad H_a: \quad \mu \neq \mu_0$$

In this example,

$$H_0: \quad \mu = 5.01 \qquad H_a: \quad \mu \neq 5.01$$

The objective of this experiment is to see if the average potency of the batch prepared with the modified procedure is different from that based on historical experience (5.01 mg). The null hypothesis takes the form of "no change," as discussed previously. To conclude that the new process has caused a change, we must demonstrate that the alternative hypothesis is true by rejecting the null hypothesis. The alternative hypothesis complements the null hypothesis. The two hypotheses are mutually exclusive and, together, in this example, cover all relevant possibilities that can result from the experiment. Either the average potency is 5.01 mg (H_0) or it is not (H_a). This is known as a *two-sided* (or *two-tailed*) test, suggesting that the average drug potency of the new batch can conceivably be smaller as well as greater than the historical process average of 5.01 mg. A *one-sided* test allows for the possibility of a difference in only one direction. Suppose that the process average of 5.01 mg suggested a preferential loss of drug during processing based on the theoretical amount added to the batch (e.g., 5.05 mg). The new procedure may have been designed to prevent this loss. Under these circumstances, one might hypothesize that the potency could only be greater (or, at least, not less) than the previous process average. Under this hypothesis, if the experiment reveals a lower potency than 5.01 mg, this result would be attributed to chance only; that is, although the average potency, in truth, is equal to or greater than 5.01 mg, chance variability may result in an experimental outcome where the observed average is "numerically" less than 5.01 mg. Such a result could occur, for example, as a result of a chance selection of tablets of low potency for the assay sample. For a one-sided test, the null and alternative hypotheses may take the following form:

$$H_0: \quad \mu = 5.01 \text{ mg} \qquad H_a: \quad \mu > 5.01 \text{ mg}$$

3. The *level of significance* is specified. This is the well-known P value associated with statements of statistical significance. The concept of the level of significance is crucial to an understanding of statistical methodology. The level of significance is defined as the probability that the statistical test results in a decision to reject H_0 (*a significant difference*) when, in fact, the treatments do not differ (H_0 is true). This concept will be clarified further when we describe the statistical test. By definition, the level of significance represents the chance of making a mistake when deciding to reject the null hypothesis. This mistake, or error, is also known as the *alpha* (α) *error* or error of the first kind (see Table 5.6). Thus, if the statistical test results in rejection of the null hypothesis, we say that the difference is significant at the α level. If α is chosen to be 0.05, the difference is significant at the 5% level. This is often expressed, equivalently, as $P < 0.05$. Figure 5.7 shows values of $\overline{X}$ which lead to rejection of H_0 for a statistical test at the 5% level if σ is known.

The *beta* (β) *error* is the probability of accepting H_0 (no treatment difference) when, in fact, some specified difference included

Table 5.6   Alpha and Beta Probabilities in Hypothesis Testing (Errors When Accepting or Rejecting H_0)

	H_0 is true	H_a (a specific alternative) is true
H_0 is rejected	Alpha (α)	1 - beta
H_0 is accepted	1 - alpha	Beta (β)

in H_a is the true difference. Although the evaluation of the β error and its involvement in sample-size determination is important, because of the complex nature of this concept, further discussion of this topic will be delayed until Chap. 6.

The choice of magnitude of α, which should be established prior to the start of the experiment, rests on the experimenter or sponsoring organization. To make this choice, one should consider the risks or consequences that will result if an α error is made, that is, the error made when declaring that a significant difference exists when the treatments are indeed equivalent. Traditionally, α is chosen as 5% (0.05). An α error of 5% means that a decision that a significant difference exists between treatments (based on the rejection of H_0) has a probability of 5% (1 in 20) of being incorrect ($P = 0.05$). Such a decision has credibility and is generally accepted as "proof" of a difference by regulatory agencies. When using the word "significant," one infers with a large degree of confidence that the experimental result does not support the null hypothesis.

An important concept is that if the statistical test results in a decision of *no significance*, the conclusion does *not* prove that H_0 is true or, in this case, that the average potency is 5.01 mg. Usually, "non-significance" is a weak statement, not carrying the clout or authority of the statement of "significance." Note that the chance of erroneously accepting H_0 is equal to β (Table 5.6). This means that β *percent* of the time, a nonsignificant result will be observed (H_0 is accepted as true), when a true difference specified by H_a truly exists. Unfortunately, most of the time when planning experiments, unlike α, β is not fixed in advance. The β level is often a result of circumstance. In most experiments, β is a consequence of the sample size, which is usually based on considerations other than the size of β. However, the sample size is best computed with the aid of a predetermined value of β (see Chap. 6). In our experiment, β was not fixed in advance. The sample of 20 tablets was chosen as a matter of tradition and convenience.

4. The *sample size*, in our example, has been fixed based on considerations that did not include β, as discussed above. However, the sample size can be calculated after α and β are specified, so that the experiment will be of sufficient size to have properties that will satisfy the choice of the α and β errors (see Chap. 6 for further details).

5. After the experiment is completed, relevant statistics are computed. In this example and most situations with which we will be concerned, mean values are to be compared. It is at this point that the *statistical test of significance* is performed as follows.

For a two-sided test, compute the ratio:

$$Z = \frac{|\bar{X} - \mu_0|}{\sqrt{\sigma^2/N}} = \frac{|\bar{X} - \mu_0|}{\sigma/\sqrt{N}} \qquad (5.4)$$

The numerator of the ratio is the absolute value of the difference between the observed and hypothetical mean. (In a two-sided test, low or negative values as well as large positive values of the mean lead to significance.) The variance of $(\bar{X} - \mu_0)$* is equal to

$$\frac{\sigma^2}{N}$$

The denominator of Eq. (5.4) is the standard deviation of the numerator. The Z ratio [Eq. (5.4)] consists of a difference, divided by its standard deviation. The ratio is exactly the Z transformation presented in Chap. 3 [Eq. (3.14)], which transforms a normal distribution with mean μ and variance σ^2 to the standard normal distribution ($\mu = 0$, $\sigma^2 = 1$).

In general, σ^2 is unknown, but it can be estimated from the sample data, and the sample estimate, S^2, is used in the denominator of Eq. (5.4). An important question is how to determine if the ratio

$$t = \frac{|\bar{X} - \mu_0|}{\sqrt{S^2/N}} \qquad (5.5)$$

leads to a decision of "significant." This prevalent situation (σ^2 unknown) will be discussed below.

As discussed above, significance is based on a probability statement defined by α. More specifically, the difference is considered to be statistically significant (H_0 is rejected) if the observed difference between the sample mean and μ_0 is sufficiently large so that the observed or larger differences are improbable (probability of α or less, e.g., $P \leqslant 0.05$) if the null hypothesis is

---

*The variance of $\bar{X} - \mu_0$ is equal to the variance of $\bar{X}$ because μ_0 is constant and has a variance of 0.

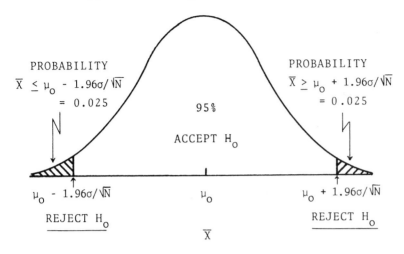

Figure 5.7 Region of rejection (critical region) in a statistical test (two-sided) at the 5% level with σ^2 known.

true (μ = 5.01 mg). In order to calculate the relevant probability, the observations are assumed to be statistically independent and normally distributed.

With these assumptions, the ratio shown in Eq. (5.4) has a normal distribution with mean equal to 0 and variance equal to 1 (the standard normal distribution). The concept of the α error is illustrated in Fig. 5.7. The values of $\overline{X}$ that lead to rejection of the null hypothesis define the "region of rejection," also known as the *critical region*. With a knowledge of the variance, the area corresponding to the critical region can be calculated using the standard normal distribution. The probability of observing a mean value in the critical region of the distribution defined by the null hypothesis is α. This region is usually taken as symmetrical areas in the tails of the distribution, with each tail containing $\alpha/2$ of the area (2-1/2% in each tail at the 5% level) for a two-tailed test. Under the null hypothesis and the assumption of normality, $\overline{X}$ is normal with mean μ_0 and variance σ^2/N. The Z ratio [Eq. (5.4)] is a standard normal deviate, as noted above. Referring to Table IV.2, the values of $\overline{X}$ that satisfy

$$\frac{\overline{X} - \mu_0}{\sigma/\sqrt{N}} \leqslant -1.96 \qquad \text{or} \qquad \frac{\overline{X} - \mu_0}{\sigma/\sqrt{N}} \geqslant +1.96 \qquad (5.6)$$

will result in rejection of H_0 at the 5% level. The values of $\overline{X}$ that lead to rejection of H_0 may be derived by rearranging Eq. (5.6).

$$\overline{X} \leqslant \mu_0 - \frac{1.96\sigma}{\sqrt{N}} \qquad \text{or} \qquad \overline{X} \geqslant \mu_0 + \frac{1.96\sigma}{\sqrt{N}} \qquad (5.7)$$

or, equivalently,

$$|\overline{X} - \mu_0| \geqslant \frac{1.96\sigma}{\sqrt{N}} \qquad (5.8)$$

If the value of $\overline{X}$ falls in the critical region, as defined in Eqs. (5.7) and (5.8), the null hypothesis is rejected and the difference is said to be significant at the α (5%) level.

The statistical test of the mean assay result from Table 5.5 may be performed: (a) assuming that σ is known ($\sigma = 0.11$) and (b) assuming that σ is unknown, but estimated from the sample (S = 0.0806).

The following examples demonstrate the procedure for applying the test of significance for a *single mean*.

(a) *One-sample test, variance known.* In this case we believe that the large quantity of historical data defines the standard deviation of the process precisely, and that this standard deviation represents the variation in the new batch. We assume, therefore, that σ^2 is known. In addition, as noted above, if the data from the sample are independent and normally distributed, the test of significance is based on the standard normal curve table (Table IV.2). The ratio as described in Eq. (5.4) is computed using the known value of the variance. If the absolute value of the ratio is greater than that which cuts off $\alpha/2$ percent of the area (defining the two tails of the rejection region, Fig. 5.7), the difference between the drug and placebo is said to be significant at the α level. *For a two-sided test, the absolute value of the difference* is used because both large positive and negative differences are considered evidence for rejecting the null hypothesis.

In this example, we will use a two-sided test, because the change in potency, if any, may occur in either direction, higher or lower. The level of significance is set at the traditional 5% level.

$$\alpha = 0.05$$

Compute the ratio [Eq. (5.4)]

$$Z = \frac{|\overline{X} - \mu_0|}{\sigma/\sqrt{N}} = \frac{|5.0655 - 5.01|}{0.11\sqrt{20}} = 2.26$$

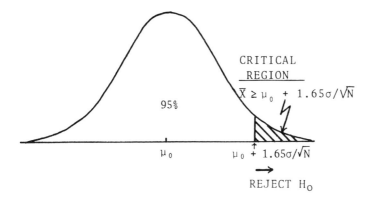

Figure 5.8   Rejection region for a one-sided test.

At the 5% level, values of $|Z| \geq 1.96$ will lead to a declaration of significance for a two-sided test [Eq. (5.6)]. Therefore, the new batch can be said to have a greater mean potency than previous batches.

The level of significance is set *before* the actual experimental results are obtained. In the previous example, a one-sided test at the 5% level may be justified if convincing evidence were available to demonstrate that the new process would only result in mean results equal to or greater than the historical mean. If such a one-sided test had been deemed appropriate, the null hypothesis would be

H_0: $\mu = 5.01$ mg   as before

The alternative hypothesis, H_a: $\mu > 5.01$ mg, eliminates the possibility that the new process can lower the mean potency. The concept is illustrated in Fig. 5.8. Now the rejection region lies only in values of $\overline{X}$ greater than 5.01 mg, as described below. An observed value of $\overline{X}$ below 5.01 mg is considered to be due only to chance.

The rejection region is defined for values of $\overline{X}$ equal to or greater than $\mu_0 + 1.65\sigma/\sqrt{N}$ [or, equivalently, $(\overline{X} - \mu_0)/(\sigma/\sqrt{N}) \geq 1.65$] because 5% of the area of the normal curve is found above this value (Table IV.2). This is in keeping with the definition of α: If the null hypothesis is true, we will erroneously reject the null hypothesis 5% of the time. Thus we can see that a *smaller* difference is needed for significance using a one-sided test; the Z ratio need only exceed 1.65 rather than 1.96 for significance at the

5% level. In the present example, values of $\overline{X} \geqslant [5.01 + 1.65(0.11)/\sqrt{20}] = 5.051$ will lead to significance for a one-sided test. Clearly, the observed mean of 5.0655 is significantly different from 5.01 ($P < 0.05$). Note that in a one-sided test, the sign of the numerator is important and the absolute value is not used.

Usually, statistical tests are two-sided tests. One-sided tests are warranted in certain circumstances. However, the choice of a one-sided test should be made a priori, and one must be prepared to defend its use. As mentioned above, in the present example, if evidence were available to show that the new process could not reduce the potency, a one-sided test would be acceptable. To have such evidence and convince others (particularly, regulatory agencies) of its validity is not always an easy task. Also, from a scientific point of view, two-sided tests are desirable because significant results in both positive and negative directions are usually of interest.

(b) *One-sample test, variance unknown.* In most experiments in pharmaceutical research, the variance is unknown. Usually, the only estimate of the variance comes from the experimental data itself. As has been emphasized in the example above, use of the cumulative standard normal distribution (Table IV.2) to determine probabilities for the comparison of a mean to a known value (μ_0) is valid only if the variance is known.

The procedure for testing the significance of the difference of an observed mean from a hypothetical value (one-sample test) when the variance is estimated from the sample data is the same as that with the variance known, with the following exceptions:

(1) The variance is computed from the experimental data. In the present example, the variance is $(0.0806)^2$; the standard deviation is 0.0806 from Table 5.5.

(2) The ratio is computed using S^2 instead of σ^2 as in Eq. (5.5). For a two-sided test, this ratio,

$$t = \frac{| \overline{X} - \mu_0 |}{S/\sqrt{N}} \tag{5.5}$$

is not distributed as a standard normal variable. If the mean is normally distributed, the ratio [Eq. (5.5)] has a t distribution. The t distribution looks like the standard normal distribution but has more area in the tails; the t distribution is more spread out. The shape of the t distribution depends on the degrees of freedom (d.f.). As the d.f. increase the t distribution looks more and more like the standard normal distribution as shown in Fig. 5.9. When the d.f. are equal to ∞, the t distribution is identical to the standard normal distribution (i.e., the variance is known).

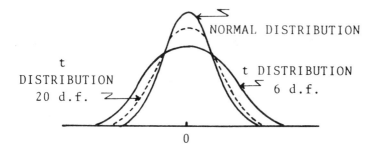

Figure 5.9   t distribution compared to the standard normal
distribution.

    The t distribution is a probability distribution that was intro-
duced in Sec. 5.1.1 and Chap. 3.   The area under the t distributions shown in Fig. 5.9 is 1.   Thus, as in the case of the normal
distribution (or any continuous distribution), areas within specified
intervals represent probabilities.   However, unlike the normal distribution, there is *no* transformation which will change all t distributions (differing d.f.'s) to one "standard" t distribution.   Clearly, a
tabulation of all possible t distributions would be impossible.   Table
IV.4 shows commonly used probability points for representative t
distributions.   The values in the table are points in the t distribution representing cumulative areas (probabilities) of 80, 90, 95, 97.5,
and 99.5%.   For example, with d.f. = 10, 97.5% of the area of the t
distribution is below a value of t equal to 2.23 (see Fig. 5.10).

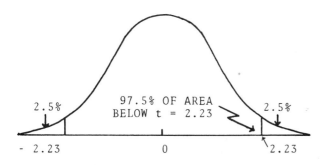

Figure 5.10   t distribution with 10 degrees of freedom.

Note that when d.f. = ∞, the t value corresponding to a cumulative probability of 97.5% (0.975) is 1.96, exactly the same value as that for the standard normal distribution. Since the t distribution is symmetrical about zero, as is the standard normal distribution, a t value of -2.23 cuts off $1 - 0.975 = 0.025$ of the area (d.f. = 10). This means that to obtain a significant difference of means at the 5% level for a two-sided test and d.f. equal to 10, the abolute value of the t ratio [Eq. (5.5)] must exceed 2.23. Thus the t values in the column headed "0.975" in Table IV.4 are values to be used for two-tailed significance tests at the 5% level (or for a two-sided 95% confidence interval). Similarly, the column headed "0.95" contains appropriate t values for significance tests at the 10% level for two-sided tests, or the 5% level for one-sided tests. The column headed "0.995" represents t values used for two-sided tests at the 1% level, or for 99% confidence intervals.

The number of d.f. used to obtain the appropriate value of t from Table IV.4 are the d.f. associated with the variance estimate in the denominator of the t ratio [Eq. (5.5)]. The d.f. for a mean is $N - 1$, or 19 (20 $-$ 1) in this example. The test is a two-sided test at the 5% level. The t ratio is

$$t = \frac{|\,\overline{X} - \mu_0\,|}{S/\sqrt{N}}$$

$$= \frac{|\,5.0655 - 5.01\,|}{0.0806/\sqrt{20}} = 3.08$$

The value of t needed for significance for a two-sided test at the 5% level is 2.09 (Table IV.4, 19 d.f.). Therefore, the new process results in a "significant" increase in potency (P < 0.05).

A 95% confidence interval for the true mean potency may be constructed as described in Sec. 5.1.1 [Eq. (5.2)]:

$$5.0655 \pm 2.09 \left(\frac{0.0806}{\sqrt{20}} \right) = 5.028 \text{ to } 5.103 \text{ mg}$$

Note that the notion of the *confidence interval* is closely associated with the *statistical test*. If the confidence interval covers the hypothetical value, the difference is not significant at the indicated level, and vice versa. In our example, the difference was significant at the 5% level, and the 95% confidence interval does *not* cover the hypothetical mean value of 5.01.

Example 4: As part of the process of new drug research, a pharmaceutical company places all new compounds through an "antihypertensive" screen. A new compound is given to a group of animals and the reduction in blood pressure measured. Experience has shown that a blood pressure reduction of more than 15 mmHg in these hypertensive animals is an indication for further testing as a new drug candidate. Since such testing is expensive, the researchers wish to be reasonably sure that the compound truly reduces the blood pressure by more than 15 mmHg before testing is continued; that is, they will continue testing only if the experimental evidence suggests that the true blood pressure reduction is greater than 15 mmHg with a high probability.

H_0: $\mu \leq 15$ mmHg reduction $\qquad$ H_a: $\mu > 15$ mmHg reduction

The null hypothesis is a statement that the new compound is unacceptable (blood pressure change is equal to or less than 15 mmHg). This is typical of the concept of the null hypothesis. A rejection of the null hypothesis means that a difference probably exists. In our example, a true difference greater than 15 mmHg means that the compound should be tested further. This is a *one-sided* test. Experimental results showing a difference of 15 mmHg or less will result in a decision to accept H_0, and the compound will be put aside. If the blood pressure reduction exceeds 15 mmHg, the reduction will be tested for significance using a t test.

$\alpha = 10\% \ (0.10)$

The level of significance of 10% was chosen in lieu of the usual 5% level for the following reason. A 5% significance level means that 1 time in 20 a compound will be chosen as effective when the true reduction is less than 15 mmHg. The company was willing to take a risk of 1 in 10 of following up an ineffective compound in order to reduce the risk of missing potentially effective compounds. Other things being equal, an increase in the α error decreases the β error; that is, there is a smaller chance of accepting H_0 when it is false. Note that the t value needed for significance is smaller at the 10% level than that at the 5% level. Therefore, a smaller reduction in blood pressure is needed for significance at the 10% level. The standard procedure in this company is to test the compound on 10 animals. The results shown in Table 5.7 were observed in a test of a newly synthesized potential antihypertensive agent.

The t test is [Eq. (5.5)]

$$t = \frac{15.9 - 15}{3.87/\sqrt{10}} = \frac{0.9}{1.22} = 0.74$$

Table 5.7   Blood Pressure Reduction
Caused by a New Antihypertensive
Compound in 10 Animals (mmHg)

15	12
18	17
14	21
8	16
20	18

$\overline{X} = 15.9$ $S = 3.87$

The value of t needed for significance is 1.38 (Table IV.4, one-sided test at the 10% level with 9 degrees of freedom).   Therefore, the compound is not sufficiently effective to be considered further. Although the average result was larger than 15 mmHg, it was not sufficiently large to encourage further testing, according to the statistical criterion.

What difference (reduction) would have been needed to show a significant reduction, assuming that the sample variance does not change?   Equation (5.5) may be rearranged as follows: $\overline{X} = t(S)/\sqrt{N} + \mu_0$.   If $\overline{X}$ is greater than or equal to $t(s)/\sqrt{N} + \mu_0$, the average reduction will be significant, where t is the table value at the α level of significance with $(N - 1)$ d.f.   In our example,

$$\frac{t(s)}{\sqrt{N}} + \mu_0 = \frac{(1.38)(3.87)}{\sqrt{10}} + 15 = 16.7$$

A blood pressure reduction of 16.7 mmHg or more (the critical region) would have resulted in a significant difference.   (See Exercise Problem 10.)

5.2.2   Case II: Comparisons of Means from Two Independent Groups (Two-Independent-Groups Test)

A preliminary discussion of this test was presented in Sec. 5.2. This most important test is commonly encountered in clinical studies (a parallel-groups design).   Table 5.8 shows a few examples of research experiments that may be analyzed by the test described here.   The data of Table 5.2 will be used to illustrate this test. The experiment consisted of a comparison of an active drug and a placebo where each treatment is tested on different patients.   The

Table 5.8 Some Examples of Experiments that May be Analyzed by the Two-Independent-Groups Test

Clinical studies	Active drug compared to a standard drug or placebo; treatments given to different persons, one treatment per person
Preclinical studies	Comparison of drugs for efficacy and/or toxicity with treatments given to different animals
Comparison of product attributes from two batches	Tablet dissolution, potency, weight, etc., from two batches

results of the study showed an average blood pressure reduction of 10 mmHg for 11 patients receiving drug, and an average reduction of 1 mmHg for 10 patients receiving placebo. The principal feature of this test (or design) is that treatments are given to two independent groups. The observations in one group are independent of those in the second group. In addition, we assume that the data within each group are normally and independently distributed.

The steps to be taken in performing the two-independent-groups test are similar to those described for the one-sample test (see Sec. 5.2.1).

1. *Patients are randomly assigned to the two treatment groups.* (For a description of the method of random assignment, see Chap. 4.) The number of patients chosen to participate in the study in this example was largely a consequence of cost and convenience. Without these restraints, a suitable sample size could be determined with a knowledge of β, as described in Chap. 6. The drug and placebo were to be randomly assigned to each of 12 patients (12 patients for each treatment). There were several dropouts, resulting in 11 patients in the drug group and 10 patients in the placebo group.

2. *The null and alternative hypotheses are*

$$H_0: \mu_1 - \mu_2 = \Delta = 0 \qquad H_a: \Delta \neq 0$$

We hypothesize no difference between treatments. A "significant" result means that treatments are considered different. This is a two-sided test. The drug treatment may be better or worse than placebo.

3. α *is set at 0.05.*
4. *The form of the statistical test depends on whether or not variances are known.* In the usual circumstances, the variances are unknown.

Two-Independent-Groups Test, Variances Known

If the variances of both groups are known, the ratio

$$Z = \frac{\overline{X}_1 - \overline{X}_2 - (\mu_1 - \mu_2)}{\sqrt{\sigma_1^2/N_1 + \sigma_2^2/N_2}} \tag{5.9}$$

has a normal distribution with mean 0 and standard deviation equal to 1 (the standard normal distribution). The numerator of the ratio is the difference between the observed difference of the means of the two groups $(\overline{X}_1 - \overline{X}_2)$ and the hypothetical difference $(\mu_1 - \mu_2$ according to $H_0)$. In the present case, and indeed in most of the examples of this test that we will consider, the hypothetical difference is zero (i.e., H_0: $\mu_1 - \mu_2 = 0$). The variability of $(\overline{X}_1 - \overline{X}_2)$* (defined as the standard deviation) is equal to

$$\sqrt{\sigma_{\overline{X}_1}^2 + \sigma_{\overline{X}_2}^2}$$

[as described in App. I, if A and B are independent, $\sigma^2(A - B) = \sigma_A^2 + \sigma_B^2$].

Thus, as in the one-sample case, the test consists of forming a ratio whose distribution is defined by the standard normal curve. In the present example (test of an antihypertensive agent), suppose that the *variances* corresponding to drug and placebo are *known* to be 144 and 100, respectively. The rejection region is defined by α. For α = 0.05, values of Z greater than 1.96 or less than −1.96 ($|Z| \geq 1.96$) will be lead to rejection of the null hypothesis. Z is defined by Eq. (5.9).

---

*The variance of $\overline{X}_1 - \overline{X}_2 - (\mu_1 - \mu_2)$ is equal to the variance of $(\overline{X}_1 - \overline{X}_2)$ because μ_1 and μ_2 are constants and have a variance equal to zero.

For a two-sided test

$$Z = \frac{|\overline{X}_1 - \overline{X}_2|}{\sqrt{\sigma_1^2/N_1 + \sigma_2^2/N_2}}$$

$\overline{X}_1 = 10$, $\overline{X}_2 = 1$, $N_1 = 11$, and $N_2 = 10$. Thus

$$Z = \frac{|10 - 1|}{\sqrt{144/11 + 100/10}} = 1.87$$

Since the absolute value of the ratio does not exceed 1.96, the difference is not significant at the 5% level. From Table IV.2, the probability of observing a value of Z greater than 1.87 is approximately 0.03. Therefore, the test can be considered significant at the 6% level [2(0.03) = 0.06 for a two-tailed test]. The probability of observing an absolute difference of 9 mmHg or more between drug and placebo, if the two products are identical, is 0.06 or 6%.

We have set α equal to 5% as defining an unlikely event from a distribution with known mean (0) and variance (144/11 + 100/10 = 23.1). An event as far or farther from the mean (0) than 9 mmHg can occur 6 times in a 100 if H_0 is true. Strictly speaking, this is not cause for rejecting H_0 because we set α at 5% a priori (i.e., before performing the experiment). In reality, there is nothing special about 5%. The use of 5% as the α level is based strongly on tradition and experience, as mentioned previously. Should significance at the 6% level result in a different decision than a level of 5%? To document efficacy, a significance level of 6% may not be adequate for acceptance by regulatory agencies. There has to be some cutoff point; otherwise, if 6% is acceptable, why not 7%, and so on? However, for internal decisions or for leads in experiments used to obtain information for further work or to verify theories, 5% and 6% may be too close to "call." Rather than closing the door on experiments that show differences at P = 0.06, one might think of such results as being of "borderline" significance, worthy of a second look. In our example, had the difference between drug and placebo been approximately 9.4 mmHg, we would have called the difference "significant," rejecting the hypothesis that the placebo treatment was equal to the drug.

P values are often presented with experimental results even though the statistical test shows nonsignificance at the predetermined α level. In this experiment, a statement that P = 0.06 ("The difference is significant at the 6% level") does not imply that the treatments are considered to be significantly different. We emphasize that if the α level is set at 5%, a decision that the treatments are different should be declared only if the experimental results show that $P \leq 0.05$. However, in practical situations, it is often useful for the experimenter and other interested parties to know the P value, particularly in the case of "borderline" significance.

Two-Independent-Groups Test, Variance Unknown

The procedure for comparing means of two independent groups when the variances are estimated from the sample data is the same as that with the variances known, with the following exceptions:

   1. *The variance is computed from the sample data.* In order to perform the statistical test to be described below, in addition to the usual assumptions of normality and independence, *we assume that the variance is the same for each group.* (If the variances differ, a modified procedure can be used as described later in this chapter.) A rule of thumb for moderate-sized samples (N equal 10 to 20) is that the ratio of the two variances should not be greater than 3 to 4. Sometimes, in doubtful situations, a test for the equality of the two variances may be appropriate (see Sec. 5.3) before performing the test of significance for means described here. To obtain an estimate of the common variance, first compute the variance of each group. The two variances are *pooled* by calculating a weighted average of the variances, the best estimate of the true common variance. The weights are equal to the degrees of freedom, d.f., $N_1 - 1$ and $N_2 - 1$, for groups 1 and 2, respectively. N_1 and N_2 are the sample sizes for the two groups. The following formula may be used to calculate the pooled variance:

$$S_p^2 = \frac{(N_1 - 1)S_1^2 + (N_2 - 1)S_2^2}{N_1 + N_2 - 2} \qquad (5.10)$$

Note that we do not calculate the pooled variance by first pooling together all of the data from the two groups. The pooled variance obtained by pooling the two *separate* variances will always be equal to or smaller than that computed from all of the data combined disregarding groups. In the latter case, the variance estimate includes the variability due to differences of means as well as that due to the variance within each group (see Exercise Problem 5). Appendix I has a further discussion of pooling variance.

   2. *The ratio that is used for the statistical test is similar to Eq. (5.9).* Because the variance, S_p^2 (pooled variance), is estimated from the sample data, the ratio

$$t = \frac{(\overline{X}_1 - \overline{X}_2) - (\mu_1 - \mu_2)}{\sqrt{S_p^2/N_1 + S_p^2/N_2}} = \frac{(\overline{X}_1 - \overline{X}_2) - (\mu_1 - \mu_2)}{S_p\sqrt{1/N_1 + 1/N_2}}$$

$$(5.11)$$

is used instead of Z [Eq. (5.9)]. The degrees of freedom for the distribution is determined from the variance estimate, S_p^2. This is equal to the d.f., pooled from the two groups, equal to $(N_1 - 1) + (N_2 - 1)$ or $N_1 + N_2 - 2$.

These concepts are explained and clarified, step by step, in the following examples.

Example 5: Two different formulations of a tablet of a new drug are to be compared with regard to rate of dissolution. Ten tablets of each formulation are tested, and the percent dissolution after 15 min in the dissolution apparatus is observed. The results are tabulated in Table 5.9. The object of this experiment is to determine if the dissolution rates of the two formulations differ. The

Table 5.9 Percent Dissolution After 15 Min for Two Tablet Formulations

	Formulation A	Formulation B
	68	74
	84	71
	81	79
	85	63
	75	80
	69	61
	80	69
	76	72
	79	80
	74	65
Average	77.1	71.4
Variance	33.43	48.71
s.d.	5.78	6.98

test for the "significance" of the observed difference is described
in detail as follows:

    1. *State the null and alternative hypotheses:*

$$H_0: \quad \mu_1 = \mu_2 \qquad\qquad H_a: \quad \mu_1 \neq \mu_2$$

μ_1 and μ_2 are the true mean 15-min dissolution values for formulations A and B, respectively. This is a two-sided test. There is no
reason to believe that one or the other formulation will have a faster
or slower dissolution, a priori.

    2. *State the significance level* $\alpha = 0.05$. The level of signifi-
cance is chosen as the traditional 5% level.

    3. *Select the samples.* Ten tablets taken at random from each
of the two pilot batches will be tested.

    4. *Compute the value of the t statistic [Eq. (5.11)].*

$$\frac{|\,\overline{X}_1 - \overline{X}_2 - (\mu_1 - \mu_2)\,|}{S_p \sqrt{1/N_1 + 1/N_2}} = t = \frac{|\,77.1 - 71.4\,|}{S_p \sqrt{1/10 + 1/10}}$$

$\overline{X}_1 = 77.1$ and $\overline{X}_2 = 71.4$ (see Table 5.9). $N_1 = N_2 = 10$ (d.f. = 9
for each group). S_p is calculated from Eq. (5.10).

$$S_p = \sqrt{\frac{9(33.43) + 9(48.71)}{18}} = 6.41$$

Note that the *pooled standard deviation* is the *square root of the
pooled variance*, where the pooled variance is a weighted average
of the variances from each group. It is *not correct to average the
standard deviations*. Although the sample variances of the two
groups are not identical, they are "reasonably" close, close enough
so that the assumption of equal variances can be considered to be
acceptable. The assumption of equal variance and independence of
the two groups is more critical than the assumption of normality of
the data, because we are comparing means. Means tend to be normally distributed even when the individual data do not have a normal distribution, according to the central limit theorem. The observed value of t (18 d.f.) is

$$\frac{|\,\overline{X}_1 - \overline{X}_2\,|}{S_p \sqrt{1/N_1 + 1/N_2}}$$

$$t = \frac{|\,77.1 - 71.4\,|}{6.4\sqrt{2/10}} = 1.99$$

Values of t equal to or greater than 2.10 (Table IV.4, d.f. = 18) lead to rejection of the null hypothesis. These values, which comprise the *critical region*, result in a declaration of "significance." In this experiment, the value of t is 1.99, and the difference is not significant at the 5% level (P > 0.05). This does not mean that the two formulations have the same rate of dissolution. The declaration of nonsignificance here probably means that the sample size was too small; that is, the same difference with a larger sample would be significant at the 5% level. Two different formulations are apt not to be identical with regard to dissolution. The question of statistical versus practical significance may be raised here. If the dissolutions are indeed different, will the difference of 5.7% (77.1% − 71.4%) affect drug absorption in vivo? A confidence interval on the difference of the means may be an appropriate way of presenting the results.

Confidence Interval for the Difference of Two Means

A confidence interval for the difference of two means can be constructed in a manner similar to that presented for a single mean as shown in Sec. 5.1 [Eq. (5.2)]. For example, a confidence interval with a confidence coefficient of 95% is

$$(\overline{X}_1 - \overline{X}_2) \pm (t)S_p \sqrt{\frac{1}{N_1} + \frac{1}{N_2}} \qquad (5.12)$$

t is the value obtained from Table IV.4 with appropriate d.f., with the probability used for a two-sided test. (Use the column labeled "0.975" in Table IV.4 for a 95% interval.) For the example discussed above (tablet dissolution), a 95% confidence interval for the difference of the mean 15-min dissolution values [Eq. (5.12)] is

$$(77.1 - 71.4) \pm 2.10(6.41)(0.447) = 5.7 \pm 6.02 = -0.32 \text{ to } 11.72\%$$

Thus the 95% confidence interval is from −0.32 to 11.72%.

Test of Significance If Variances of
the Two Groups are Unequal

If the two groups can be considered not to have equal variances and the variances are estimated from the samples, the usual t test procedure is not correct. This problem has been solved and is often denoted as the Behrens-Fisher procedure. Special tables are needed for the solution, but a good approximate test for the equality of two means can be performed using Eq. (5.13) [2].

$$t' = \frac{|\bar{X}_1 - \bar{X}_2|}{\sqrt{S_1^2/N_1 + S_2^2/N_2}} \tag{5.13}$$

If $N_1 = N_2 = N$, then the critical t is taken from Table IV.4 with $N - 1$ instead of the usual $2(N - 1)$ d.f. If N_1 and N_2 are not equal, then the t value needed for significance is a weighted average of the appropriate t values from Table IV.4 with $N_1 - 1$ and $N_2 - 1$ d.f.

Weighted average of t values $= (w_1 t_1 + w_2 t_2)/(w_1 + w_2)$

where the weights are: $w_1 = S_1^2/N_1$ $w_2 = S_2^2/N_2$

To make the calculation clear, assume that the means of two groups of patients treated with an antihypertensive agent showed the following reduction in blood pressure (mmHg).

	Group A	Group B
Mean	10.7	7.2
Variance (S^2)	51.8	5.3
N	20	15

We have reason to believe that the variances differ, and for a two-sided test, we first calculate t' according to Eq. (5.13):

$$t' = \frac{|10.7 - 7.2|}{\sqrt{51.8/20 + 5.3/15}} = 2.04$$

The critical value of t' is obtained using the weighting procedure. At the 5% level, t with 19 d.f. = 2.09 and t with 14 d.f. = 2.14. The weighted average t value is

$$\frac{(51.8/20)(2.09) + (5.3/15)(2.14)}{(51.8/20) + (5.3/15)} = 2.10$$

Since t' is less than 2.10, the difference is considered to be not significant at the 5% level.

Overlapping Confidence Intervals and
Statistical Significance

When comparing two independent treatments for statistical significance, sometimes people erroneously make conclusions based on the
confidence intervals constructed from each treatment separately. In
particular, if the confidence intervals overlap, the treatments are
considered not to differ. This reasoning is not necessarily correct.
The fallacy can be easily seen from the following example. Consider
two independent treatments, A and B, representing two formulations
of the same drug with the following dissolution results:

Treatment	N	Average	s.d.
A	6	37.5	6.2
B	6	47.4	7.4

For a two-sided test, the two sample t test results in a t value
of

$$t = \frac{|47.4 - 37.5|}{6.83 \sqrt{1/6 + 1/6}} = 2.51$$

Since 2.51 exceeds the critical t value with 10 d.f. (2.23), the results shows significance at the 5% level.
Computation of the 95% confidence intervals for the two treatments results in the following:

Treatment A: $37.5 \pm (2.57)(6.2) \sqrt{1/6} = 30.99$ to 44.01

Treatment B: $47.4 \pm (2.57)(7.4) \sqrt{1/6} = 39.64$ to 55.16

Clearly, in this example, the individual confidence intervals
overlap (the values between 39.64 and 44.01 are common to both
intervals), yet the treatments are significantly different. The 95%
confidence interval for the difference of the two treatments is

$(47.4 - 37.5) \pm 8.79 = 1.1$ to 18.19

As has been noted earlier in this section, if the 95% confidence
interval does not cover 0, the difference between the treatments
is significant at the 5% level.

Summary of t-Test Procedure and Design for
Comparison of Two Independent Groups

The t-test procedure is essentially the same as the test using the
normal distribution (Z test). The t test is used when the variance(s)
are unknown and estimated from the sample data. The t distribuion
with ∞ d.f. is identical to the standard normal distribution. Therefore, the t distribution with ∞ d.f. can be used for normal distribution tests (e.g., comparison of means with variance known). When
using the t test, it is necessary to compute a pooled variance.
[With variances known, a pooled variance is not computed; see Eqs.
(5.10) and (5.11).] An assumption underlying the use of this t test
is that the variances of the comparative groups are the same. Other
assumptions when using the t test are that the data from the two
groups are independent and normally distributed. If the variances
are considered to be unequal, use the approximate Behrens-Fisher
method.

If H_0 is rejected (the difference is "significant"), one accepts
the alternative, H_a: $\mu_1 \neq \mu_2$ or $\mu_1 - \mu_2 \neq 0$. The best estimate of
the true difference between the means is the observed difference.
A confidence interval gives a range for the true difference (see
above). If the confidence interval covers 0, the statistical test is
not significant at the corresponding alpha level.

*Planning an experiment to compare the means of two independent
groups usually requires the following considerations*:

1. *Define the objective*. For example, in the example above,
the objective was to determine if the two formulations differed with
regard to rates of dissolution.

2. Determine the *number of samples* (experimental units) to be
included in the experiment. We have noted that statistical methods
may be used to determine the sample size (Chap. 6). However,
practical considerations such as cost and time constraints are often
predominating factors. The *sample size* of the two groups *need not
be equal* in this type of design, also known as a *parallel-groups* or
one-way analysis of variance design. If the primary interest is the
comparison of means of the two groups, equal sample sizes are
optimal (assuming that the variances of the two groups are equal).
That is, given the total number of experimental units available
(patients, tablets, etc.), the most powerful comparison will be obtained by dividing the total number of experimental units into two
equal groups. The reason for this is that $(1/N_1) + (1/N_2)$, which
is in the denominator of the test ratio, is maximized when $N_1 =
N_2 = N_t/2$ (N_t is the total sample size). In many circumstances
(particularly in clinical studies), observations are lost due to
errors, patient dropouts, and so on. The analysis described here
is still valid, but some power will be lost. *Power* is the ability of
the test to discriminate between the treatment groups. (Power is

discussed in detail in Chap. 6.) Sometimes, it is appropriate to use different sample sizes for the two groups. In a clinical study where a new drug treatment is to be compared to a standard or placebo treatment, one may wish to obtain data on adverse experiences due to the new drug entity in addition to comparisons of efficacy based on some relevant mean outcome. In this case, the design may include more patients on the new drug than the comparative treatment. Also, if the variances of two groups are known to be unequal, the otpimal sample sizes will not be equal [4].

3. *Choose the samples.* It would seem best in many situations to be able to apply treatments to randomly chosen experimental units (e.g., patients). Often, practical considerations make this procedure impossible, and some compromise must be made. In clinical trials, it is usually not possible to select patients at random according to the strict definition of "random." We usually choose investigators who assign treatments to the patients available to the study in a random manner.

4. *Observations are made* on the samples. Every effort should be made to avoid bias. Blinding techniques and randomizing the order of observations (e.g., assays) are examples of ways to avoid bias. Given a choice, objective measurements, such as body weights, blood pressure, and blood assays, are usually preferable to subjective measurements, such as degree of improvement, psychological traits, and so on.

5. The *statistical analysis*, as described above, is then applied to the data. The statistical methods and probability levels (e.g., α) should be established prior to the experiment. However, one should not be immobilized because of prior commitments. If experimental conditions differ from that anticipated, and alternative analyses are warranted, a certain degree of flexibility is desirable. However, statistical theory (and common sense) shows that it is not fair to examine the data to look for all possible effects not included in the objectives. The more one looks, the more one will find. In a large data set, any number of unusual findings will be apparent if the data are examined with a "fine-tooth comb." If such unexpected results are of interest, it is best to design a new experiment to explore and define these effects. Otherwise, large data sets can be incorrectly used to demonstrate a large number of unusual, but inadvertent, random, and inconsequential "statistically" significant differences.

5.2.3 Test for Comparison of Means of Related Samples (Paired–Sample t Test)

Experiments are often designed so that comparisons of two means are made on related samples. This design is usually more *sensitive*

Table 5.10   Examples of Related Samples

Clinical studies	Each patient takes each drug on different occasions (e.g., crossover study)
	Each patient takes each drug simultaneously, such as in skin testing; for example, an ointment is applied to different parts of the body
	Matched pairs: two patients are matched for relevant characteristics (age, sex, disease state, etc.) and two drugs randomly assigned, one to each patient
Preclinical studies	Drugs assigned randomly to littermates
Analytical development	Same analyst assays all samples
	Each laboratory assays all samples in collaborative test
	Each method is applied to a homogeneous sample
Stability studies	Assays over time from material from same container

than the two-independent-groups t test. A test is more sensitive if the experimental variability is smaller. With smaller variability, smaller differences can be detected as statistically significant. In clinical studies, a paired design is often described as one in which each patient acts as his or her own "control." A bioequivalance study, in which each subject takes each of a test and reference drug product, is a form of paired design (see Sec. 11.4).

In the paired-sample experiment, the two treatments are applied to experimental units which are closely related. If the same person takes both treatments, the relationship is obvious. Table 5.10 shows common examples of related samples used in paired tests.

The paired t test is identical in its implementation to the one-sample test described in Sec. 5.2.1. In the paired test, the single sample is obtained by taking differences between the data for the two treatments for each experimental unit (patient or subject, for example). With N pairs of individuals, there are N data points (i.e., N differences). The N differences are designated as δ. Example 4, concerning the average reduction in blood pressure in a preclinical screen, was a paired-sample test in disguise. The paired data consisted of pre- and post-drug blood pressure readings for each animal. We were interested in the difference of pre and post values (δ), the blood pressure reduction.

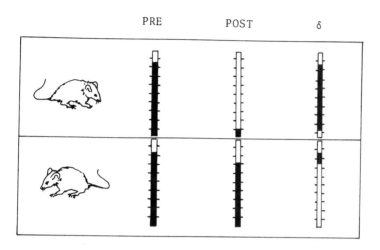

In paired tests, treatments should be assigned either in random order, or in some designed way, as in the crossover design. In the crossover design, usually one-half of the subjects receive the two treatments in the order A –B, and the remaining half of the subjects receive the treatments in the opposite order, where A and B are the two treatments. The crossover design is discussed in detail in Chap. 11. With regard to blood pressure reduction, it is obvious that the order cannot be randomized. The pretreatment reading occurs before the posttreatment reading. The inflexibility of this ordering can create problems in interpretation of such data. The conclusions based on these data could be controversial because of the lack of a "control" group. If extraneous conditions that could influence the experimental outcome are different at the times of the initial and final observation (pre- and posttreatment), the treatment effect is "confounded" with the differences in conditions at the two points of observation. Therefore, randomization of the order of treatment given to each subject is important for the validity of this statistical test. For example, consider a study to compare two hypnotic drugs with regard to sleep-inducing effects. If the first drug were given to all patients before the second drug, and the initial period happened to be associated with hot and humid weather conditions, any observed differences between drugs (or lack of difference) would be "tainted" by the effect of the weather on the therapeutic response.

An important feature of the paired design is that the experimental units receiving the two treatments are, indeed, related.

Table 5.11   Results of a Bioavailability Study Comparing a New Formulation (A) to a Marketed Form (B) with Regard to the Area Under the Blood-Level Curve

Animal	A	B	δ = B $-$ A	A/B = R
1	136	166	30	0.82
2	168	184	16	0.91
3	160	193	33	0.83
4	94	105	11	0.90
5	200	198	-2	1.01
6	174	197	23	0.88
			$\overline{\delta}$ = 18.5	$\overline{R}$ = 0.89
			S_{δ} = 13.0	S_R = 0.069

Sometimes, this is not as obvious as the example of the same patient taking both treatments. One can think of the concept of relatedness in terms of the paired samples being more alike than samples from members of different pairs. Pairs may be devised in clinical trials by pairing patients with similar characteristics, such as age, sex, severity of disease, and so on.

Example 6: A new formulation of a marketed drug is to be tested for bioavailability, comparing the extent of absorption to the marketed form on six laboratory animals. Each animal received both formulations in random order on two different occasions. The results, the area under the blood level versus time curve (AUC), are shown in Table 5.11.

$$H_0: \Delta = 0^* \qquad H_a: \Delta \neq 0$$

This is a two-sided test, with the null hypothesis of equality of means of the paired samples. (The true difference is zero.) Before the experiment, it was not known which formulation would be more or less bioavailable if, indeed, the formulations are different. The significance level is set at 5%. From Table 5.11, the average difference is 18.5 and the standard deviation of the differences (δ values) is 13.0. The t test is

---

*Δ is the hypothetical difference, and $\overline{\delta}$ is the observed average difference.

$$t = \frac{\bar{\delta} - \Delta}{S/\sqrt{N}} \tag{5.14}$$

The form of the test is the same as the one-sample t test [Eq. (5.5)]. In our example, a two-sided test,

$$t = \frac{|18.5 - 0|}{13/\sqrt{6}} = 3.48$$

For a two-sided test at the 5% level, a t value of 2.57 is needed for significance (d.f. = 5; there are six pairs). Therefore, the difference is significant at the 5% level. Formulation B appears to be more bioavailable.

In many kinds of experiments, *ratios* are more meaningful than differences as a practical expression of the results. In comparative bioavailability studies, the ratio of the AUCs of the two competing formulations is more easily interpreted than is their difference. The ratio expresses the *relative* absorption of the formulations. From a statistical point of view, if the AUCs for formulations A and B are normally distributed, the difference of the AUCs is also normally distributed. It can be proven that the ratio of the AUCs will *not* be normally distributed and the assumption of normality for the t test is violated. However, if the variability of the ratios is not great and the sample size is sufficiently "large," analyzing the ratios should give conclusions similar to that obtained from the analysis of the differences. Another alternative for the analysis of such data is the logarithmic transformation (see Chap. 10), where the differences of the logarithms of the AUCs are analyzed. For purposes of illustration, we will analyze the data in Table 5.11 using the ratio of the AUCs for formulations A and B. The ratios are calculated in the last column in Table 5.11.

The null and alternative hypotheses in this case are

$$H_0: \quad R_0 = 1 \qquad H_a: \quad R_0 \neq 1$$

where R_0 is the true ratio. If the products are identical, we would expect to observe an average ratio close to 1 from the experimental data. For the statistical test, we choose α equal to 0.05 for a two-sided test. Applying Eq. (5.5), where $\bar{X}$ is replaced by the average ratio $\bar{R}$:

$$t = \frac{|\bar{R} - 1|}{S/\sqrt{6}} = \frac{|0.89 - 1|}{0.069/\sqrt{6}} = +3.85$$

Note that this is a one-sample test. We are testing the mean of a single sample of ratios versus the hypothetical value of 1. Because this is a two-sided test, negative or positive values can lead to significant differences. As in the analysis of the differences, the value of t is significant at the 5% level. (According to Table IV.4, at the 5% level, t must exceed 2.57 for significance.)

A *confidence interval* for the average ratio (or difference) of the AUCs can be computed in a manner similar to that presented earlier in this chapter [Eq. (5.2)]. A 95% confidence interval for the true ratio A/B is

$$\overline{R} \pm \frac{t(S)}{\sqrt{N}}$$

$$0.89 \pm \frac{2.57(0.069)}{\sqrt{6}} = 0.89 \pm 0.07 = 0.82 \text{ to } 0.96$$

Again, the fact that the confidence interval does not cover the value specified by H_0 (1) means that the statistical test is significant at the 5% level.

5.2.4 Normal Distribution Tests for Proportions (Binomial Tests)

The tests described thus far in this chapter (normal distribution and t tests as well as confidence intervals) can also be applied to data that are binomially distributed. To apply tests for binomial variables based on the normal distribution, a conservative rule is that the sample sizes should be sufficiently large so that both $N\hat{p}$ and $N\hat{q}$ are larger than or equal to 5. Where $\hat{p}$ is the observed proportion and $\hat{q} = 1 - \hat{p}$. For symmetric distributions ($p \stackrel{\sim}{=} 0.5$), this constraint may be relaxed somewhat. The binomial tests are based on the normal approximation to the binomial and, therefore, we use normal curve probabilities when making decisions in these tests. To obtain the probabilities for tests of significance, we can use the t table with ∞ d.f. or the standard normal distribution (Tables IV.4 and IV.2, respectively). We will also discuss the application of the χ^2 (chi-square) distribution to the problem of comparing the "means" of binomial populations.

Test to Compare the Proportion of a Sample
to a Known or Hypothetical Proportion

This test is equivalent to the normal test of the mean of a single population. The test is

$$Z = \frac{\hat{p} - p_0}{\sqrt{p_0 q_0 / N}} \qquad (5.15)$$

where

$\hat{p}$ = observed proportion

p_0 = hypothetical proportion under the null hypothesis
$H_0: \; p' = p_0$

The test procedure is analogous to the one-sample tests described in Sec. 5.2.1. Because of the discrete nature of binomial data, a correction factor is recommended to improve the normal approximation. The correction, often called the *Yates continuity correction*, consists of subtracting $1/(2N)$ from the absolute value of the numerator of the test statistic [Eq. (5.15)]:

$$Z = \frac{|\hat{p} - p_0| - 1/(2N)}{\sqrt{p_0 q_0 / N}} \qquad (5.16)$$

For a two-tailed test, the approximation can be improved as described by Snedecor and Cochran [5]. The correction is the same as the Yates correction if np is "a whole number or ends in 0.5." Otherwise, the correction is somewhat less than $1/2N$ (see Ref. 5 for details). In the examples presented here, we will use the Yates correction. This results in probabilities very close to those which would be obtained by using exact calculations based on the binomial theorem. Some examples should make the procedure clear.

Example 7: Two products are to be compared for preference with regard to some attribute. The attribute could be sensory (taste, smell, etc.) or therapeutic effect as examples. Suppose that an ointment is formulated for rectal itch and is to be compared to a marketed formulation. Twenty patients try each product under "blind" conditions and report their preference. The null hypothesis and alternative hypothesis are

$$H_0: \; p_a = p_b \qquad \text{or} \qquad H_0: \; p_a = 0.5 \qquad H_a: \; p_a \neq 0.5$$

Where p_a and p_b are the hypothetical preferences for A and B, respectively. If the products are truly equivalent, we would expect one-half of the patients to prefer either product A or B. Note that is is a *one-sample* test. There are two possible outcomes that can result from each observation: a patient prefers A or prefers B $(p_a + p_b = 1)$.

We observe the proportion of preferences (successes) for A, where A is the new formulation. This is a two-sided test; very few or very many preferences for A would suggest a significant difference in preference for the two products. Final tabulation of results showed that 15 of 20 patients found product A superior (5 found B superior). Does this result represent a "significant" preference for product A? Applying Eq. (5.16), we have

$$Z = \frac{|\,15/20 - 0.5\,| - 1/40}{\sqrt{(0.5)(0.5)/20}} = 2.01$$

Note the correction for continuity, $1/(2N)$. Also note that the denominator uses the value of pq based on the null hypothesis ($p_a = 0.5$), not the sample proportion ($0.75 = 15/20$). This procedure may be rationalized if one verbalizes the nature of the test. We assume that the preferences are equal for both products ($p_a = 0.5$). We then observe a sample of 20 patients to see if the results conform with the hypothetical preference. Thus the test is based on a hypothetical binomial distribution with the expected number of preferences equal to 10 ($p_a \times 20$). See Fig. 5.11, which illustrates the rejection region in this test. The value of $Z = 2.01$ (15 preferences in a sample of 20) is sufficiently large to reject the null hypothesis. A value of 1.96 or greater is significant at the 5% level (Table IV.2). The test of $p_0 = 0.5$ is common in statistical procedures. The sign test described in Chap. 15 is a test of equal proportions (i.e., $p_0 = q_0 = 0.5$).

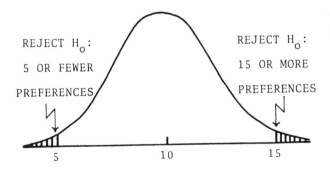

REJECT H_o:
5 OR FEWER
PREFERENCES

REJECT H_o:
15 OR MORE
PREFERENCES

5   10   15

NUMBER OF PREFERENCES

Figure 5.11   Rejection region for the test of $p_a = 0.5$ for a sample of 20 patients ($\alpha = 0.05$, two-sided test).

Example 8: A particularly lethal disease is known to result in 95% fatality if not treated. A new treatment is given to 100 patients and 10 survive. Does the treatment merit serious consideration as a new therapeutic regimen for the disease? We can use the normal approximation because the expected number of successes and failures both are $\geqslant 5$, i.e., $Np_0 = 5$ and $Nq_0 = 95$ ($p_0 = 0.05$, $N = 100$). A one-sided test is performed because evidence supports the hypothesis that the treatment cannot worsen the chances of survival. The α level is set at 0.05. Applying Eq. (5.16), we have

$$H_0: \quad p_0 = 0.05 \qquad H_a: \quad p_0 > 0.05$$

$$Z = \frac{|0.10 - 0.05| - 1/200}{\sqrt{(0.05)(0.95)/100}} = 2.06$$

Table IV.2 shows that a value of Z equal to 1.65 would result in significance at the 5% level (one-sided test). Therefore, the result of the experiment is strong evidence that the new treatment is effective ($P < 0.05$).

If either Np_0 or Nq_0 is less than 5, the normal approximation to the binomial may not be justified. Although this rule is conservative, if in doubt, in these cases, probabilities must be calculated by enumerating all possible results which are equally or less likely to occur than the observed result under the null hypothesis. This is a tedious procedure, but in some cases it is the only way to obtain the probability for significance testing. Fortunately, most of the time, the sample sizes of binomial experiments are sufficiently large to use the normal approximation.

Tests for the Comparison of Proportions from Two Independent Groups

Experiments commonly occur in the pharmaceutical and biological sciences which involve the comparison of proportions from two independent groups. These experiments are analogous to the comparison of means in two independent groups using the t or normal distributions. For proportions, the form of the test is similar. With a sufficiently large sample size, the normal approximation to the binomial can be used, as in the single-sample test. For the hypothesis: $H_0: p_a = p_b$ ($p_a - p_b = 0$), the test using the normal approximation is:

$$Z = \frac{\hat{p}_a - \hat{p}_b}{\sqrt{p_0 q_0 (1/N_1 + 1/N_2)}} \tag{5.17}$$

Table 5.12   Sample Calculation for Pooling
Proportions from Two Groups

Group I	Group II
N = 20	N = 30
$\hat{p}_1 = 0.8$	$\hat{p}_2 = 0.6$
$p_0 = \text{pooled } p = \dfrac{20 \times 0.8 + 30 \times 0.6}{20 + 30} = 0.68$	

where $\hat{p}_a$ and $\hat{p}_b$ are the observed proportions in groups A and B,
respectively, and N_1 and N_2 are the sample sizes for groups A and
B, respectively, p_0 and q_0 are the "pooled" proportion of successes
and failures. The pooled proportion, p_0, is similar to the pooled
standard deviation in the t test. For proportions, the results of
the two comparative groups are pooled together and the "overall"
observed proportion is equal to p_0. Under the null hypothesis,
the probability of success is the same for both groups, A and B.
Therefore, the best estimate of the common probability for the two
groups is the estimate based on the combination of data from the
entire experiment. An example of this calculation is shown in
Table 5.12. The pooled proportion, p_0, is a weighted average of
the two proportions. This is exactly the same as adding up the
total number of "successes" and dividing this by the total number
of observations. In the example in Table 5.12, the total number of
successes is 34, 16 in group I and 18 in group II. The total number of observations is 50, 30 + 20. The following examples illustrate
the computations.
   Example 9: In a clinical study designed to test the safety and
efficacy of a new therapeutic agent, the incidence of side effects
are compared for two groups of patients, one taking the new drug
and the other group taking a marketed standard agent. Headache
is a known side effect of such therapy. Of 212 patients on the new
drug, 35 related that they had experienced severe headaches. Of
196 patients on the standard therapy, 46 suffered from severe headaches. Can the new drug be claimed to result in fewer headaches
than the standard drug at the 5% level of significance? The null
and alternative hypotheses are

$$H_0:\ p_1 = p_2\ (p_1 - p_2 = 0) \qquad H_a:\ p_1 \neq p_2$$

This is a two-sided test. Before performing the statistical test, the following computations are necessary:

$$\hat{p}_1 = \frac{35}{212} = 0.165$$

$$\hat{p}_2 = \frac{46}{196} = 0.235$$

$$p_0 = \frac{81}{408} = 0.199 \ (q_0 = 0.801)$$

Applying Eq. (5.17), we have

$$Z = \frac{|0.235 - 0.165|}{\sqrt{(0.199)(0.801)(1/212 + 1/196)}} = \frac{0.07}{0.0395} = 1.77$$

Since a Z value of 1.96 is needed for significance at the 5% level, the observed difference between the two groups with regard to the side effect of "headache" is not significant ($P > 0.05$).

Example 10: In a preclinical test, the carcinogenicity potential of a new compound is determined by administering several doses to different groups of animals. A control group (placebo) is included in the study as a reference. One of the dosage groups showed an incidence of the carcinoma in 9 of 60 animals (15%). The control group exhibited 6 carcinomas in 65 animals (9.2%). Is there a difference in the proportion of animals with the carcinoma in the two groups ($\alpha = 5\%$)? Applying Eq. (5.17), we have

$$H_0: \ p_1 = p_2 \qquad H_a: \ p_1 \neq p_2$$

$$Z = \frac{|9/60 - 6/65|}{\sqrt{(15/125)(110/125)(1/60 + 1/65)}} = \frac{0.0577}{0.058} = 0.99$$

Note that $\hat{p}_1 = 0.15$, $\hat{p}_2 = 6/65 = 0.092$, and $p_0 = 15/125 = 0.12$.

Since Z does not exceed 1.96, the difference is not significant at the 5% level. This test could have been a one-sided test (a priori) if one were certain that the new compound could not lower the risk of carcinoma. However, the result is not significant at the 5% level for a one-sided test; a value of Z equal to 1.65 or greater is needed for significance for a one-sided test.

Example 11: A new operator is assigned to a tablet machine. A sample of 1000 tablets from this machine showed 8% defects. A random sample of 1000 tablets from the other tablet presses used

during this run showed 5.7% defects. Is there reason to believe
that the new operator produced more defective tablets than that
produced by the more experienced personnel? We will perform a
two-sided test at the 5% level, using Eq. (5.17).

$$Z = \frac{|0.08 - 0.057|}{\sqrt{(0.0685)(0.9315)(2/1000)}} = \frac{0.023}{0.0113} = 2.04$$

Since the value of Z (2.04) is greater than 1.96, the difference is
significant at the 5% level. We can conclude that the new operator
is responsible for the larger number of defective tablets produced
at his station. (See also Exercise Problem 19.) If a continuity
correction is used, the equivalent chi-square test with a correction
as described below is recommended.*

There is some controversy about the appropriateness of a continuity correction in these tests. D'Agostino et al. [6] examined
various alternatives and compared the results to exact probabilities.
They concluded that for small sample sizes (N_1 and N_2 < 15), the
use of the Yates continuity correction resulted in too conservative
probabilities (i.e., probabilities were too high which may lead to a
lack of rejection of H_0 in some cases). They suggest that in these
situations a correction should not be used. They also suggest an
alternative analysis that is similar to the t test.

$$t = \frac{|p_1 - p_2|}{s.d. \sqrt{1/N_1 + 1/N_2}} \tag{5.18}$$

where s.d. is the pooled standard deviation computed from the data
considering a success equal to 1 and a failure equal to 0. The
value of t is compared to the appropriate t value with $N_1 + N_2 - 2$
d.f. The computation for the example in Table 5.12 follows:

For Group 1, $s_1^2 = (16 - 16^2/20)/19 = 0.168$

For Group 2, $s_2^2 = (18 - 18^2/30)/29 = 0.248$

---

*The continuity correction can make a difference when making de-
cisions based on the α level, when the statistical test is "just significant" (e.g., P = 0.04 for a test at the 5% level). The correction makes the test "less significant."

(Note for Group 1 that the number of successes is 16 and the number of failures is 4. Thus, we have 16 values equal to 1 and 4 values equal to 0. The variance is calculated from these 20 values.) The pooled variance is:

$$(19 \times 0.168 + 29 \times 0.248)/48 = 0.216$$

The pooled standard deviation is 0.465.
From Eq. (5.18),

$$t = \frac{|0.8 - 0.6|}{0.465\sqrt{1/20 + 1/30}} = 1.49$$

The t value with 48 d.f. for significance at the 5% level for a two-sided test is 2.01. Therefore the results fail to show a significant difference at the 5% level.

Fleiss [7] advocates the use of the Yates continuity correction. He states "Because the correction for continuity brings probabilities associated with χ^2 and Z into close agreement with the exact probabilities, the correction should always be used."

5.2.5 Chi-Square Tests for Proportions

An alternative method of comparing proportions is the chi-square (χ^2) test. This test results in identical conclusions as the binomial test in which the normal approximation is used as described above. The chi-square distribution is frequently used in statistical tests involving counts and proportions, as discussed in Chap. 15. Here we will show the application to fourfold tables (2 × 2 tables), the comparison of proportions in two independent groups.

The chi-square distribution is appropriate where the normal approximation to the distribution of discrete variables can be applied. In particular, when comparing two proportions, the chi-square distribution with 1 d.f. can be used to approximate probabilities. (The values for the χ^2 distribution with one d.f. are exactly the square of the corresponding normal deviates. For example, the "95%" cutoff point for the chi-square distribution with 1 d.f. 3.84, equal to 1.96^2.)

The use of the chi-square distribution to test for differences of proportions in two groups has two advantages: (a) the computations are easy and (b) a continuity correction can be easily applied. The reader may have noted that a continuity correction was not used in the examples for the comparison of two independent groups described above. The correction was not included because the computation of the correction is somewhat complicated. In the

Table 5.13   Results of the Experiment Shown in
Table 5.12 in the Form of a Fourfold Table

| | Group | | |
	I	II	Total
Number of successes	16	18	34
Number of failures	4	12	16
Total	20	30	50

chi-square test, however, the continuity correction is relatively
simple. The correction is most easily described in the context of an
example. We will demonstrate the chi-square test using the data in
Table 5.12. We can think of these data as resulting from a clinical
trial where groups I and II represent two comparative drugs. The
same results are presented in the *fourfold table* shown in Table
5.13.

The chi-square statistic is calculated as follows:

$$\chi^2 = \Sigma \frac{(O - E)^2}{E} \qquad (5.19)$$

where

O = observed number in a cell (there are four cells in the experiment in Table 5.13; a cell is the intersection of a row
and column; the upper left-hand cell, number of successes
in group I, has the value 16 contained in it)

E = expected number in a cell

The expected number is the number that would result if each group
had the same proportion of successes and failures. The best estimate of the common p (proportion of successes) is the pooled value,
as calculated in the test using the normal approximation above [Eq.
(5.17)]. The pooled, p, p_0, is 0.68 (34/50). With a probability
of success of 0.68 (34/50), we would expect "13.6" successes for
group I (20 × 0.68). The expected number of failures is
20 × 0.32 = 6.4. The expected number of failures can also be obtained by subtracting 13.6 from the total number of observations in
group I, 20 − 13.6 = 6.4. Similarly, the expected number of successes in group II is 30 × 0.68 = 20.4. Again the number, 20.4,
could have been obtained by subtracting 13.6 from 34.

Table 5.14   Expected Values for the Experiment Shown in Table 5.13

	Group		
	I	II	Total
Expected number of successes	13.6	20.4	34
Expected number of failures	6.4	9.6	16
Total	20.0	30.0	50

This concept (and calculation) is illustrated in Table 5.14, which shows the expected values for Table 5.13. The marginal totals (34, 16, 20, and 30) in the "expected value" table are the same as in the original table, Table 5.13. In order to calculate the expected values, multiply the two marginal totals for a cell and divide this value by the grand total. This simple way of calculating the expected values will be demonstrated for the upper left-hand cell, where the observed value is 16. The expected value is

$$\frac{(20)(34)}{(50)} = 13.6$$

Once the expected value for one cell is calculated, the expected values for the remaining cells can be obtained by subtraction.

Expected successes in group II = 34 − 13.6 = 20.4

Expected failures in group I = 20 − 13.6 = 6.4

Expected failures in group II = 16 − 6.4 = 9.6

Given the marginal totals and the value for any *one* cell, the values for the other three cells can be calculated. Once the expected values have been calculated, the chi-square statistic is evaluated according to Eq. (5.19).

$$\Sigma \frac{(O - E)^2}{E} = \frac{(16 - 13.6)^2}{13.6} + \frac{(18 - 20.4)^2}{20.4} + \frac{(4 - 6.4)^2}{6.4}$$

$$+ \frac{(12 - 9.6)^2}{9.6} = 2.206$$

The numerator of each term is $(\pm 2.4)^2 = 5.76$.   Therefore, the computation of χ^2 can be simplified as follows:

$$\chi^2 = (O - E)^2 \left(\frac{1}{E_1} + \frac{1}{E_2} + \frac{1}{E_3} + \frac{1}{E_4} \right) \tag{5.20}$$

where E_1 through E_4 are the expected values for each of the four cells.

$$\chi^2 = (2.4)^2 \left(\frac{1}{13.6} + \frac{1}{20.4} + \frac{1}{6.4} + \frac{1}{9.6} \right) = 2.206$$

One can show that this computation is exactly equal to the square of the Z value using the normal approximation to the binomial. (See Exercise Problem 11.)

The degrees of freedom for the test described above (the four-fold table) is equal to 1. In general, the degrees of freedom for an $R \times C$ contingency table, where R is the number of rows and C is the number of columns, is equal to $(R - 1)(C - 1)$. The analysis of $R \times C$ tables is discussed in Chap. 15.

Table IV.5, a table of points in the cumulative chi-square distribution, shows that a value of 3.84 is needed for significance at the 5% level (1 degree of freedom). Therefore, the test in this example is not significant; that is, the proportion of successes in group I is not significantly different from that in group II, 0.8 and 0.6, respectively.

To illustrate further the computations of the chi-square statistic and the application of the continuity correction, we will analyze the data in Example 10, where the normal approximation to the binomial was used for the statistical test. Table 5.15 shows the observed and expected values for the results of this preclinical study.

Table 5.15   Observed and Expected Values for Preclinical Carcinogenicity Study[a]

	Drug	Placebo	Total
Animals with carcinoma	9 (7.2)	6 (7.8)	15
Animals without carcinoma	51 (52.8)	59 (57.2)	110
Total	60	65	125

[a]Parenthetical values are expected values.

The uncorrected chi-square analysis results in a value of 0.98 $(0.99)^2$. (See Exercise Problem 18.) The continuity correction is applied using the following rule: If the fractional part of the difference $(O - E)$ is larger than 0 but $\leqslant 0.5$, delete the fractional part. If the fractional part is greater than 0.5 or exactly 0, "reduce the fractional part to 0.5." Some examples should made the application of this rule clearer.

$O - E$	Corrected for continuity
3.0	2.5
3.2	3.0
3.5	3.0
3.9	3.5
3.99	3.5
4.0	3.5

In the example above, $O - E = \pm 1.8$. Therefore, correct this value to ± 1.5. The corrected chi-square statistic is [Eq. (5.20)]

$$(1.5)^2 \left(\frac{1}{7.2} + \frac{1}{7.8} + \frac{1}{52.8} + \frac{1}{57.2} \right) = 0.68$$

In this example, the result is not significant using either the corrected or uncorrected values. However, when chi-square is close to significance at the α level, the continuity correction can make a difference. The continuity correction is more apparent in its effect on the computation of chi-square in small samples. With large samples, the correction makes less of a difference.

The chi-square test, like the normal approximation, is an approximate test, applying a continuous distribution to discrete data. The test is valid (close to correct probabilities) when the expected value in each cell is at least 5. This is an approximate rule. Because the rule is conservative, in some cases, an expected value in one or more cells of less than 5 can be tolerated. However, one should be cautious in applying this test if the expected values are too small.

5.2.6 Confidence Intervals for Proportions

Examples of the formation of a confidence interval for a proportion have been presented earlier in this chapter (Example 3). Although the confidence interval for the binomial is calculated using the standard deviation of the binomial based on the sample proportion, we should understand that in most cases, the s.d. is unknown. The sample standard deviation is an estimate of the true standard deviation, which for the binomial depends on the true value of the proportion or probability. However, when we use the sample estimate of the s.d. for the calculations, the confidence interval and statistical tests are valid using criteria based on the normal distribution (Table IV.2). We do not use the t distribution as in the procedures discussed previously.

The confidence interval for the true proportion or binomial probability, p_0 is

$$\hat{p} \pm Z \sqrt{\frac{\hat{p}\hat{q}}{N}} \tag{5.3}$$

where $\hat{p}$ is the observed proportion in a sample of size N. The value of Z depends on the confidence coefficient (e.g., 1.96 for a 95% interval). Of 500 tablets inspected, 20 were found to be defective ($\hat{p} = 20/500 = 0.04$). A 95% confidence interval for the true proportion of defective tablets is

$$\hat{p} \pm 1.96 \sqrt{\frac{\hat{p}\hat{q}}{N}} = 0.04 \pm 1.96 \sqrt{\frac{(0.04)(0.96)}{500}}$$

$$= 0.04 \pm 0.017 = 0.023 \text{ to } 0.057$$

To obtain a *confidence interval for the difference of two proportions* (two independent groups), use the following formula:

$$(\hat{p}_1 - \hat{p}_2) \pm Z \sqrt{\frac{\hat{p}_1\hat{q}_1}{N_1} + \frac{\hat{p}_2\hat{q}_2}{N_2}} \tag{5.21}$$

where $\hat{p}_1$ and $\hat{p}_2$ are the observed proportions in groups 1 and 2, respectively, and N_1 and N_2 are the respective sample sizes of the two groups. Z is the appropriate normal deviate (1.96 for a 95% confidence interval).

In the example of incidence of headaches in two groups of patients, the proportion of headaches observed in group 1 was $35/212 = 0.165$ and the proportion in group 2 was $46/196 = 0.235$. A 95% confidence interval for the difference of the two proportions, calculated from Eq. (5.21), is

$$(0.235 - 0.165) \pm 1.96 \sqrt{\frac{(0.165)(0.835)}{212} + \frac{(0.235)(0.765)}{196}}$$

$$= 0.07 \pm 0.078 = 0.148 \text{ to } -0.008$$

The difference between the two proportions was not significant at the 5% level in a two-sided test (see "Test for Comparison of Proportions from Two Independent Groups" in Sec. 5.2.4). Note that 95% confidence interval covers 0, the difference specified in the null hypothesis (H_0: $p_1 - p_2 = 0$).*

Hauck and Anderson [8] recommend the use of a continuity correction for the construction of confidence intervals that give better results than that obtained without a correction [Eq. (5.21)]. If a 90% or 95% interval is used, the Yates correction works well if N_1p_1, N_1q_1, N_2p_2, and N_2q_2 are all greater than or equal to 3. The 99% interval is good for N_1p_1, N_1q_1, N_2p_2, and N_2q_2 all greater than or equal to 5. The correction is $1/2N_1 + 1/2N_2$. Applying the correction to the previous example, a 95% confidence interval is:

$$0.235 - 0.165 - (1/424 + 1/392) \pm 1.96 \sqrt{\frac{(0.165)(0.835)}{212} + \frac{(0.235)(0.765)}{196}}$$

$$= 0.065 \pm 0.078 = 0.143 \text{ to } -0.013$$

5.3 COMPARISON OF VARIANCES IN INDEPENDENT SAMPLES

Most of the statistical tests presented in this book are concerned with means. However, situations arise where variability is important as a measure of a process or product performance. For example, when mixing powders for tablet granulations, one may be interested in measuring the homogeneity of the mix as may be indicated in validation procedures. The "degree" of homogeneity can be determined by assaying different portions of the mix, and calculating the standard deviation or variance. (Sample weights equal to that in the final dosage form are most convenient.) A small variance would be associated with a relatively homogeneous mix, and vice versa. Variability is also often of interest when assaying drug blood levels in a bioavailability study or when determining a clinical response to drug therapy. We will describe statistical tests appropriate for two situations: the comparison of two variances from independent samples, and the comparison of variances in related (paired) samples. The test for related samples will be presented in

---

*The form of the confidence interval Eq. (5.21) differs from the form of the statistical test in that the latter uses the pooled variance [Eq. (5.17)]. Therefore, this relationship will not always hold for the comparison of two proportions.

Chap. 7 because methods of calculation involve material presented there. The test for the comparison of variances in independent samples described here assumes that the data in each sample are independent and normally distributed.

The notion of significance tests for two variances is similar to the tests for means (e.g., the t test). The null hypothesis is usually of the form

$$H_0: \quad \sigma_1^2 = \sigma_2^2$$

For a two-sided test, the alternative hypothesis admits the possibility of either variance being larger or smaller than the other:

$$H_a: \quad \sigma_1^2 \neq \sigma_2^2$$

The statistical test consists of calculating the ratio of the two sample variances. The ratio has an F distribution with $(N_1 - 1)$ d.f. in the numerator and $(N_2 - 1)$ d.f. in the denominator. To determine if the ratio is "significant" (i.e., the variances differ), the observed ratio is compared to appropriate table values of F at the α level. The F distribution is not symmetrical and, in general, to make statistical decisions, we would need F tables with both upper and lower cutoff points.

Referring to Fig. 5.12, if the F ratio falls between F_L and F_U, the test is not significant. We do not reject the null hypothesis of equal variances. If the F ratio is below F_L or above F_U, we reject the null hypothesis and conclude that the variances differ (at the 5% level, the shaded area in the example of Fig. 5.12). The F table to test the equality of two variances is the same as that used

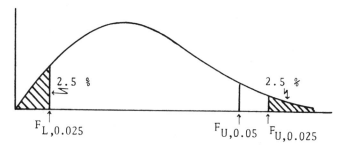

Figure 5.12 Example of two-sided cutoff points in an F distribution.

to determine significance in analysis of variance tests to be presented in Chap. 8 (Table IV.6). However, F tables for ANOVA usually give only the upper cutoff points (F_U, 0.05 in Fig. 5.12, for example).

Nevertheless, it is possible to perform a two-sided test for two variances using the one-tailed F table (Table IV.6) by forming the ratio with the *larger variance in the numerator*. Thus the ratio will always be equal to or greater than 1. The ratio is then referred to the usual ANOVA F table, but the level of significance is twice that stated in the table. For example, the values that must be exceeded for significance in Table IV.6 represent cutoff points at the 10% or 2% level if the larger variance is in the numerator. For significance at the 5% level, use Table 5.16, a brief table of the upper 0.025 cutoff points for some F distributions.

To summarize, for a two-sided test at the 5% level, calculate the ratio of the comparative variances with the larger variance in the numerator. (Clearly, if the variances in the two groups are identical, there is no need to perform a test of significance.) To be significant at the 5% level, the ratio must be equal to or greater than the tabulated upper 2.5% cutoff points (see Table 5.16). For significance at the 10% level, for a two-sided test, use the upper 5% points in Table IV.6.

For a *one-sided test*, if the null hypothesis is

$$H_0: \quad \sigma_A^2 \geqslant \sigma_B^2 \qquad H_a: \quad \sigma_A^2 < \sigma_B^2$$

Perform the test only if S_A^2 is smaller than S_B^2, with S_B^2 in the numerator. (If S_A^2 is equal to or greater than S_B^2, we cannot reject the null hypothesis.) Refer the ratio to Table IV.6 for significance at the 5% (or 1%) level.

One should appreciate that this statistical test is particularly sensitive to departures from the assumptions of normality and independence of the two comparative groups.

An example should clarify the procedure. Two granulations were prepared by different procedures. Seven random samples of powdered mix of equal weight (equal to the weight of the final dosage form) were collected from each batch and assayed for active material, with the results shown in Table 5.17. The test is to be performed at the 5% level: $H_0: \quad \sigma_1^2 = \sigma_2^2; \quad H_a: \quad \sigma_1^2 \neq \sigma_2^2.$ For a two-sided test, we form the ratio of the variances with S_B^2, the larger variance in the numerator.

$$F = \frac{1.297}{0.156} = 8.3$$

Table 5.16   Brief Table of Upper 0.025 Cutoff Points of the F Distribution

Degrees of freedom in denominator	Degrees of freedom in numerator											
	2	3	4	5	6	8	10	15	20	25	30	∞
2	39.0	39.2	39.3	39.3	39.3	39.4	39.4	39.4	39.5	39.5	39.5	39.5
3	16.0	15.4	15.1	14.9	14.7	14.5	14.4	14.3	14.2	14.1	14.1	13.9
4	10.6	10.0	9.6	9.4	9.2	9.0	8.8	8.7	8.6	8.5	8.5	8.3
5	8.4	7.8	7.4	7.2	7.0	6.8	6.6	6.4	6.3	6.3	6.2	6.0
6	7.3	6.6	6.2	6.0	5.8	5.6	5.5	5.3	5.2	5.1	5.1	4.9
7	6.5	5.9	5.5	5.3	5.1	4.9	4.8	4.6	4.5	4.4	4.4	4.1
8	6.1	5.4	5.1	4.8	4.7	4.4	4.3	4.1	4.0	3.9	3.9	3.7
9	5.7	5.1	4.7	4.5	4.3	4.1	4.0	3.8	3.7	3.6	3.6	3.3
10	5.5	4.8	4.5	4.2	4.1	3.9	3.7	3.5	3.4	3.4	3.3	3.1
15	4.8	4.2	3.8	3.6	3.4	3.2	3.1	2.9	2.8	2.7	2.6	2.4
20	4.5	3.9	3.5	3.3	3.1	2.9	2.8	2.6	2.5	2.4	2.4	2.1
24	4.3	3.7	3.4	3.2	3.0	2.8	2.6	2.4	2.3	2.3	2.2	1.9
30	4.2	3.6	3.3	3.0	2.9	2.7	2.5	2.3	2.2	2.1	2.1	1.8
40	4.1	3.5	3.1	2.9	2.7	2.5	2.4	2.2	2.1	2.0	1.9	1.6
∞	3.7	3.1	2.8	2.6	2.4	2.2	2.1	1.8	1.7	1.6	1.6	1.0

Table 5.17 Assays from Samples from Two Granulations

Granulation A		Granulation B	
20.6	20.7	20.2	19.0
20.9	19.8	21.5	21.8
20.6	20.4	18.9	20.4
21.0		21.0	
$\overline{X} = 20.57$	$S^2 = 0.156$	$\overline{X} = 20.4$	$S^2 = 1.297$

The tabulated F value with 6 d.f. in the numerator and denominator (Table 5.16) is 5.8. Therefore, the variances can be considered significantly different ($P < 0.05$); granulation B is more variable than granulation A. If the test were performed at the 10% level, we would refer to the upper 5% points in Table IV.6, where a value greater than 4.28 would be significant.

If the test were *one-sided, at the 5% level*, for example, with the null hypothesis:

$$H_0: \quad \sigma_A^2 = \sigma_B^2 \qquad H_a: \quad \sigma_A^2 < \sigma_B^2$$

the ratio $1.297/0.156 = 8.3$ would be referred to Table IV.6 for significance. Now, a value greater than 4.28 would be significant at the 5% level.

If more than two variances are to be compared, the F test discussed above is not appropriate. Bartlett's test is the procedure commonly used to test the equality of more than two variances [1].

5.4 TEST OF EQUALITY OF MORE THAN TWO VARIANCES

The test statistic computation is shown in Eq. (5.22).

$$\chi^2 = \Sigma(N_i - 1)\ln S^2 - \Sigma[(N_i - 1)\ln S_i^2] \tag{5.22}$$

where S^2 is the pooled variance and S_i^2 is the variance of the ith sample.

Table 5.18   Results of Variability of Assays of Granulation at Six Locations in a Mixer

Location	N	N − 1	Variance (S^2)	ln S^2
A	3	2	3.6	1.2809
B	3	2	4.7	1.5476
C	3	2	2.9	1.0647
D	5	4	8.3	2.1163

The computations are demonstrated for the data of Table 5.18. In this example, samples of a granulation were taken at 4 different locations in a mixer.   Three samples were analyzed in each of 3 of the locations, and 5 samples analyzed in the 4th location.   The purpose of this experiment was to test the homogeneity of the mix in a validation experiment.   Part of the statistical analysis requires an estimate of the variability within each location.   The statistical test (analysis of variance, Chap. 8) assumes homogeneity of variance within the different locations.   Bartlett's test allows us to test for the homogeneity of variance (Table 5.18).

The pooled variance is calculated as the weighted average of the variances, where the weights are the d.f. ($N_i − 1$).

$$\text{Pooled } S^2 = [2 \times 3.6 + 2 \times 4.7 + 2 \times 2.9 + 4 \times 8.3]/$$

$$[2 + 2 + 2 + 4] = 5.56$$

$$\Sigma\ N_i - 1 = 10$$

$$\Sigma[(N_i - 1)\ \ln S_i^2 = 2(1.2809) + 2(1.5476) + 2(1.0647)$$

$$+ 4(2.1163) = 16.2516$$

$$\chi^2 = 10 \times \ln (5.56) - 16.2516 = 0.904$$

To test χ^2 for significance, compare the result to the tabulated value of χ^2 (Table IV.5) with 3 d.f. (1 less than the number of variances being compared) at the appropriate significance level.   A value of 7.81 is needed for significance at the 5% level.   Therefore, we conclude that the variances do not differ.   A significant value of χ^2 means that the variances are not all equal.   This test is very sensitive to nonnormality. That is, if the variances come from non-normal populations, the conclusions of the test may be erroneous.

See Exercise Problem 22 for another example where Bartlett's test can be used to test the homogeneity of variances.

Table 5.19 summarizes tests discussed in this chapter.

Table 5.19 Summary of Tests

Test		Section
Mean of single population	$t = \dfrac{\overline{X} - \mu}{S\sqrt{1/N}}$	5.2.1
Comparison of means from two independent populations (variances known)	$Z = \dfrac{\overline{X}_1 - \overline{X}_2}{\sqrt{\sigma_1^2/N_1 + \sigma_2^2/N_2}}$	5.2.2
Comparisons of means from two independent populations (variance unknown)	$t = \dfrac{\overline{X}_1 - \overline{X}_2}{S_p\sqrt{1/N_1 + 1/N_2}}$	5.2.2
Comparison of means from two related samples (variance unknown)[a]	$t = \dfrac{\overline{\delta}}{S\sqrt{1/N}}$	5.2.3
Proportion from a single population[b]	$Z = \dfrac{\hat{p} - p_0}{\sqrt{p_0 q_0/N}}$	5.2.4
Comparison of two proportions from independent groups[b]	$Z = \dfrac{\hat{p}_1 - \hat{p}_2}{\sqrt{p_0 q_0(1/N_1 + 1/N_2)}}$	5.2.4
Comparison of variances (two-sided test)	$F = \dfrac{S_1^2}{S_2^2}$ $(S_1^2 > S_2^2)$	5.3

[a]If the variance is known, use the normal distribution.

[b]A continuity correction may be used (5.24 and 5.25).

KEY TERMS

Alpha level
Alternative hypothesis
Bartlett's test
Behrens-Fisher test
Beta error
Bias
Binomial trials
Blinding
Cells
Chi-square test
Confidence interval
Continuity correction
Critical region
Crossover design
Cumulative normal distribution
Degrees of freedom
Delta
Error
Error of first kind
Estimation
Expected values
Experimental error
Fourfold table
F test
Hypothesis testing
Independence
Independent groups
Level of significance

Marginal totals
Nonsignificance
Normal curve test
Null hypothesis
One-sample test
One-sided test
One-way analysis of variance
Paired-sample t test
Parallel-groups design
Parameters
Pooled proportion
Pooled variance
Power
Preference tests
Randomization
Region of rejection
Sample size
Sensitive
Significance
t distribution
t test
Two-by-two table
Two-independent-groups t test
Two-tailed (sided) test
Uncontrolled study
Variance
Yates correction
Z transformation

EXERCISES

1. Calculate the probability of finding a value of 49.8 or less if $\mu = 54.7$ and $\sigma = 2$.
2. If the variance of the population of tablets in Table 5.1 were known to be 4.84, compute a 99% confidence interval for the mean.
3. (a) Six analysts perform an assay on a portion of the same homogeneous material with the following results: 5.8, 6.0, 5.7, 6.1, 6.0, and 6.1. Place 95% confidence limits on the true mean.
   (b) A sample of 500 tablets show 12 to be defective. Place a 95% confidence interval on the percent defective in the lot.

(c) Place a 95% confidence interval on the difference between two products in which 50 of 60 patients responded to product A, and 25 of 50 patients responded to product B.

4. (a) Quality control records show the average tablet weight to be 502 mg with a standard deviation of 5.3. There are sufficient data so that these values may be considered known parameter values. A new batch shows the following weights from a random sample of six tablets: 500, 499, 504, 493, 497, and 495 mg. Do you believe that the new batch has a different mean from the process average?

(b) Two batches of tablets were prepared by two different processes. The potency determinations made on five tablets from each batch were as follows: batch A: 5.1, 4.9, 4.6, 5.3, 5.5; batch B: 4.8, 4.8, 5.2, 5.0, 4.5. Test to see if the means of the two batches are equal.

(c) Answer part (a) if the variance were unknown. Place a 95% confidence interval on the true average weight.

5. (a) In part (b) of Problem 4, calculate the variance and the standard deviation of the 10 values as if they were one sample. Are the values of the s.d. and s^2 smaller or larger than the values calculated from "pooling"?

(b) Calculate the pooled s.d. above by "averaging" the s.d.'s from the two samples. Is the result different from the "pooled" s.d. as described in the text?

6.

Batch 1 (drug)	Pass/fail (improve, worsen)	Batch 2 (placebo)	Pass/fail (improve, worsen)
10.1	P	9.5	F
9.7	F	8.9	F
10.1	P	9.4	F
10.5	P	10.4	P
12.3	P	9.9	F
11.8	P	10.1	P
9.6	F	9.0	F
10.0	F	9.7	F
11.2	P	9.9	F
11.3	P	9.8	F

(a) What are the mean and s.d. of each batch? Test for difference between the two batches using a t test.

(b) What might be the "population" corresponding to this sample? Do you think that the sample size is large enough? Why? Ten objects were selected from each batch for this test. Is this a good design for comparing the average results from two batches?

(c) Consider values above 10.0 a success and values 10.00 or
    less a failure. What is the proportion of successes for
    batch 1 and batch 2? Is the proportion of successes in
    batch 1 different from the proportion in batch 2 (5% level)?

(d) Put 95% confidence limits on the proportion of successes
    with all data combined.

7. A new analytical method is to be compared to an old method.
   The experiment is performed by a single analyst. She selects
   four batches of product at random and obtains the following
   results.

Batch	Method 1	Method 2
1	4.81	4.93
2	5.44	5.43
3	4.25	4.30
4	4.35	4.47

(a) Do you think that the two methods give different results
    on the average?

(b) Place 95% confidence limits on the true difference of the
    methods.

8. The following data for blood protein (g/100 ml) were observed
   for the comparison of two drugs. Both drugs were tested on
   each person in random order.

Patient	Drug A	Drug B
1	8.1	9.0
2	9.4	9.9
3	7.2	8.0
4	6.3	6.0
5	6.6	7.9
6	9.3	9.0
7	7.6	7.9
8	8.1	8.3
9	8.6	8.2
10	8.3	8.9
11	7.0	8.3
12	7.7	8.8

(a) Perform a statistical test for drug differences at the 5%
    level.

(b) Place 95% confidence limits on the average difference be-
    tween drugs A and B.

9. For examples 10 and 11, calculate the pooled p and q (p_0 and q_0).

10. In Example 4, perform a t test if the mean were 16.7 instead of 15.9.

11. Use the normal approximation and chi-square test (with and without continuity correction) to answer the following problem. A placebo treatment results in 8 patients out of 100 having elevated blood urea nitrogen (BUN) values. The drug treatment results in 16 of 100 patients having elevated values. Is this significantly different from the placebo?

12. Quality control records show that the average defect rate for a product is 2.8%. Two hundred items are inspected and 5% are found to be defective in a new batch. Should the batch be rejected? What would you do if you were the director of quality control? Place confidence limits on the *percent* defective and the *number* defective (out of 200).

**13. In a batch size of 1,000,000, 5000 tablets are inspected and 50 are found defective.
    (a) Put 95% confidence limits on the true number of defectives in the batch.
    (b) At $\alpha = 0.05$, do you think that there could be more than 2% defective in the batch?
    **(c) If you wanted to estimate the true proportion of defectives within ±0.1% with 95% confidence, how many tablets would you inspect?

14. In a clinical test, 60 people received a new drug and 50 people received a placebo. Of the people on the new drug, 40 of the 60 showed a positive response and 25 of the 50 people on placebo showed a positive response. Perform a statistical test to determine if the new drug shows more of an effect than the placebo. Place a 95% confidence interval on the difference of proportion of positive response in the two test groups.

15. In a paired preference test, each of 100 subjects was asked to choose the preference between A and B. Of these 100, 60 showed no preference, 30 preferred A, and 10 preferred B. Is A significantly preferred to B?

16. Over a long period of time, a screening test has shown a response rate for a control of 20%. A new chemical shows 9 positive results in 20 observations (45%). Would you say that this candidate is better than the control? Place 99% confidence limits on the true response rate for the new chemical.

17. Use the chi-square test with the continuity correction to see if there is a significant difference in the following comparison. Two batches of tablets were made using different excipients.

In batch A, 10 of 100 tablets sampled were chipped. In batch B, 17 of 95 tablets were chipped. Compare the two batches with respect to proportion chipped at the 5% level.

18. Show that the uncorrected value of chi-square for the data in Table 5.15 is 0.98.

19. Use the chi-square test, with continuity correction, to test for significance (5% level) for the data in Example 11.

20. Perform a statistical test to compare the variances in the two groups in Problem 6. H_0: $\sigma_1^2 = \sigma_2^2$; H_a: $\sigma_1^2 \neq \sigma_2^2$. Perform the test at the 10% level.

21. Compute the value of the corrected χ^2 statistic for data of Example 11 in 5.2.4. Compute the t value as recommended by D'agostino et al. Compare the uncorrected value of Z with these results.

22. The homogeneity of a sample taken from a mixer was tested after 5, 10, and 15 minutes. The variances of 6 samples taken at each time were 16.21, 1.98, 2.02. Based on the results of Bartlett's test for homogeneity of variances, what are your conclusions?

REFERENCES

1. Westlake, W. J., *Biometrics*, 32, 741−744, 1976.
2. Westlake, W. J., Bioavailability and bioequivalence of pharmaceutical formulations, in *Statistical Issues in Drug Research and Development*, (K. E. Peace, ed.), Marcel Dekker, New York, 1990.
3. Snedecor, G. W. and Cochran, W. G., *Statistical Methods*, 6th ed., Iowa State University Press, Ames, Iowa, 1967.
4. Cochran, W. G., *Sampling Techniques*, 3rd ed., Wiley, New York, 1967.
5. Snedecor, G. W. and Cochran, W. G., *Statistical Methods*, 7th ed., Iowa State University Press, Ames, Iowa, 1980.
6. D'Agostino, R. B., Chase, W., and Belanger, A., *The American Statistician*, 42, 198, 1988.
7. Fleiss, J., *Statistical Methods for Rates and Proportions*, 2nd ed., Wiley, New York, 1981.
8. Hauck, W. and Anderson, S., *The American Statistician*, 40, 318, 1986.

6
Sample Size and Power

The question of the size of the sample, the number of observations, to be used in scientific experiments is of extreme importance. Most experiments beg the question of sample size. Particularly when time and cost are critical factors, one wishes to use the minimum sample size to achieve the experimental objectives. Even when time and cost are less crucial, the scientist wishes to have some idea of the number of observations needed to yield sufficient data to answer the objectives. An elegant experiment will make the most of the resources available, resulting in a sufficient amount of information from a minimum sample size. For simple comparative experiments, where one or two groups are involved, the calculation of sample size is relatively simple. A knowledge of the α level (level of significance), β level ($1 -$ power), the standard deviation, and a meaningful "practically significant" difference is necessary in order to calculate the sample size.

Power is defined as $1 - \beta$ (i.e., $\beta = 1 -$ power). Power is the ability of a statistical test to show significance if a specified difference truly exists. The magnitude of power depends on the level of significance, the standard deviation, and the sample size. Thus power and sample size are related.

In this chapter we present methods for computing the sample size for relatively simple situations for normally distributed and binomial data. The concept and calculation of power are also introduced.

6.1   INTRODUCTION

The question of sample size is a major consideration in the planning of experiments, but may not be answered easily from a scientific point of view. In some situations, the choice of sample size is

limited. Sample size may be dictated by official specifications, regulations, cost constraints, and/or the availability of sampling units
such as patients, manufactured items, animals, and so on. The
USP content uniformity test is an example of a test in which the
sample size is fixed and specified [1].

The sample size is also specified in certain quality control sampling plans such as those described in MIL-STD-105D [2]. These
sampling plans are used when sampling products for inspection for
attributes such as product defects, missing labels, specks in tablets, or ampul leakage. The properties of these plans have been
thoroughly investigated and defined as described in the document
cited above. The properties of the plans include the chances
(probability) of rejecting or accepting batches with a known proportion of rejects in the batch (Sec. 12.3).

Sample-size determination in comparative clinical trials is a
factor of major importance. Since very large experiments will detect very small, perhaps clinically insignificant, differences as
being statistically significant, and small experiments will often find
large, clinically significant differences as statistically insignificant,
the choice of an appropriate sample size is critical in the design of
a clinical program to demonstrate safety and efficacy. When cost is
a major factor in implementing a clinical program, the number of
patients to be included in the studies may be limited by lack of
funds. With fewer patients, a study will be less sensitive. Decreased sensitivity means that the comparative treatments will be
relatively more difficult to distinguish statistically if they are, in
fact, different.

The problem of choosing a "correct" sample size is related to
experimental objectives and the risk (or probability) of coming to
an incorrect decision when the experiment and analysis are completed. For simple comparative experiments, certain prior information is required in order to compute a sample size that will satisfy
the experimental objectives. The following considerations are essential when estimating sample size.

1. The α level must be specified which, in part, determines
the difference needed to represent a statistically significant result.
To review, the α level is defined as the risk of concluding that
treatments differ when, in fact, they are the same. The level of
significance is usually (but not always) set at the traditional value
of 5%.

2. The β error must be specified for some specified treatment
difference, Δ. Beta, β, is the risk (probability) of erroneously
concluding that the treatments are not significantly different when,
in fact, a difference of size Δ or greater exists. The assessment
of β and Δ, the "practically significant" difference, *prior* to the
initiation of the experiment, is not easy. Nevertheless, an educated

guess is required. β is often chosen to be between 5 and 20%. Hence one may be willing to accept a 20% (1 in 5) chance of not arriving at a statistically significant difference when the treatments are truly different by an amount equal to (or greater than) Δ. The consequences of committing a β error should be considered carefully. If a true difference of practical significance is missed and the consequence is costly, β should be made very small, perhaps as small as 1%. Costly consequences of missing an effective treatment should be evaluated not only in monetary terms, but should also include public health issues, such as the possible loss of an effective treatment in a serious disease.

3. The difference to be detected, Δ (that difference considered to have practical significance), should be specified as described in (2) above. This difference should not be arbitrarily or capriciously determined, but should be considered carefully with respect to meaningfulness from both a scientific and commercial marketing standpoint. For example, when comparing two formulas for time to 90% dissolution, a difference of 1 or 2 min might be considered meaningless. A difference of 10 or 20 min, however, may have practical consequences in terms of in vivo absorption characteristics.

4. A knowledge of the standard deviation (or an estimate) for the significance test is necessary. If no information on variability is available, an educated guess, or results of studies reported in the literature using related compounds, may be sufficient to give an estimate of the relevant variability. The assistance of a statistician is recommended when estimating the standard deviation for purposes of determining sample size.

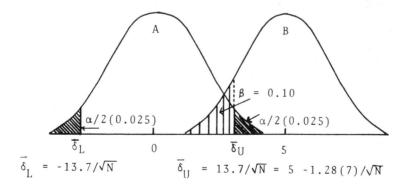

Figure 6.1 Scheme to demonstrate calculation of sample size based on α, β, Δ, and σ: $\alpha = 0.05$, $\beta = 0.10$, $\Delta = 5$, $\sigma = 7$; H_0: $\Delta = 0$, H_a: $\Delta = 5$.

To compute the sample size in a comparative experiment, (a) α, (b) β, (c) Δ, and (d) σ must be specified. The computations to determine sample size are described below (see also Fig. 6.1).

6.2 DETERMINATION OF SAMPLE SIZE FOR SIMPLE COMPARATIVE EXPERIMENTS FOR NORMALLY DISTRIBUTED VARIABLES

The calculation of sample size will be described with the aid of Fig. 6.1. This explanation is based on normal distribution or t tests. The derivation of sample-size determination may appear complex. The reader not requiring a "proof" can proceed directly to the appropriate formulas below.

6.2.1 Paired-Sample and Single-Sample Tests

We will first consider the case of a paired-sample test where the null hypothesis is that the two treatment means are equal: H_0: $\Delta = 0$. In the case of an experiment comparing a new antihypertensive drug candidate and a placebo, an average difference of 5 mmHg in blood pressure reduction might be considered of sufficient magnitude to be interpreted as a difference of "practical significance" ($\Delta = 5$). The standard deviation for the comparison was known, equal to 7, based on a large amount of experience with this drug.

In Fig. 6.1, the normal curve labeled A represents the distribution of differences with mean equal to 0 and σ equal to 7. This is the distribution under the null hypothesis (i.e., drug and placebo are identical). Curve B is the distribution of differences when the alternative, H_a: $\Delta = 5$,* is true (i.e., the difference between drug and placebo is equal to 5). Note that curve B is identical to curve A except that B is displaced 5 mmHg to the the right. Both curves have the same standard deviation, 7.

With the standard deviation, 7, known, the statistical test is performed at the 5% level as follows [Eq. (5.4)]:

$$Z = \frac{\bar{\delta} - \Delta}{\sigma/\sqrt{N}} = \frac{\bar{\delta} - 0}{7/\sqrt{N}} \tag{6.1}$$

---

*Δ is considered to be the *true* mean difference, similar to μ.
$\bar{\delta}$ will be used to denote the *observed* mean difference.

For a two-tailed test, if the absolute value of Z is 1.96 or greater, the difference is significant. According to Eq. (6.1), to obtain significance

$$| \bar{\delta} | \geq \frac{\sigma Z}{\sqrt{N}} = \frac{7(1.96)}{\sqrt{N}} = \frac{13.7}{\sqrt{N}} \qquad (6.2)$$

Therefore, values of $\bar{\delta}$ equal to or greater than $13.7/\sqrt{N}$ (or equal to or less than $-13.7/\sqrt{N}$) will lead to a declaration of significance. These points are designated as $\bar{\delta}_L$ and $\bar{\delta}_U$ in Fig. 6.1, and represent the cutoff points for statistical significance at the 5% level; that is, observed differences equal to or more remote from the mean than these values result in "statistically significant differences."

If curve B is the true distribution (i.e., $\Delta = 5$), an observed mean difference greater than $13.7/\sqrt{N}$ (or less than $-13.7/\sqrt{N}$) will result in the correct decision; H_0 will be rejected and we conclude that a difference exists. If $\Delta = 5$, observations of a mean difference between $13.7/\sqrt{N}$ and $-13.7/\sqrt{N}$ will lead to an *incorrect decision*, the acceptance of H_0 (no difference) (see Fig. 6.1). By definition, the probability of making this *incorrect* decision is equal to β.

In the present example, β will be set at 10%. In Fig. 6.1, β is represented by the area in curve B below $13.7/\sqrt{N}$ (δ_U), equal to 0.10. (This area, β, represents the probability of accepting H_0 if $\Delta = 5$.)

We will now compute that value of $\bar{\delta}$ which cuts off 10% of the area in the lower tail of the normal curve with a mean of 5 and a standard deviation of 7 (curve B in Fig. 6.1). Table IV.2 shows that 10% of the area in the standard normal curve is below -1.28. The value of $\bar{\delta}$ (mean difference in blood pressure between the two groups) which corresponds to a given value of Z (-1.28, in this example) is obtained from the formula for the Z transformation [Eq. (3.14)] as follows:

$$Z_{\beta} = \frac{\bar{\delta} - \Delta}{\sigma / \sqrt{N}} \qquad (6.3)$$

$$\bar{\delta} = \Delta + Z_{\beta} \left(\frac{\sigma}{\sqrt{N}} \right)$$

Applying Eq. (6.3) to our present example, $\bar{\delta} = 5 - 1.28(7/\sqrt{N})$. The value of $\bar{\delta}$ in Eqs. (6.2) and (6.3) is identically the same, equal to $\bar{\delta}_U$. This is illustrated in Fig. 6.1.

From Eq. (6.2), $\bar{\delta}_U = 13.7/\sqrt{N}$, satisfying the definition of α.
From Eq. (6.3), $\bar{\delta}_U = 5 - 1.28(7)/\sqrt{N}$, satisfying the definition of

Table 6.1 Sample Size as a Function
of Beta with $\Delta = 5$ and $\sigma = 7$:
Paired Test ($\alpha = 0.05$)

Beta	Sample size, N
1%	36
5%	26
10%	21
20%	16

β. We have two equations in two unknowns($\bar{\delta}_U$ and N), and N is
evaluated as follows:

$$\frac{13.7}{\sqrt{N}} = 5 - \frac{1.28(7)}{\sqrt{N}}$$

$$N = \frac{(13.7 + 8.96)^2}{5^2} = 20.5 \cong 21$$

In general, Eqs. (6.2) and (6.3) can be solved for N to yield the
following equation:

$$N = \left(\frac{\sigma}{\Delta}\right)^2 (Z_\alpha + Z_\beta)^2 \tag{6.4}$$

where Z_α and Z_β* are the appropriate normal deviates obtained
from Table IV.2. In our example, $N = (7/5)^2(1.96 + 1.28)^2 \cong 21$.
A sample size of 21 will result in a statistical test with 90% power
($\beta = 10$%) against an alternative of 5, at the 5% level of significance.
Table 6.1 shows how the choice of β can affect the sample size for
a test at the 5% level with $\Delta = 5$ and $\sigma = 7$.

The formula for computing the sample size if the standard deviation is known [Eq. (6.4)] is appropriate for a paired-sample test
or for the test of a mean from a *single population*. For example,
consider a test to compare the mean drug content of a sample of
tablets to the labeled amount, 100 mg. The two-sided test is to be
performed at the 5% level. Beta is designated as 10% for a difference

---

*Z_β is taken as the positive value of Z in this formula.

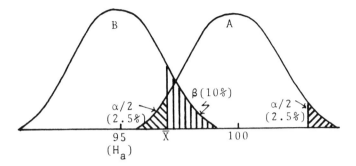

Figure 6.2 Illustration of the calculation of N for tablet assays. $\overline{X} = 95 + \sigma Z_\beta / \sqrt{N} = 100 - \sigma Z_\alpha / \sqrt{N}$.

of -5 mg (95 mg potency or less). That is, we wish to have a power of 90% to detect a difference from 100 mg if the true potency is 95 mg or less. If σ is equal to 3, how many tablets should be assayed? Applying Eq. (6.4), we have

$$N = \left(\frac{3}{5}\right)^2 (1.96 + 1.28)^2 = 3.8$$

Assaying four tablets will satisfy the α and β probabilities. Note that $Z = 1.28$ cuts off 90% of the area under curve B (the "alternative" curve) in Fig. 6.2, leaving 10% (β) of the area in the upper tail of the curve. Table 6.2 shows values of Z_α and Z_β for various levels of α and β to be used in Eq. (6.4).

Equation (6.4) is correct for computing the sample size for a paired- or one-sample test if the standard deviation is known.

In most situations, the standard deviation is unknown and a prior estimate of the standard deviation is necessary in order to calculate sample size requirements. In this case, the estimate of the standard deviation replaces σ in Eq. (6.4), but the calculation results in an answer that is slightly too small. The underestimation occurs because the values of Z_α and Z_β are smaller than the corresponding t values which should be used in the formula when the standard deviation is unknown. The situation is somewhat complicated by the fact that the value of t depends on the sample size (d.f.), which is yet unknown. The problem can be solved by an iterative method, but for practical purposes, one can use the appropriate values of Z to compute the sample size [as in Eq. (6.4)] and add on a few extra samples (patients, tablets, etc.) to compensate for the use of Z rather than t. Guenther has shown

Table 6.2   Values of Z_α and Z_β for Sample-Size Calculations

	Z_α		$Z_\beta{}^a$
	One-sided	Two-sided	
1%	2.32	2.58	2.32
5%	1.65	1.96	1.65
10%	1.28	1.65	1.28
20%	0.84	1.28	0.84

[a]The value of β is for a single specified alternative. For a two-sided test, the probability of rejection of the alternative, if true, (accept H_0) is virtually all contained in the tail nearest the alternative mean.

that the simple addition of $0.5Z_\alpha{}^2$, which is equal to approximately 2 for a two-sided test at the 5% level, results in a very close approximation to the correct answer [3]. In the problem illustrated above (tablet assays), if the standard deviation were *unknown* but *estimated* as being equal to 3 based on previous experience, a better estimate of the sample size would be $N + 0.5Z_\alpha{}^2 = 3.8 + 0.5(1.96)^2 \cong 6$ tablets.

6.2.2   Determination of Sample Size for Comparison of Means in Two Groups

For a two-independent-groups test (parallel design), with the standard deviation known and equal number of observations per group, the formula for N (where N is the sample size for each group) is

$$ N = 2 \left(\frac{\sigma}{\Delta}\right)^2 (Z_\alpha + Z_\beta)^2 \tag{6.5} $$

If the standard deviation is unknown and a prior estimate is available (s.d.), substitute s.d. for σ in Eq. (6.5) and compute the sample size; but add on $0.25Z_\alpha{}^2$ to the sample size for each group.

Example 1: This example illustrates the determination of the sample size for a two-independent-groups (two-sided test) design. Two variations of a tablet formulation are to be compared with regard to dissolution time. All ingredients except for the lubricating agent were the same in these two formulations. In this case, a decision was made that if the formulations differed by 10 min or more to 80% dissolution, it would be extremely important that the experiment show a statistically significant difference between the formulations. Therefore, the pharmaceutical scientist decided to fix the β error at 1% in a statistical test at the traditional 5% level. Data were available from dissolution tests run during the development of formulations of the drug and the standard deviation was *estimated* as 5 min. With the information presented above, the sample size can be determined from Eq. (6.5). We will add on $0.25Z_\alpha^2$ samples to the answer because the standard deviation is unknown.

$$N = 2\left(\frac{5}{10}\right)^2 (1.96 + 2.32)^2 + 0.25(1.96)^2 = 10.1$$

The study was performed using 12 tablets from each formulation rather than the 10 or 11 suggested by the answer in the calculation above. Twelve tablets were used because the dissolution apparatus could accommodate six tablets per run.

Example 2: A bioequivalence study was being planned to compare the bioavailability of a final production batch to a previously manufactured pilot-sized batch of tablets which were made for clinical studies. Two parameters resulting from the blood-level data would be compared: area under the plasma level versus time curves (AUC) and peak plasma concentration (C_{max}). The study was to have 80% power ($\beta = 0.20$) to detect a difference of 20% or more between the formulations. The test is done at the usual 5% level of significance. Estimates of the standard deviations of the *ratios* of the values of each of the parameters [(final product)/(pilot batch)], were determined from a small pilot study. The standard deviations were different for the parameters. Since the researchers could not agree that one of the parameters was clearly critical in the comparison, they decided to use a "maximum" number of patients based on the variable with the largest relative variability. In this example, C_{max} was most variable, the ratio having a standard deviation of approximately 0.30. Since the design and analysis of the bioequivalence study is a variation of the paired t test, Eq. (6.4) was used to calculate the sample size, adding on $0.5Z_\alpha^2$, as recommended previously.

$$N = \left(\frac{\sigma}{\Delta}\right)^2 (Z_\alpha + Z_\beta)^2 + 0.5 (Z_\alpha^2) \tag{6.6}$$

$$= \left(\frac{0.3}{0.2}\right)^2 (1.96 + 0.84)^2 + 0.5(1.96)^2 = 19.6$$

Table 6.3 Sample Size Needed for Two-Sided t Test with Standard Deviation Estimated

	One-sample test								Two-sample test with N units per group							
	Alpha = 0.05				Alpha = 0.01				Alpha = 0.05				Alpha = 0.01			
	Beta =				Beta =				Beta =				Beta =			
Estimated S/Δ	0.01	0.05	0.10	0.20	0.01	0.05	0.10	0.20	0.01	0.05	0.10	0.20	0.01	0.05	0.10	0.20
4.0	296	211	170	128	388	289	242	191	588	417	337	252	770	572	478	376
2.0	76	54	44	34	100	75	63	51	148	106	86	64	194	145	121	96
1.5	44	32	26	20	58	54	37	30	84	60	49	37	110	82	69	55
1.0	21	16	13	10	28	22	19	16	38	27	23	17	50	38	32	26
0.8	14	11	9	8	19	15	13	11	25	18	15	12	33	25	21	17
0.67	11	8	7	6	15	12	11	9	18	13	11	9	24	18	15	13
0.5	7	6	5	4	10	8	8	7	11	8	7	6	14	11	10	8
0.4	6	5	4	4	8	7	6	6	8	6	5	4	10	8	7	6
0.33	5	4	4	3	7	6	6	5	6	5	4	4	8	6	6	5

Twenty subjects were used for the comparison of the bioavailabilities of the two formulations.

Sometimes the sample sizes computed to satisfy the desired α and β errors can be inordinately large when time and cost factors are taken into consideration. Under these circumstances, a compromise must be made — most easily accomplished by relaxing the α and β requirements* (see Table 6.1). The consequence of this compromise is that probabilities of making an incorrect decision based on the statistical test will be increased. Other ways of reducing the required sample size are (a) to increase the precision of the test by improving the assay methodology or carefully controlling extraneous conditions during the experiment, for example, or (b) to compromise by increasing Δ, that is, accepting a larger difference which one considers to be of practical importance.

Table 6.3 gives the sample size for some representative values of the ratio σ/Δ, α, and β, where the s.d. (s) is estimated.

6.3 DETERMINATION OF SAMPLE SIZE FOR BINOMIAL TESTS

The formulas for calculating the sample size for comparative binomial tests are similar to those described for normal curve or t tests. The major difference is that the value of σ^2, which is assumed to be the same under H_0 and H_a in the two-sample independent-groups t or Z tests, is different for the distributions under H_0 and H_a in the binomial case. This difference occurs because σ^2 is dependent on p, the probability of success, in the binomial. The value of p will be different depending on whether H_0 or H_a represents the true situation. The appropriate formulas for determining sample size for the one- and two-sample tests are:

One-sample test:

$$N = 1/2 \left[\frac{p_0 q_0 + p_1 q_1}{\Delta^2} \right] (Z_\alpha + Z_\beta)^2 \tag{6.7}$$

where $\Delta = p_1 - p_0$; p_1 is the proportion that would result in a meaningful difference, and p_0 is the hypothetical proportion under the null hypothesis.

---

*In practice, α is often fixed by regulatory considerations and β is determined as a compromise.

Two-sample test:

$$N = \left[\frac{\frac{p_1 q_1 + p_2 q_2}{2}}{\Delta^2} \right] (Z_\alpha + Z_\beta)^2 \qquad (6.8)$$

where $\Delta = p_1 - p_2$; p_1 and p_2 are prior estimates of the proportions in the experimental groups. The values of Z_α and Z_β are the same as those used in the formulas for the normal curve or t tests. N is the sample size for each group. If it is not possible to estimate p_1 and p_2 prior to the experiment, one can make an educated guess of a meaningful value of Δ and set p_1 and p_2 both equal to 0.5 in the *numerator* of Eq. (6.8). This will maximize the sample size, resulting in a conservative estimate of sample size.

Fleiss [5] gives a fine discussion of an approach to estimating Δ, the practically significant difference, when computing the sample size. For example, one approach is first to estimate the proportion for the more well-studied treatment group. In the case of a comparative clinical study, this could very well be a standard treatment. Suppose this treatment has shown a success rate of 50%. One might argue that if the comparative treatment is additionally successful for 30% of the patients who do not respond to the standard treatment, then the experimental treatment would be valuable. Therefore the success rate for the experimental treatment should be 50% + 0.3 (50%) = 65% to show a practically significant difference. Thus, p_1 would be equal to 0.5 and p_2 would be equal to 0.65.

Example 3: A reconciliation of quality control data over several years showed that the proportion of unacceptable capsules for a stable encapsulation process was 0.8% (p_0). A sample size for inspection is to be determined so that if the true proportion of unacceptable capsules is equal to or greater than 1.2% ($\Delta = 0.4\%$), the probability of detecting this change is 80% ($\beta = 0.2$). The comparison is to be made at the 5% level using a *one-sided* test. According to Eq. (6.7),

$$N = \frac{1}{2} \left[\frac{0.008 \cdot 0.992 + 0.012 \cdot 0.988}{(0.008 - 0.012)^2} \right] (1.65 + 0.84)^2$$

$$= \frac{7670}{2} = 3835$$

The large sample size resulting from this calculation is typical of that resulting from binomial data. If 3835 capsules are too many to inspect, α, β, and/or Δ must be increased. In the example above, management decided to increase α. This is a conservative decision in that more good batches would be "rejected" if α is increased; that is, the increase in a α results in an increased probability of rejecting good batches, those with 0.8% unacceptable or less.

Example 4: Two antibiotics, a new product and a standard
product, are to be compared with respect to the 2-week cure rate
of a urinary tract infection, where a cure is bacteriological evidence that the organism no longer appears in urine. From previous
experience the cure rate for the standard product is estimated as
80%. From a practical point of view, if the new product shows an
85% or better cure rate, the new product can be considered superior. The marketing division of the pharmaceutical company felt
that this difference would support claims of better efficacy for the
new product. This is an important claim. Therefore, β is chosen
to be 1% (power = 99%). A two-sided test will be performed at the
5% level to satisfy FDA guidelines. The test is two-sided because,
a priori, the new product is not known to be better or worse than
the standard. The calculation of sample size to satisfy the conditions above makes use of Eq. (6.8); here $p_1 = 0.8$ and $p_2 = 0.85$.

$$N = \left[\frac{0.08 \cdot 0.2 + 0.85 \cdot 0.15}{(0.80 - 0.85)^2} \right] (1.96 + 2.32)^2 = 2107$$

The trial would have to include 4214 patients, 2107 on each drug,
to satisfy the α and β risks of 0.05 and 0.01, respectively. If
this number of patients is greater than can be accommodated, the
β error can be increased to 5 or 10%, for example. A sample size
of 1499 per group is obtained for a β of 5%, and 1207 patients per
group for β equal to 10%

Although Eq. (6.8) is adequate for computing the sample size
for most situations, the calculation of N can be improved by considering the continuity correction [5]. This would be particularly
important for small sample sizes.

$$N' = [N/4] [1 + \sqrt{1 + 8/(N |p_2 - p_1|)}]^2$$

where N is the sample size computed from Eq. (6.8) and N' is the
corrected sample size. In the example, for $\alpha = 0.05$ and $\beta = 0.01$,
the corrected sample size is:

$$N' = [2107/4] [1 + \sqrt{1 + 8/(2107 |0.80 - 0.85|)}]^2 = 2186$$

6.4   DETERMINATION OF SAMPLE SIZE TO
OBTAIN A CONFIDENCE INTERVAL
OF SPECIFIED WIDTH

The problem of estimating the number of samples needed to estimate the mean with a known precision by means of the confidence

interval is easily solved using the formula for the confidence interval (see Sec. 5.1). This approach has been used as an aid in
predicting election results based on preliminary polls where the
samples are chosen by simple random sampling. For example, one
may wish to estimate the proportion of voters who will vote for
candidate A within 1% of the actual proportion.

We will consider the application of this problem to the estimation
of proportions. In quality control, one can closely estimate the
true proportion of percent defects to any given degree of precision.
In a clinical study, a suitable sample size may be chosen to estimate the true proportion of successes within certain specified limits.
According to Eq. (5.3), a two-sided confidence interval with confidence coefficient P for a proportion is

$$\hat{p} \pm Z_p \sqrt{\frac{\hat{p}\hat{q}}{N}} \tag{5.3}$$

To obtain a 99% confidence interval with a width of 0.01 (i.e., construct an interval that is within ±0.005 of the observed proportion,
$\hat{p} \pm 0.005$),

$$Z_p \sqrt{\frac{\hat{p}\hat{q}}{N}} = 0.005$$

or

$$N = \frac{Z_p^2(\hat{p}\hat{q})}{(W/2)^2} \quad \text{where } W = \text{width of interval} \tag{6.9}$$

$$N = \frac{(2.58)^2(\hat{p}\hat{q})}{(0.005)^2}$$

A more exact formula for the sample size for small values of N is
given in Ref. 4.

Example 5: A quality control supervisor wishes to have an
estimate of the proportion of tablets in a batch which weigh between 195 and 205 mg, where the proportion of tablets in this
interval is to be estimated within ±0.05 (W = 0.10). How many
tablets should be weighed? Use a 95% confidence interval.

To compute N, we must have an estimate of $\hat{p}$ [see Eq. (6.9)].
If $\hat{p}$ and $\hat{q}$ are chosen to be equal to 0.5, N will be at a maximum.
Thus, if one has no inkling as to the magnitude of the outcome,
using $\hat{p} = 0.5$ in Eq. (6.9) will result in a sufficiently large sample

size (probably, too large). Otherwise, estimate $\hat{p}$ and $\hat{q}$ based on previous experience and knowledge. In the present example from previous experience, approximately 80% of the tablets are expected to weigh between 195 and 205 mg ($\hat{p}$ = 0.8). Applying Eq. (6.9),

$$N = \frac{(1.96)^2(0.8)(0.2)}{(0.10/2)^2} = 245.9$$

A total of 246 tablets should be weighed. In the actual experiment, 250 tablets were weighed, and 195 of the tablets (78%) weighed between 195 and 205 mg. The 95% confidence interval for the true proportion, according to Eq. (5.3), is

$$p \pm 1.96 \sqrt{\frac{\hat{p}\hat{q}}{N}} = 0.78 \pm 1.96 \sqrt{\frac{(0.78)(0.22)}{250}} = 0.78 \pm 0.051$$

The interval is slightly greater than ±5% because p is somewhat less than 0.8 (pq is larger for p = 0.78 than for p = 0.8). Although 5.1% is acceptable, to ensure a sufficient sample size, in general, one should estimate p closer to 0.5 in order to cover possible poor estimates of p.

If $\hat{p}$ had been chosen equal to 0.5, we would have calculated

$$N = \frac{(1.96)^2(0.5)(0.5)}{(0.10/2)^2} = 384.2$$

Example 6: A new vaccine is to undergo a nationwide clinical trial. An estimate is desired of the proportion of the population that would be afflicted with the disease after vaccination. A good guess of the expected proportion of the population diseased without vaccination is 0.003. Pilot studies show that the incidence will be about 0.001 (0.1%) after vaccination. What size sample is needed so that the width of a 99% confidence interval for the proportion diseased in the vaccinated population should be no greater than 0.0002? To ensure that the sample size is sufficiently large, the value of p to be used in Eq. (6.9) is chosen to be 0.0012, rather than the expected 0.0010.

$$N = \frac{(2.58)^2(0.9988)(0.0012)}{(0.0002/2)^2} = 797,809$$

The trial will have to include approximately 800,000 subjects in order to yield the desired precision.

6.5   POWER

Power is the probability that the statistical test results in rejection of H_0 when a specified alternative is true.   The "stronger" the power, the better the chance that the null hypothesis will be rejected (i.e., the test results in a declaration of "significance") when, in fact, H_0 is false.   The larger the power, the more sensitive is the test.   *Power* is defined as $1 - \beta$.   The larger the β error, the weaker is the power.   Remember that β is an error resulting from *accepting H_0 when H_0 is false*.   Therefore, $1 - \beta$ is the probability of *rejecting H_0 when H_0 is false*.

From an idealistic point of view, the power of a test should be calculated *before* an experiment is conducted.   In addition to defining the properties of the test, power is used to help compute the sample size, as discussed above.   Unfortunately, most experiments proceed without consideration of power (or β).   This results from the difficulty of choosing an appropriate value of β.   There is no traditional value of β to use, as is the case for α, where 5% is usually used.   Thus the power of the test is often computed after the experiment has been completed.

Power is best described by diagrams such as those shown previously in this chapter (Figs. 6.1 and 6.2).   In these figures, β is the area of the curves represented by the alternative hypothesis which is included in the region of acceptance defined by the null hypothesis.   The concept of power is also illustrated in Fig. 6.3. To illustrate the calculation of power, we will use data presented for the test of a new antihypertensive agent (Sec. 6.2), a paired sample test, with $\sigma = 7$ and H_0: $\Delta = 0$.   The test is performed at the 5% level of significance.   Let us suppose that the sample size is limited by cost.   The sponsor of the test had sufficient funds to

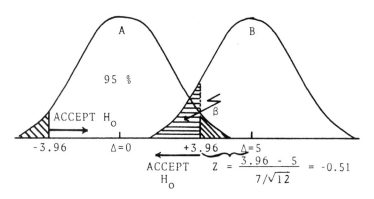

Figure 6.3   Illustration of beta or power $(1 - \beta)$.

pay for a study which included only *12 subjects*. The design described earlier in this chapter (Sec. 6.2) used 26 patients with β specified equal to 0.05 (power = 0.95). With 12 subjects, the power will be considerably less than 0.95. The following discussion shows how power is calculated.

The cutoff points for statistical significance (which specify the critical region) are defined by α, N, and σ. Thus the values of $\bar{\delta}$ that will lead to a significant result for a two-sided test are as follows:

$$Z = \frac{|\bar{\delta}|}{\sigma/\sqrt{N}}$$

$$\bar{\delta} = \frac{\pm Z\sigma}{\sqrt{N}}$$

In our example, Z = 1.96 (α = 0.05), σ = 7, and N = 12.

$$\bar{\delta} = \frac{\pm(1.96)(7)}{\sqrt{12}} = \pm 3.96$$

Values of $\bar{\delta}$ greater than 3.96 or less than -3.96 will lead to the decision that the products differ at the 5% level. Having defined the values of $\bar{\delta}$ that will lead to rejection of H_0, we obtain the power for the alternative, H_a: $\Delta = 5$, by computing the probability that an average result, $\bar{\delta}$, will be less than 3.96, if H_a is true (i.e., $\Delta = 5$).

This concept is illustrated in Fig. 6.3. Curve B is the distribution with mean equal to 5 and σ = 7. If curve B is the true distribution, the probability of observing a value of $\bar{\delta}$ below 3.96 is the probability of accepting H_0 if the alternative hypothesis is true ($\Delta = 5$). This is the definition of β. This probability can be calculated using the Z transformation.

$$Z = \frac{3.96 - 5}{7/\sqrt{12}} = -0.51$$

Referring to Table IV.2, the area below +3.96 (Z = -0.51) for curve B is approximately 0.31. The power is $1 - \beta = 1 - 0.31 =$ 0.69. The use of 12 subjects results in a power of 0.69 to "detect" a difference of +5 compared to the 0.95 power to detect such a difference when 26 subjects were used. A power of *0.69* means that if the *true difference were 5 mmHg*, the statistical test will result in *significance with a probability of 69%*; 31% of the time, such a test will result in acceptance of H_0.

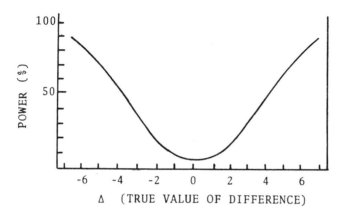

Figure 6.4   Power curve for N = 12, α = 0.05, σ = 7, and H_0: Δ = 0.

A *power curve* is a plot of the power, $1 - \beta$, versus alternative values of Δ. Power curves can be constructed by computing β for several alternatives and drawing a smooth curve through these points. For a two-sided test, the power curve is symmetrical around the hypothetical mean, Δ = 0, in our example. The power is equal to α when the alternative is equal to the hypothetical mean under H_0. Thus the power is 0.05 when Δ = H_0 (Fig. 6.4) in the power curve. The power curve for the present example is shown in Fig. 6.4.

The following conclusions may be drawn concerning the *power* of a test if α is kept constant:

1. The larger the sample size, the larger the power.
2. The larger the difference to be detected (H_a), the larger the power. A large sample size will be needed in order to have strong power to detect a small difference.
3. The larger the variability (s.d.), the weaker the power.
4. If α is increased, power is increased (β is decreased) (see Fig. 6.3). An increase in α (e.g., 10%) results in a smaller Z. The cutoff points are shorter, and the area of curve B below the cutoff point is smaller.

Power is a function of N, Δ, σ, and α.

A simple way to compute the approximate power of a test is to use the formula for sample size [Eqs. (6.4) and (6.5), for example] and solve for Z_β. In the previous example, a single sample or a paired test, Eq. (6.4) is appropriate:

$$N = \left(\frac{\sigma}{\Delta}\right)^2 (Z_\alpha + Z_\beta)^2 \qquad (6.4)$$

$$Z_\beta = \frac{\Delta}{\sigma} \sqrt{N} - Z_\alpha \qquad (6.10)$$

Once having calculated Z_β, the probability determined directly from Table IV.2 is equal to the power, $1 - \beta$. See the discussion and examples below.

In the problem discussed above, applying Eq. (6.10) with $\Delta = 5$, $\sigma = 7$, $N = 12$, and $Z_\alpha = 1.96$:

$$Z_\beta = \frac{5}{7} \sqrt{12} - 1.96 = 0.51$$

According to the notation used for Z (see Table 6.2), β is the area above Z_β. Power is the area below Z_β (power = $1 - \beta$). In Table IV.2, the area above $Z = 0.51$ is approximately 31%. The power is $1 - \beta$. Therefore, the power is 69%.*

If N is small and the variance is unknown, appropriate values of t should be used in place of Z_α and Z_β. Alternatively, we can adjust N by subtracting $0.5Z_\alpha^2$ or $0.25Z_\alpha^2$ from the actual sample size for a one- or two-sample test, respectively. The following examples should make the calculations clearer.

Example 7: A bioavailability study has been completed in which the ratio of the AUCs for two comparative drugs was submitted as evidence of bioequivalence. The FDA asked for the power of the test as part of their review of the submission. The null hypothesis for the comparison is H_0: $R = 1$, where R is the true average ratio. The test was two-sided with α equal to 5%. Eighteen subjects took each of the two comparative drugs in a paired-sample design. The standard deviation was calculated from the final results of the study, and was equal to 0.3. The power is to be determined for a difference of 20% for the comparison. This means that if the test product is truly more than 20% greater or smaller

---

*The value corresponding to Z in Table IV.2 gives the power directly. In this example, the area in the table corresponding to a Z of 0.51 is approximately 0.69.

than the reference product, we wish to calculate the probability
that the ratio will be judged to be significantly different from 1.0.
The value of Δ to be used in Eq. (6.10) is 0.2.

$$Z_\beta = \frac{0.2\sqrt{16}}{0.3} - 1.96 = 0.707$$

Note that the value of N is taken as 16. This is the inverse of the
procedure for determining sample size, where $0.5Z_\alpha^2$ was added to
N. Here we subtract $0.5Z_\alpha^2$ (approximately 2) from N; $18 - 2 = 16$.
According to Table IV.2, the area corresponding to $Z = 0.707$ is
approximately 0.76. Therefore, the power of this test is 76%.
That is, if the true difference between the formulations is 20%, a
significant difference will be found between the formulations 76% of
the time. This is very close to the 80% power that is recommended
for bioavailability tests (where $\Delta = 0.2$).

Example 8: A drug product is prepared by two different methods. The average tablet weights of the two batches are to be compared, weighing 20 tablets from each batch. The average weights
of the two 20-tablet samples were 507 and 511 mg. The pooled
standard deviation was calculated to be 12 mg. The director of
quality control wishes to be "sure" that if the average weights
truly differ by 10 mg or more, the statistical test will show a significant difference. When he was asked, "How sure?", he said 95%
sure. This can be translated into a β of 5% or a power of 95%.
This is a *two-independent-groups* test. Solving for Z_β from Eq.
(6.5), we have

$$Z_\beta = \frac{\Delta}{\sigma} \sqrt{\frac{N}{2}} - Z_\alpha \qquad\qquad (6.11)$$

$$= \frac{10}{12} \sqrt{\frac{19}{2}} - 1.96 = 0.609$$

As discussed above, the value of N is taken as 19 rather than 20,
by subtracting $0.25Z_\alpha^2$ from N for the two-sample case. Referring
to Table IV.2, we note that the power is approximately 73%. The
experiment does not have sufficient power according to the director's standards. To obtain the desired power, we can increase
the sample size (i.e., weigh more tablets). (See Exercise Problem 10.)

KEY TERMS

Alpha level

Attribute

Beta error

Confidence interval

Delta

Power

Power curve

"Practical" significance

Sample size

Sampling plan

Sensitivity

Z transformation

EXERCISES

1. Two diets are to be compared with regard to weight gain of weanling rats. If the weight gains due to the diets differ by 10 g or more, we would like to be 80% sure that we obtain a significant result. How many rats should be in each group if the s.d. is estimated to be 5 and the test is performed at the 5% level?

2. How many rats per group would you use if the standard deviation were known to be equal to 5 in Problem 1?

3. In Example 3 where two antibiotics are being compared, how many patients would be needed for a study with $\alpha = 0.05$, $\beta = 0.10$, using a parallel design, and assuming that the new product must have a cure rate of 90% to be acceptable as a better product than the standard? (Cure rate for standard = 80%.)

4. It is hypothesized that the difference between two drugs with regard to success rate is 0 (i.e., the drugs are not different). What size sample is needed to show a difference of 20% significant at the 5% level with a β error of 10%? (Assume that the response rate is about 50% for both drugs, a *conservative* estimate.) The study is a two-independent-samples design (parallel groups).

5. How many observations would be needed to estimate a response rate of about 50% within ±15% (95% confidence limits)? How many observations would be needed to estimate a response rate of 20 ± 15%?

6. Your boss tells you to make a new tablet formulation which should have a dissolution time (90% dissolution) of 30 min. The previous formulation took 40 min to 90% dissolution. She tells you that she wants an α level of 5% and that if the new formulation really has a dissolution time of 30 min or less, she wants to be 99% sure that the statistical comparison will show significance. (This means that the β error is 1%.) The s.d. is approximately 10. What size sample would you use to test the new formulation?

7. In a clinical study comparing the effect of two drugs on blood pressure, 20 patients were to be tested on each drug (two groups). The change in blood pressure from baseline measurements was to be determined. The s.d., measured as the difference among individuals' responses, is *estimated* from past experience to be 5.

   (a) If the statistical test is done at the 5% level, what is the power of the test against an alternative of 3 mmHg difference between the drugs (H_0: $\mu_1 = \mu_2$ or $\mu_1 - \mu_2 = 0$). This means: What is the probability that the test will show significance if the true difference between the drugs is 3 mmHg or more (H_a: $\mu_1 - \mu_2 = 3$)?

   (b) What is the power if there are 50 people per group? α is 5%.

8. A tablet is produced with a labeled potency of 100 mg. The standard deviation is known to be 10. What size sample should be assayed if we want to have 90% power to detect a difference of 3 mg from the target? The test is done at the 5% level.

9. In a bioequivalence study, the ratio of AUCs are to be compared. A sample size of 12 subjects is used in a paired design. The standard deviation resulting from the statistical test is 0.25. What is the power of this test against a 20% difference if α is equal to 0.05?

10. How many samples would be needed to have 95% power for Example 8?

11. In a bioequivalence study, the maximum blood level is to be compared for two drugs. This is a crossover study (paired design) where each subject takes both drugs. Eighteen subjects entered the study with the following results. The observed difference is 10 $\mu g/ml$. The s.d. (from this experiment) is 40. A practical difference is considered to be 15 $\mu g/ml$. What is the power of the test for a 15-$\mu g/ml$ difference for a two-sided test at the 5% level?

12. How many observations would you need to estimate a proportion within ±5% (95% confidence interval) if the expected proportion is 10%?

13. A parallel design is used to measure the effectiveness of a new antihypertensive drug. One group of patients receives the drug and the other group receives placebo. A difference of 6 mmHg is considered to be of practical significance. The standard deviation (difference from baseline) is unknown but is estimated as 5 based on some preliminary data. Alpha is set at 5% and β at 10%. How many patients should be used in each group?

14. From Table 6.3, find the number of samples needed to determine the difference between the dissolution of two formulations for

$\alpha = 0.05$, $\beta = 0.10$, $S = 25$, for a "practical" difference of 25 (minutes).

REFERENCES

1. *United States Pharmacopeia*, 20th rev., and *National Formulary*, 15th ed., USP Pharmacopeial Convention, Inc., Rockville, Md., 1980.
2. MIL-STD-105D, Military Sampling Procedures and Tables for Inspection by Attributes, U.S. Government Printing Office, Washington, D.C.
3. Guenther, W. C., Sample Size Formulas for Normal Theory Tests, *Am. Stat.*, *35*, 243, 1981.
4. Dixon, W. J. and Massey, F. J., Jr., *Introduction to Statistical Analysis*, 3rd ed., McGraw-Hill, New York, 1969.
5. Fleiss, J., *Statistical Methods for Rates and Proportions*, 2nd ed., Wiley, New York, 1981.

7
Linear Regression and Correlation

Simple linear regression analysis is a statistical technique that defines the functional relationship between two variables, X and Y, by the "best-fitting" straight line. A straight line is described by the equation, $Y = A + BX$, *where Y is the dependent variable* (ordinate), *X is the independent variable* (abscissa), and *A and B* are the *Y intercept* and *slope of the line*, respectively (see Fig. 7.1).* Applications of regression analysis in pharmaceutical experimentation are numerous. This procedure is commonly used:

1. To describe the relationship between variables where the functional relationship is known to be linear, such as in Beer's law plots, where optical density is plotted against drug concentration

2. When the functional form of a response is unknown, but where we wish to represent a trend or rate as characterized by the slope (e.g., as may occur when following a pharmacological response over time)

3. When we wish to describe a process by a relatively simple equation that will relate the response, Y, to a fixed value of X, such as in stability prediction (concentration of drug versus time).

In addition to the specific applications noted above, regression analysis is used to define and characterize dose-response relationships, for fitting linear portions of pharmacokinetic data, and in obtaining the best fit to linear physical–chemical relationships.

---

*The notation $Y = A + BX$ is standard in statistics. We apologize for any confusion that may result from the reader's familiarity with the equivalent, $Y = mX + b$, used frequently in analytical geometry.

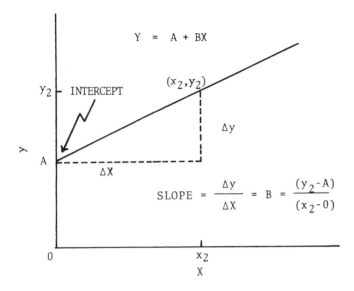

Figure 7.1 Straight-line plot.

Correlation is a procedure commonly used to characterize quantitatively the relationship between variables. Correlation is related to linear regression, but its application and interpretation are different. This topic is introduced at the end of this chapter.

7.1 INTRODUCTION

Straight lines are constructed from sets of data pairs, X and Y. Two such pairs (i.e., two points) uniquely define a straight line. As noted previously, a straight line is defined by the equation

$$Y = A + BX \tag{7.1}$$

where A is the Y intercept (the value of Y when X = 0) and B is the slope ($\Delta Y / \Delta X$). $\Delta Y / \Delta X$ is $(Y_2 - Y_1)/(X_2 - X_1)$ for any two points on the line (see Fig. 7.1). The slope and intercept define the line; once A and B are given, the line is specified. In the elementary example of only two points, a statistical approach to define the line is clearly unnecessary.

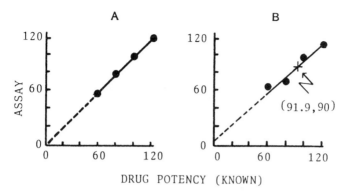

Figure 7.2   Plot of assay recovery versus known amount: theoretical and actual data.

In general, with more than two X, y points,* a plot of y versus X will not *exactly* describe a straight line, even when the relationship is known to be linear.   The failure of experimental data derived from truly linear relationships to lie exactly on a straight line is due to errors of observation (experimental variability).   Figure 7.2 shows the results of four assays of drug samples of different, but known potency.   The assay results are plotted against the known amount of drug.   If the assays are performed without error, the plot results in a 45° line (slope = 1) which, if extended, passes through the origin; that is, the Y intercept, A, is 0 (Fig. 7.2A). In this example, the equation of the line $Y = A + BX$ is $Y = 0 + 1(X)$, or $Y = X$.   Since there is no error in this experiment, the line passes exactly through the four X, Y points.

Real experiments are not error free, and a plot of X, y data rarely exactly fits a straight line, as shown in Fig. 7.2B).   We will examine the problem of obtaining a line to fit data that are not error free.   In these cases, the line does not go exactly through all of the points.   A "good" line, however, should come "close" to the experimental points.   When the variability is small, a line drawn by eye will probably be very close to that constructed more exactly by

---

*In the rest of this chapter, y denotes the experimentally observed point, and Y denotes the corresponding point on the least squares "fitted" line (or the true value of Y, according to context).

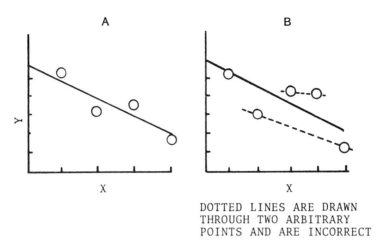

DOTTED LINES ARE DRAWN
THROUGH TWO ARBITRARY
POINTS AND ARE INCORRECT

Figure 7.3   Fit of line with variable data.

a statistical approach (Fig. 7.3A). With large variability, the "best" line is not obvious. What single line would you draw to best fit the data plotted in Fig. 7.3B? Certainly, lines drawn through any two arbitrarily selected points will not give the best (or a unique) line to fit the totality of data.

Given N pairs of variables, X, y, we can define the best straight line describing the relationship of X and y as that line which minimizes the sum of squares of the vertical distances of each point from the fitted line. The definition of "sum of squares of the vertical distances of each point from the fitted line" (see Fig. 7.4) is written mathematically as $\Sigma (y - Y)^2$, where y represents the experimental points and Y represents the corresponding points on the fitted line. The line constructed according to this definition is called the *least squares* line. Applying techniques of calculus, the slope and intercept of the least squares line can be calculated from the sample data as follows:

$$\text{Slope} = b = \frac{\Sigma (X - \overline{X})(y - \overline{y})}{\Sigma (X - \overline{X})^2} \qquad (7.2)$$

$$\text{Intercept} = a = \overline{y} - b\overline{X} \qquad (7.3)$$

Remember that the slope and intercept uniquely define the line.

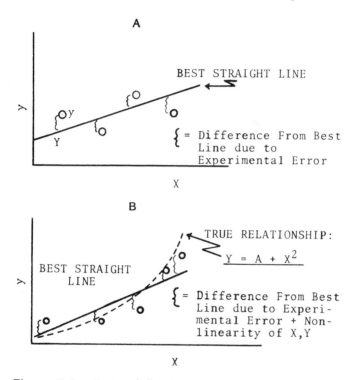

Figure 7.4   Lack of fit due to (A) experimental error and (B) non-linearity.

Remember that the slope and intercept uniquely define the line.

There is a shortcut computing formula for the slope, similar to that described previously for the standard deviation:

$$b = \frac{N \sum Xy - (\sum X)(\sum y)}{N \sum X^2 - (\sum X)^2} \qquad (7.4)$$

where N is the number of X, y pairs. The calculation of the slope and intercept is relatively simple, and can usually be quickly computed with a hand calculator. Some calculators have a built-in program for calculating the regression parameter estimates, a and b.*

---

*a and b are the sample estimates of the true parameters, A and B.

Table 7.1 Raw Data from Fig. 7.2A to Calculate the Least Squares Line

Drug potency, X	Assay, y	Xy
60	60	3,600
80	80	6,400
100	100	10,000
120	120	14,400
Σ X = 360	Σ y = 360	Σ Xy = 34,400
Σ X^2 = 34,400		

For the example shown in Fig. 7.2A, the line that exactly passes through the four data points has a slope of 1 and an intercept of 0. The line, Y = X, is clearly the best line for these data, an exact fit. The least squares line, in this case, is exactly the same line, Y = X. The calculation of the intercept and slope using the least squares formulas, Eqs. (7.3) and (7.4), is illustrated below. Table 7.1 shows the raw data used to construct the line in Fig. 7.2A.

According to Eq. (7.4) (N = 4, Σ X^2 = 34,400, Σ Xy = 34,400, Σ X = Σ y = 360),

$$b = \frac{(4)(3600 + 6400 + 10,000 + 14,400) - (360)(360)}{4(34,400) - (360)^2} = 1$$

a is computed from Eq. (7.3); a = $\overline{y} - b\overline{X}$ ($\overline{y} = \overline{X} = 90$, b = 1). a = 90 − 1(90) = 0. This represents a situation where the assay results exactly equal the known drug potency (i.e., there is no error).

The actual experimental data depicted in Fig. 7.2B are shown in Table 7.2. The slope b and the intercept a are calculated from Eqs. (7.4) and (7.3). According to Eq. (7.4),

$$b = \frac{4(33,600) - (360)(353)}{4(34,400) - (360)^2} = 0.915$$

According to Eq. (7.3),

$$a = \frac{353}{4} - 0.915(90) = 5.9$$

Table 7.2 Raw Data from Fig. 7.2B Used to Calculate the Least Squares Line

Drug potency, X	Assay, y	Xy
60	63	3,780
80	75	6,000
100	99	9,900
120	116	13,920
Σ X = 360	Σ y = 353	Σ Xy = 33,600
Σ X^2 = 34,400	Σ y^2 = 32,851	

A perfect assay (no error) has a slope of 1 and an intercept of 0, as shown above. The actual data exhibit a slope close to 1, but the intercept appears to be too far from 0 to be attributed to random error. Exercise Problem 2 addresses the interpretation of these results as they relate to assay method characteristics.

This example suggests several questions and problems regarding linear regression analysis. The line that best fits the experimental data is an estimate of some true relationship between X and Y. In most circumstances, we will fit a straight line to such data only if we believe that the true relationship between X and Y is linear. The experimental observations will not fall exactly on a straight line because of variability (e.g., error associated with the assay). This situation (true linearity associated with experimental error) is different from the case where the underlying true relationship between X and Y is not linear. In the latter case, the lack of fit of the data to the least squares line is due to a combination of experimental error and the lack of linearity of the X, Y relationship (see Fig. 7.4). Elementary techniques of simple linear regression will not differentiate these two situations: (a) experimental error with true linearity and (b) experimental error and nonlinearity. (A design to estimate variability due to both nonlinearity and experimental error is given in App. II.)

We will discuss some examples relevant to pharmaceutical research which make use of least squares linear regression procedures. The discussion will demonstrate how variability is estimated and used to construct estimates and tests of the line parameters A and B.

7.2 ANALYSIS OF STANDARD CURVES IN DRUG ANALYSIS: APPLICATION OF LINEAR REGRESSION

The assay data discussed previously can be considered as an example of the construction of a *standard curve* in drug analysis. Known amounts of drug are subjected to an assay procedure, and a plot of percentage recovered (or amount recovered) versus amount added is constructed. Theoretically, the relationship is usually a straight line. A knowledge of the line parameters A and B can be used to predict the amount of drug in an unknown sample based on the assay results. In most practical situations, A and B are unknown. The least squares estimates a and b of these parameters are used to compute drug potency (X) based on the assay response (y). For example, the least squares line for the data in Fig. 7.2B and Table 7.2 is

$$Assay \; result \; = \; 5.9 = 0.915 \; (potency) \qquad (7.5)$$

Rearranging Eq. (7.5), an unknown sample which has an assay value of 90 can be predicted to have a true potency of

$$Potency \; = \; X \; = \; \frac{y - 5.9}{0.915}$$

$$Potency \; = \; \frac{90 - 5.9}{0.915} \; = \; 91.9$$

This point (91.9, 90) is indicated in Fig. 7.2B by a cross.

7.2.1 Line Through the Origin

Many calibration curves (lines) are known to pass through the origin; that is, the assay response must be zero if the concentration of drug is zero. The calculation of the slope is simplified if the line is forced to go through the point (0, 0). In our example, if the intercept is *known* to be zero, the slope is (see also Table 7.2)

$$b \; = \; \frac{\Sigma \; Xy}{\Sigma \; X^2} \qquad (7.6)$$

$$= \; \frac{33,600}{60^2 + 80^2 + 100^2 + 120^2} \; = \; 0.977$$

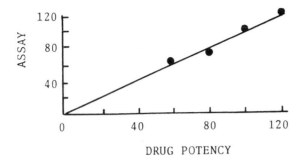

Figure 7.5   Plot of data in Table 7.2 with known (0,0) intercept.

The least squares line fitted with the zero intercept is shown in Fig. 7.5. If this line were to be used to predict actual concentrations based on assay results, we would obtain answers which are different from those predicted from the line drawn in Fig. 7.2B. However, both lines have been constructed from the same raw data. "Is one of the lines correct?", or "Is one line better than the other?" Although one cannot say with certainty which is the better line, a thorough knowledge of the analytical method will be important in making a choice. For example, a nonzero intercept suggests either non-linearity over the range of assays or the presence of an interfering substance in the sample being analyzed. The decision of which line to use can also be made on a statistical basis. A statistical test of the intercept can be performed under the null hypothesis that the intercept is 0 (H_0: A = 0, Sec. 7.4.1). Rejection of the hypothesis would be strong evidence that the line with the positive intercept best represents the data.

7.3 ASSUMPTIONS IN TESTS OF HYPOTHESES IN LINEAR REGRESSION

Although there are no prerequisites for fitting a least squares line, the testing of statistical hypotheses in linear regression depends on the validity of several assumptions.

1.   *The X variable is measured without error.* Although not always *exactly* true, X is often measured with *relatively* little error and, under these conditions this assumption can be considered to be satisfied. In the present example, X is the potency of drug in the "known" sample. If the drug is weighed on a

sensitive balance, the error in drug potency will be very small. Another example of an X variable that is often used, which can be precisely and accurately measured, is "time."

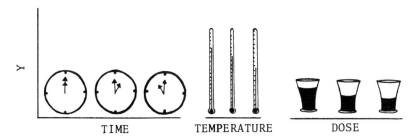

Examples of variables measured with no (or little error).

2. *For each X, y is independent and normally distributed.* We will often use the notation Y.x to show that the value of Y is a function of X.
3. *The variance of y is assumed to be the same at each X.* If the variance of y is not constant, but is either known or related to X in some way, other methods [see Sec. 7.7] are available to estimate the intercept and slope of the line [1].
4. *A linear relationship exists between X and Y.* Y = A + BX, where A and B are the true parameters. Based on theory or experience, we have reason to believe that X and Y are linearly related.

These assumptions are depicted in Fig. 7.6. Except for location (mean), the distribution of y is the same at every value of X; that

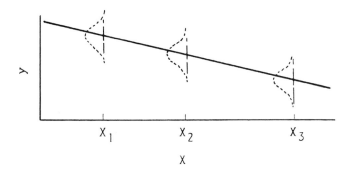

Figure 7.6 Normality and variance assumptions in linear regression.

is, y has the same variance at every value of X. In the example in Fig. 7.6, the mean of the distribution of y's decreases as X increases (the slope is negative).

7.4 ESTIMATE OF THE VARIANCE: VARIANCE OF SAMPLE ESTIMATES OF THE PARAMETERS

If the assumptions noted in Sec. 7.3 hold, the distributions of *sample estimates* of the slope and intercept, b and a, are normal with means equal to B and A, respectively.* Because of this important result, statistical tests of the parameters A and B can be performed using normal distribution theory. Also, one can show that the sample estimates are unbiased estimates of the true parameters (similar to the sample average, $\overline{X}$, being an unbiased estimate of the true mean, μ). The variances of the estimates, a and b, are calculated as follows:

$$\sigma_a^2 = \sigma_{Y.x}^2 \left[\frac{1}{N} + \frac{\overline{X}^2}{\Sigma (X - \overline{X})^2} \right] \tag{7.7}$$

$$\sigma_b^2 = \frac{\sigma_{Y.x}^2}{\Sigma (X - \overline{X})^2} \tag{7.8}$$

$\sigma_{Y.x}^2$ is the variance of the response variable, y. An estimate of $\sigma_{Y.x}^2$ can be obtained from the closeness of the data to the least squares line. If the experimental points are far from the least squares line, the estimated variability is larger than that in the case where the experimental points are close to the least squares line. This concept is illustrated in Fig. 7.7. If the data exactly fit a straight line, the experiment shows no variability. In real experiments the chance of an exact fit with more than two X, Y pairs is very small. An unbiased estimate of $\sigma_{Y.x}^2$ is obtained from the sum of squares of deviations of the observed points from the fitted line as follows:

---

*a and b are calculated as linear combinations of the normally distributed response variable, y, and thus can be shown to be also normally distributed.

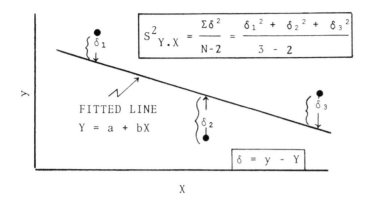

Figure 7.7 Variance calculation from least squares line.

$$S_{Y.x}^2 = \frac{\Sigma (y - Y)^2}{N - 2} = \frac{\Sigma (y - \bar{y})^2 - b^2[\Sigma (X - \bar{X})^2]}{N - 2} \qquad (7.9)$$

where y is the observed value and Y is the predicted value of Y from the least squares line (Y = a + bX) (see Fig. 7.7). The variance estimate, $S_{Y.x}^2$, has N − 2 rather than (N − 1) d.f. because two parameters are being estimated from the data (i.e., the slope and intercept).

When $\sigma_{Y.x}^2$ is unknown, the variances of a and b can be estimated substituting $S_{Y.x}^2$ for $\sigma_{Y.x}^2$ in the formulas for the variances [Eqs. (7.7) and (7.8)]. Equations (7.10) and (7.11) are used as the variance estimates, S_a^2 and S_b^2, when testing hypotheses concerning the parameters A and B. This procedure is analogous to using the sample estimate of the variance in the t test to compare sample means.

$$S_a^2 = S_{Y.x}^2 \left[\frac{1}{N} + \frac{\bar{X}^2}{\Sigma (X - \bar{X})^2} \right] \qquad (7.10)$$

$$S_b^2 = \frac{S_{Y.x}^2}{\Sigma (X - \bar{X})^2} \qquad (7.11)$$

7.4.1   Test of the Intercept, A

The background and formulas introduced previously are prerequisites
for the construction of tests of hypotheses of the regression parameters A and B. We can now address the question of the "significance"
of the Y intercept (a) for the line shown in Fig. 7.2B and Table 7.2.
The procedure is analogous to that of testing means with the t test.
In this example, the null hypothesis is H_0: A = 0. The alternative
hypothesis is H_a: A $\neq$ 0. Here the test is two-sided; a priori, if
the intercept is not equal to 0, it could be either positive or negative. A t test is performed as shown in Eq. (7.12). $S_{Y.x}^2$ and S_a^2
are calculated from Eqs. (7.9) and (7.10), respectively.

$$t_{d.f.} = t_2 = \frac{|a - A|}{\sqrt{S_a^2}} \tag{7.12}$$

where $t_{d.f.}$ is the t statistic with N $-$ 2 degrees of freedom, a is
the observed value of the intercept, and A is the hypothetical value
of the intercept. From Eq. (7.10)

$$S_a^2 = S_{Y.x}^2 \left[\frac{1}{N} + \frac{\overline{X}^2}{\Sigma (X - \overline{X})^2} \right] \tag{7.10}$$

From Eq. (7.9)

$$S_{Y.x}^2 = \frac{1.698.75 - (0.915)^2 (2000)}{2} = 12.15$$

$$S_a^2 = 12.15 \left[\frac{1}{4} + \frac{(90)^2}{2000} \right] = 52.245$$

From Eq. (7.12)

$$t_2 = \frac{|5.9 - 0|}{\sqrt{52.245}}$$

Note that this t test has two (N $-$ 2) degrees of freedom. This is a
weak test, and a large intercept must be observed to obtain statistical significance. To define the intercept more precisely, it
would be necessary to perform a larger number of assays. If there
is no reason to suspect a non-linear relationship between X and Y,

a nonzero intercept, in this example, could be interpreted as being due to some interfering substance(s) in the product (the "blank"). If the presence of a nonzero intercept is suspected, one would probably want to run a sufficient number of assays to establish its presence. A precise estimate of the intercept is necessary if this linear calibration curve is used to evaluate potency.

7.4.2 Test of the Slope, B

The test of the slope of the least squares line is usually of more interest than the test of the intercept. Sometimes, we may only wish to be assured that the fitted line has a slope other than zero. (A horizontal line has a slope of zero.) In our example, there seems to be little doubt that the slope is greater than zero (Fig. 7.2B). However, the magnitude of this slope has a special physical meaning. A slope of 1 indicates that the amount recovered (assay) is equal to the amount in the sample, after correction for the blank (i.e., subtract the Y intercept from the observed reading of y). An observation of a slope other than 1 indicates that the amount recovered is some constant percentage of the sample potency. Thus we may be interested in a test of the slope versus 1.

$$H_0: \quad B = 1 \qquad H_a: \quad B \neq 1$$

A t test is performed using the estimated variance of the slope, as follows:

$$t = \frac{b - B}{\sqrt{S_b^2}} \tag{7.13}$$

In the present example, from Eq. (7.11),

$$S_b^2 = \frac{S_{y \cdot x}^2}{\Sigma (X - \overline{X})^2} \tag{7.11}$$

$$= \frac{12.15}{2000} = 0.006075$$

Applying Eq. (7.13), for a two-sided test, we have

$$t = \frac{|0.915 - 1|}{\sqrt{0.006075}} = 1.09$$

This t test has two $(N - 2)$ degrees of freedom (the variance estimate has 2 d.f.). There is insufficient evidence to indicate that
the slope is significantly different from 1 at the 5% level. Table
IV.4 shows that a t of 4.30 is needed for significance at $\alpha = 0.05$
and d.f. = 2. The test in this example has very weak power. A
slope very different from 1 would be necessary to obtain statistical
significance. This example again emphasizes the weakness of the
statement "nonsignificant," particularly in small experiments such as
this one. The reader interested in learning more details of the use
and interpretation of regression in analytical methodology is encouraged to read Chap. 5 in Ref. 2.

7.5   A DRUG STABILITY STUDY: A SECOND
EXAMPLE OF THE APPLICATION OF
LINEAR REGRESSION

The measurement of the rate of drug decomposition is an important
problem in drug formulation studies. Because of the significance of
establishing an expiration date defining the shelf life of a pharmaceutical product, stability data are routinely subjected to statistical
analysis. Typically, the drug, alone and/or formulated, is stored
under varying conditions of temperature, humidity, light intensity,
and so on, and assayed for intact drug at specified time intervals.
The pharmaceutical scientist is assigned the responsibility of recom-
mending the expiration date based on scientifically derived stability
data. The physical conditions of the stability test (e.g., temperature, humidity), the duration of testing, assay schedules, as well
as the number of lots, bottles, and tablets that should be sampled
must be defined for stability studies. Careful definition and implementation of these conditions are important because the validity and
precision of the final recommended expiration date depends on how
the experiment is conducted.

The rate of decomposition can often be determined from plots of
potency (or log potency) versus storage time, where the relationship of potency and time is either known or assumed to be linear.
The current good manufacturing practices (CGMP) regulations [3]
state that statistical criteria, including sample size and test (i.e.,
observation or measurement) intervals for each attribute examined,
be used to assure statistically valid estimates of stability (211.166).
The expiration date should be "statistically valid" (211.137, 201.17,
211.62).

The mechanics of determining shelf life may be quite complex,
particularly if extreme conditions are used, such as those recommended for "accelerated" stability studies (e.g., high-temperature
and high-humidity conditions). In these circumstances, the

statistical techniques used to make predictions of shelf life at ambient conditions are quite advanced and beyond the scope of this
book [4]. Although extreme conditions are commonly used in stability testing in order to save time and obtain a tentative expiration
date, all products must eventually be tested for stability under the
recommended commercial storage conditions. The FDA has suggested
that at least three batches of product be tested to determine an expiration date. One should understand that different batches may
show somewhat different stability characteristics, particularly in situations where additives affect stability to a significant extent. In
these cases variation in the quality and quantity of the additives
(excipients) between batches could affect stability. One of the purposes of using several batches for stability testing is to ensure that
stability characteristics are similar from batch to batch.

The time intervals chosen for the assay of storage samples will
depend to a great extent on the product characteristics and the
anticipated stability. A "statistically" optimal design for a stability
study would take into account the planned "storage" times when the
drug product will be assayed. This problem has been addressed in
the pharmaceutical literature [5]. However, the designs resulting
from such considerations are usually cumbersome or impractical. For
example, from a statistical point of view, the slope of the potency
versus time plot (the rate of decomposition) is obtained most precisely if half of the total assay points are performed at time 0, and
the other half at the final testing time. Note that $\Sigma (X - \bar{X})^2$, the
denominator of the expression defining the variance of a slope [Eq.
(7.8)], is maximized under this condition, resulting in a minimum
variability of the slope. This "optimal" approach to designating assay sampling times is based on the assumption that the plot is linear
during the time interval of the test. In a practical situation, one
would want to see data at points between the initial and final assay
in order to assess the magnitude of the decomposition as the stability
study proceeds, as well as to verify the linearity of the decomposition. Also, management and regulatory requirements are better satisfied with multiple points during the course of the study. A reasonable schedule of assays at ambient conditions is 0, 3, 6, 9, 12,
18, and 24 months and at yearly intervals thereafter [6].

The example of the data analysis which will be presented here
will be for a single batch. If the stability of different batches is
not different, the techniques described here may be applied to data
from more than one batch. In general, a statistician should be consulted for the analysis of multibatch data which will require analysis
of variance techniques [6,7].

Consider an example of a tablet formulation which is the subject
of a stability study. Three randomly chosen tablets are assayed
at each of six time periods: 0, 3, 6, 9, 12, and 18 months after

Table 7.3   Tablet Assays from the
Stability Study

Time, X (months)	Assay,[a] y (mg)	Average
0	51, 51, 53	51.7
3	51, 50, 52	51.0
6	50, 52, 48	50.0
9	49, 51, 51	50.3
12	49, 48, 47	48.0
18	47, 45, 49	47.0

[a]Each assay represents a different
tablet.

production, at ambient storage conditions.   The data are shown in
Table 7.3 and Fig. 7.8.

Given these data, the problem is to establish an expiration date
defined as that time when a tablet contains 90% of the labeled drug
potency.   The product in this example has a label of 50 mg potency
and is prepared with a 4% overage (i.e., the product is manufactured
with a target weight of 52 mg of drug).

Figure 7.8 shows that the data are variable.   A careful examination of this plot suggests that a straight line would be a

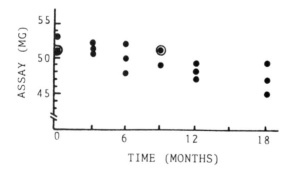

Figure 7.8   Pilot of stability data from Table 7.3.

reasonable representation of these data. The application of least squares line fitting is best justified in situations where a theoretical model exists showing that the decrease in concentration is linear with time (a zero-order process in this example). The kinetics of drug loss in solid dosage forms is complex and a theoretical model is not easily derived. In the present case, we will assume that concentration and time are truly linearly related:

$$C = C_0 - Kt \qquad\qquad (7.14)$$

where

C = concentration at time t

C_0 = concentration at time 0 (Y intercept, A)

K = rate constant ($-$slope, $-B$)

t = time (storage time)

With the objective of estimating the shelf life, the simplest approach to the analysis of these data is to estimate the slope and intercept of the least squares line, using Eqs. (7.4) and (7.3). (An interesting exercise would be to first try and estimate the slope and intercept by eye from Fig. 7.8.) When performing the least squares calculation, note that each value of the time (X) is associated with three values of drug potency (y). When calculating C_0 and K, each "time" value is counted three times and N is equal to 18. From Table 7.3,

$$\Sigma\ X = 144 \qquad\qquad \Sigma\ y = 894 \qquad\qquad \Sigma\ Xy = 6984$$

$$\Sigma\ X^2 = 1782 \qquad\qquad \Sigma\ y^2 = 44,476 \qquad\qquad N = 18$$

$$\overline{X} = 8 \qquad\qquad \Sigma\ (X - \overline{X})^2 = 630 \qquad\qquad \Sigma\ (y - \overline{y})^2 = 74$$

From Eqs. (7.4) and (7.3), we have

$$b = \frac{N\ \Sigma\ Xy - \Sigma\ X\ \Sigma\ y}{N\ \Sigma\ X^2 - (\Sigma\ X)^2} \qquad\qquad (7.4)$$

$$= \frac{18(6984) - 144(894)}{18(1782) - (144)^2} = \frac{-3024}{11,340} = 0.267 \text{ mg/month}$$

$$a = \overline{y} - b\overline{X} \qquad\qquad (7.3)$$

$$= \frac{894}{18} - (-0.267)\ \frac{144}{18} = 51.80$$

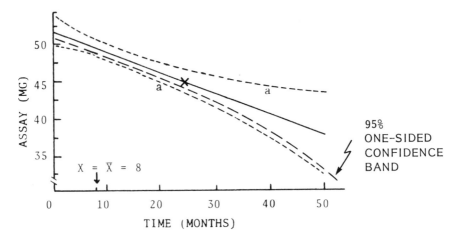

Figure 7.9   95% confidence band for "stability" line.

The equation of the straight line best fitting the data in Fig. 7.8 is

$$C = 51.8 - 0.267t \qquad\qquad (7.15)$$

The variance estimate, $S_{Y.x}^2$, represents the variability of tablet potency at a fixed time, and is calculated from Eq. (7.9):

$$S_{Y.x}^2 = \frac{\Sigma\, y^2 - (\Sigma\, y)^2/N - b^2\, \Sigma\, (X - \overline{X})^2}{N - 2}$$

$$= \frac{44,476 - (894)^2/18 - (-0.267)^2(630)}{18 - 2} = 1.825$$

To calculate the time at which the tablet potency is 90% of the labeled amount, 45 mg, solve Eq. (7.15) for t when C equals 45 mg.

$$45 = 51.80 - 0.267t$$

$$t = 25.5 \text{ months}$$

The best estimate of the time needed for these tablets to retain 45 mg of drug is 25.5 months (see the point marked with a cross in Fig. 7.9). This is an average result based on the data from 18 tablets. For any single tablet, the time for decomposition to 90% of the labeled amount will vary, depending, for example, on the amount of drug present at time zero. Nevertheless, the shelf-life estimate is based on the average result.

7.6 CONFIDENCE INTERVALS IN REGRESSION ANALYSIS

A more detailed analysis of the stability data is warranted if one understands that 25.5 months is not the true shelf life, but only an estimate of the true value. A confidence interval for the estimate of time to 45 mg potency would give a range that probably includes the true value. The concept of a confidence interval in regression is similar to that previously discussed for means. Thus the interval for the shelf life probably contains the true shelf life — that time when the tablets retain 90% of their labeled potency, on the average. The lower end of this confidence interval would be considered a conservative estimate of the true shelf life. Before giving the solution to this problem we will address the calculation of a confidence interval for Y (potency) at a given X (time). The width of the confidence interval for Y (potency) is not constant, but depends on the value of X, since Y is a function of X. In the present example, one might wish to obtain a range for the potency at 25.5 months' storage time.

Confidence Interval for Y at a Given X

We will construct a confidence interval for the true mean potency (Y) at a given time (X). The confidence interval can be shown to be equal to

$$ Y \pm t(S_{Y.x}) \sqrt{\frac{1}{N} + \frac{(X - \overline{X})^2}{\Sigma (X - \overline{X})^2}} \qquad (7.16) $$

t is the appropriate value (N − 2 degrees of freedom, Table IV.4) for a confidence interval with confidence coefficient P. For example, for a 95% confidence interval, use t values in the column headed 0.975 in Table IV.4.

In the linear regression model, y is assumed to have a normal distribution with variance $\sigma^2_{Y.x}$ at each X. As can be seen from Eq. (7.16), confidence limits for Y at a specified value of X depend on the *variance, degrees of freedom, number of data points* used to fit the line, and $X - \overline{X}$ the *distance of the specified X* (time, in this example) *from* $\overline{X}$, the average time used in the least squares line fitting. The confidence interval is smallest for the Y that corresponds to the value of X equal to $\overline{X}$ [the term, $X - \overline{X}$, in Eq. (7.16) will be zero]. As the value of X is farther from $\overline{X}$, the confidence interval for Y corresponding to the specified X is wider. Thus the estimate of Y is less precise, as the X corresponding to Y is farther away from $\overline{X}$. A plot of the confidence interval for every Y on the line results in a continuous confidence "band" as shown in Fig. 7.9. The curved, hyperbolic shape of the confidence band illustrates the varying width of the confidence interval at different values of X, Y. For example, the 95% confidence interval for Y at X = 25.5 months [Eq. (7.16)] is

$$45 \pm 2.12(1.35) \sqrt{\frac{1}{18} + \frac{(25.5 - 8)^2}{630}} = 45 \pm 2.1$$

Thus the result shows that the true value of the potency at 25.5 months is probably between 42.9 and 47.1 mg (45 ± 2.1).

A Confidence Interval for X at a Given
Value of Y

Although the interval for the potency may be of interest, as noted above, this confidence interval does not directly answer the question about the possible variability of the shelf-life estimate. A careful examination of the two-sided confidence band for the line (Fig. 7.9) shows that 90% potency (45 mg) may occur between approximately 20 and 40 months, the points marked "a" in Fig. 7.9. To obtain this range for X (time to 90% potency), using the approach of graphical estimation as described above requires the computation of the confidence band for a sufficient range of X. Also, the graphical estimate is relatively inaccurate. The confidence interval for the true X at a given Y can be directly calculated, although the formula is more complex than that used for the Y confidence interval [Eq. (7.16)].

This procedure of estimating X for a given value of Y is often called "inverse prediction." The complexity results from the fact that the solution for X, $X = (Y - a)/b$, is a quotient of variables. $(Y - a)$ and b are random variables; both have error associated with their measurement. The ratio has a more complicated distribution than a linear combination of variables such as is the case for $Y = a + bX$. The calculation of the confidence interval for the true X at a specified value of Y is

$$\frac{(X - g\overline{X}) \pm [t(S_{Y.x})/b]\left[\sqrt{(1 - g)/N + (X - \overline{X})^2/\Sigma(X - \overline{X})^2}\right]}{1 - g}$$

$$(7.17)$$

where

$$g = \frac{t^2(S_{Y.x}^2)}{b^2 \, \Sigma \, (X - \overline{X})^2}$$

t is the appropriate value for a confidence interval with confidence coefficient equal to P; for example, for a two-sided 95% confidence interval, use values of t in the column headed 0.975 in Table IV.4.

A 95% confidence interval for X will be calculated for the time to 90% of labeled potency. The potency is 45 mg (Y) when 10% of the labeled amount decomposes. The corresponding time (X) has been calculated above as 25.5 months. For a two-sided confidence interval, applying Eq. (7.17), we have

$$g = \frac{(2.12)^2(1.825)}{(-0.267)^2(630)} = 0.183$$

$$X = 25.5 \qquad \overline{X} = 8 \qquad N = 18$$

The confidence interval is

$$\frac{[25.5 - 0.183(8)] \pm [2.12(1.35)/(-0.267)] \left[\sqrt{0.817/18 + (17.5)^2/630} \, \right]}{0.817}$$

$$= \quad 19.8 \text{ to } 39.0 \text{ months}$$

Thus, using a two-sided confidence interval, the true time to 90% of labeled potency is probably between 19.8 and 39.0 months. A conservative estimate of the shelf life would be the lower value, 19.8 months.

The Food and Drug Administration has suggested that a one-sided confidence interval may be more appropriate than a two-sided interval to estimate the expiration date. For most drug products, drug potency can only decrease with time, and only the lower confidence band of the potency vs. time curve may be considered relevant. (An exception may occur in the case of liquid products where evaporation of the solvent could result in an increased potency with time.) The 95% one-sided confidence limits for the time to reach a potency of 45 is computed using Eq. (7.17). Only the lower limit is computed using the appropriate t value that cuts off 5% of the area in a single tail. For 16 d.f., this value is 1.75 (Table IV.4). The calculation is

$$\frac{[25.5 - 0.183(8)] + [1.75(1.35)/(-0.267)][\sqrt{0.817/18 + (17.5)^2/630]}}{0.817}$$

$$= \ 21.5 \ \text{months}$$

The one-sided 95% interval for X can be interpreted to mean that the time to decompose to a potency of 45 is probably greater than 21.5 months. Note that the shelf life based on the one-sided interval is longer than that based on a two-sided interval (see Fig. 7.9).

Prediction Intervals

The confidence limits for Y and X discussed above are limits for the *true values*, having specified a value of Y (potency or concentration, for example) corresponding to some value of X, or an X (time, for example) corresponding to a specified value of Y. An important application of confidence intervals in regression is to obtain confidence intervals for *actual future measurements* based on the least squares line.

1. We may wish to obtain a confidence interval for a value of Y to be actually measured at some value of X (some future time, for example).
2. In the example of the calibration (Sec. 7.2), having observed a new value, y, after the calibration line has been established, we would want to use the information from the fitted calibration line to predict the concentration, or potency, X, and establish the confidence limits for the concentration at this newly observed value of y. This is an example of inverse prediction.

For the example of the stability study, we may wish to obtain a confidence interval for an actual assay (y) to be performed at some given future time, after having performed the experiment used to fit the least squares line (case 1 above).

The formulas for calculating a "prediction interval," a confidence interval for a future determination, are similar to those presented in Eqs. (7.16) and (7.17), with one modification. In Eq. (7.16) we add 1 to the sum under the square root portion of the expression. Similarly, for the inverse problem, Eq. (7.17) the expression $(1 - g)/N$ is replaced by $(N + 1)(1 - g)/N$. Thus the prediction interval for Y at a given X is

$$Y \ \pm \ t(S_{Y.x}) \ \sqrt{1 + \frac{1}{N} + \frac{(X - \overline{X})^2}{\Sigma \ (X - \overline{X})^2}} \qquad (7.18)$$

The prediction interval for X at a specified Y is

$$(X - g\overline{X}) \pm [t(S)/b] \frac{\left[\sqrt{(N + 1)(1 - g)/N + (X - \overline{X})^2/\Sigma \, (X - \overline{X})^2} \right]}{1 - g}$$

(7.19)

The following examples should clarify the computations. In the stability study example, suppose that one wishes to construct a 95% confidence (prediction) interval for *an assay to be performed* at 25.5 months. (An actual measurement is obtained at 25.5 months.) This interval will be larger than that calculated based on Eq. (7.16), because the uncertainty now includes assay variability for the proposed assay in addition to the uncertainty of the least squares line. Applying Eq. (7.18) (Y = 45), we have

$$45 \pm 2.12(1.35) \sqrt{1 + \frac{1}{18} + \frac{17.5^2}{630}} = 45 \pm 3.55 \text{ mg}$$

In the example of the calibration line, consider an unknown sample which is analyzed and shows a value (y) of 90. A prediction interval for X is calculated using Eq. (7.19). X is predicted to be 91.9 (see Sec. 7.2).

$$g = \frac{(4.30)^2(12.15)}{(0.915)^2(2000)} = 0.134 \ (2 \text{ d.f.}) \quad 1 - g = 0.866$$

$$\frac{[91.9 - 0.134(90)] \pm (4.3)(3.49)/0.915 \left[\sqrt{5(0.866)/4 + (1.9)^2/2000} \right]}{0.866}$$

$$= 72.5 \text{ to } 111.9$$

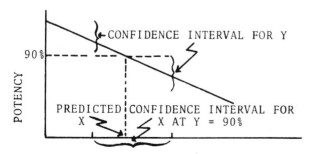

Depiction of the uncertainty in prediction in regression analysis

The relatively large uncertainty of the estimate of the true value is due to the small number of data points (four) and the relatively large variability of the points about the least squares line ($S^2_{Y.x}$ = 12.15).

Confidence Intervals for Slope (B) and Intercept (A)

A confidence interval can be constructed for the slope and intercept in a manner analogous to that for means [Eq. (6.2)]. The confidence interval for the slope is

$$ b \pm t(S_b) = b \pm \frac{t(S_{Y.x})}{\sqrt{\Sigma\ (X - \overline{X})^2}} \tag{7.20}$$

A confidence interval for the intercept is

$$ a \pm t(S_a) = a \pm t(S_{Y.x}) \sqrt{\frac{1}{N} + \frac{\overline{X}^2}{\Sigma\ (X - \overline{X})^2}} \tag{7.21}$$

A 95% confidence interval for the slope of the line in the stability example is [Eq. (7.20)]

$$ (-0.267) \pm \frac{2.12(1.35)}{\sqrt{630}} = -0.267 \pm 0.114 $$
$$ = -0.381 \text{ to } -0.153 $$

A 90% confidence interval for the intercept in the calibration line example (Sec. 7.2) is [Eq. (7.21)]

$$ 5.9 \pm 2.93(3.49) \sqrt{\frac{1}{4} + \frac{90^2}{2000}} = 5.9 \pm 21.2 = -15.3 \text{ to } 27.1 $$

(Note that the appropriate value of t with 2 d.f. for a 90% conficence interval is 2.93.)

7.7 WEIGHTED REGRESSION

One of the assumptions implicit in the applications of statistical inference to regression procedures is that the variance of y be the same at each value of X. Many situations occur in practice when this assumption is violated. One common occurrence is the variance of y being approximately proportional to X. This occurs in situations where y has a constant coefficient of variation (CV) and y is proportional to X (y = BX), commonly observed in instrumental methods of analysis in analytical chemistry. Two approaches to this problem are (a) a transformation of y to make the variance homogeneous, such as the log transformation (see Chap. 10), and (b) a weighted regression analysis.

Below is an example of weighted regression analysis in which we assume a constant CV and the variance of y proportional to X as noted above. This suggests a weighted regression, weighting each value of Y by a factor that is inversely proportional to the variance, $1/X^2$. Table 7.4 shows data for the spectrophotometric analysis of a drug performed at 5 concentrations in duplicate.

Equation (7.22) is used to compute the slope for the weighted regression procedure.

$$b = \frac{\Sigma\, wXy - \Sigma\, wX\; \Sigma\, wy/\Sigma\, w}{\Sigma\, wX - (\Sigma\, wX)^2/\Sigma\, w} \tag{7.22}$$

The computations follow:

$$\Sigma\, w = 0.04 + 0.04 + \ldots + 0.0001 + 0.0001 = 0.1042$$

$$\Sigma\, wXy = (0.04)(5)(0.105) + (0.04)(5)(0.098) + \ldots$$
$$(0.0001)(100)(1.964) + (0.0001)(100)(2.013) = 0.19983$$

$$\Sigma\, wX = 2(0.04)(5) + 2(0.01)(10) + \ldots + 2(0.0001)(100) = 0.74$$

Table 7.4 Analytical Data for a Spectrophotometric Analysis

Concentration (X)	Optical density (y)		CV	Weight (w)
5	0.105	0.098	0.049	0.04
10	0.201	0.194	0.025	0.01
25	0.495	0.508	0.018	0.0016
50	0.983	1.009	0.018	0.0004
100	1.964	2.013	0.017	0.0001

Σ wy = (0.04)(0.105) + (0.04)(0.098) + . . . +
(0.0001)(1.964) + (0.0001)(2.013) = 0.0148693

Σ wX^2 = 2(0.04)(5) + 2(0.01)(10) . . . + 2(0.0001)(100) = 10

Therefore, the slope b =

$$\frac{0.19983 - (0.74)(0.0148693)/0.1042}{10 - (0.74)^2/0.1042} = 0.01986$$

The intercept is

$$a = \overline{y}_w - b \, (\overline{X}_w) \tag{7.23}$$

where $\overline{y}_w = \Sigma wy/\Sigma w$ and $\overline{X}_w = \Sigma wX/\Sigma w$

$$a = 0.0148693/0.1042 - 0.01986(0.74/0.1042) = 0.00166$$

The weighted least squares line is shown in Fig. 7.10.

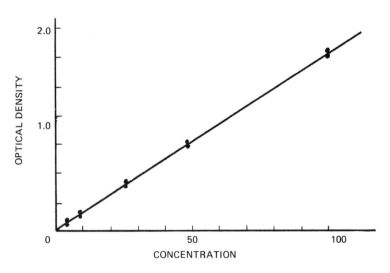

Figure 7.10   Weighted regression plot for data from Table 7.4.

7.8   ANALYSIS OF RESIDUALS

Emphasis is placed elsewhere in this book on the importance of carefully examining and graphing data prior to performing statistical
analyses.   The approach to examining data in this context is commonly known as Exploratory Data Analysis (EDA) [8].   One aspect
of EDA is the examination of residuals.   Residuals can be thought
of as deviations of the observed data from the fit to the statistical
model.   Examination of residuals can reveal problems such as variance
heterogeneity or nonlinearity.   This brief introduction to the prin-
ciple of residual analysis uses the data from the regression analysis
in Sec. 7.7.

The residuals from a regression analysis are obtained from the
differences between the observed and predicted values.   Table 7.5
shows the residuals from an unweighted least squares fit of the
data of Table 7.4.   Note that the fitted values are obtained from
the least squares equation $y = 0.001789 + 0.019874(X)$.

If the linear model and the assumptions in the least squares
analysis are valid, the residuals should be approximately normally
distributed, and no trends should be apparent.

Figure 7.11 shows a plot of the residuals as a function of X.
The fact that the residuals show a fan-like pattern, getting larger
as X increases, suggest the use of a log transformation or weighting
procedure to reduce the variance heterogeneity.   In general, the

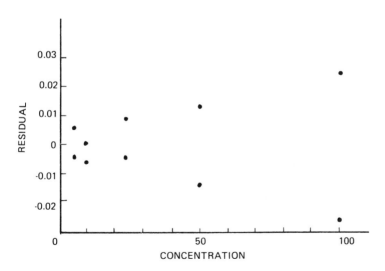

Figure 7.11   Residual plot for unweighted analysis of data of
Table 7.5.

Table 7.5   Residuals from Least Squares Fit of Analytical Data (Table 7.4)

	Unweighted			Log transform	
Actual	Predicted value	Residual	Actual	Predicted value	Residual
0.105	0.101	+0.00384	−2.254	−2.298	+0.044
0.201	0.201	+0.00047	−1.604	−1.6073	+0.0033
0.495	0.499	−0.00364	−0.703	−0.695	−0.008
0.983	0.995	−0.0126	−0.017	−0.0004	−0.0166
1.964	1.989	−0.025	+0.675	+0.6863	−0.0113
0.098	0.101	−0.00316	−2.323	−2.298	−0.025
0.194	0.201	−0.00653	−1.640	−1.6073	−0.0033
0.508	0.499	+0.00936	−0.677	−0.6950	+0.018
1.009	0.995	+0.0135	+0.009	−0.0042	+0.0132
2.013	1.989	+0.00238	+0.700	0.6863	+0.0137

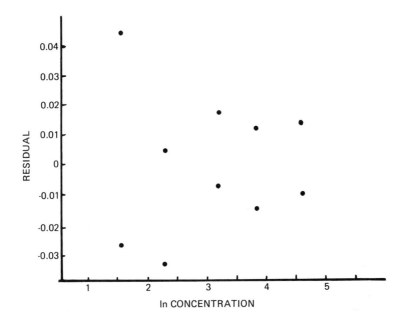

Figure 7.12   Residual plot for analysis of ln transformed data of
Table 7.5.

the intelligent interpretation of residual plots requires knowledge
and experience. In addition to the appearance of patterns in the
residual plots that indicate relationships and character of data, outliers usually become obviously apparent [11].

   Figure 7.12 shows the residual plot after a log (ln) transformation of X and Y. Much of the variance heterogeneity has been
removed.

   For readers who desire more information on this subject, the
book *Graphical Exploratory Data Analysis* [12] is recommended.

7.9   NONLINEAR REGRESSION**

Linear regression applies to the solution of relationships where the
function of Y is linear in the parameters. For example, the equation

---

**This is a more advanced topic.

$$Y = A + BX$$

is linear in A and B, the parameters. Similarly, the equation

$$Y = A + Be^{-X}$$

is also linear in the parameters. One should also appreciate that a linear equation can exist in more than two dimensions. The equation

$$Y = A + BX + CX^2$$

an example of a quadratic equation, is linear in the parameters, A, B, and C. These parameters can be estimated by using methods of multiple regression [1].

An example of a relationship that is nonlinear in this context is

$$Y = A + e^{BX}$$

Here the parameter B is not in a linear form.

If a linearizing transformation can be made, then this approach to estimating the parameters would be easiest. For example, the simple first-order kinetic relationship

$$Y = Ae^{-BX}$$

is not linear in the parameters, A and B. However, a log transformation results in a linear equation

$$\ln Y = \ln A - BX$$

Using the least squares approach, we can estimate ln A (A is the antilog) and B, where ln A is the intercept and B is the slope of the straight line when ln Y is plotted vs. X. If statistical tests and other statistical estimates are to be made from the regression analysis, the assumptions of normality of Y (now ln Y) and variance homogeneity of Y at each X are necessary. If Y is normal and the variances of Y at each X are homogeneous to start with, the ln transformation will invalidate the assumptions. (On the other hand, if Y is lognormal with constant coefficient of variation, the log transformation will be just what is needed to validate the assumptions.)

Some relationships cannot be linearized. For example, in pharmacokinetics, the one-compartment model with first order absorption and excretion has the following form

Table 7.6 Data from a Stability
Study

Time (t)	Concentration mg/L (C)
1 hour	63
2 hours	34
3 hours	22

$$C = D (e^{-ket} - e^{-kat})$$

where D, ke, and ka are constants (parameters). This equation
cannot be linearized. The use of nonlinear regression methods can
be used to estimate the parameters in these situations as well as the
situations in which Y is normal with homogeneous variance prior to
a transformation, as noted above.

The solutions to nonlinear regression problems require more advanced mathematics relative to most of the material in this book. A
knowledge of elementary calculus is necessary, particularly the application of Taylor's theorem. Also, a knowledge of matrix algebra
is useful in order to solve these kinds of problems. A simple example will be presented to demonstrate the principles. The general
matrix solutions to linear and multiple regression will also be
demonstrated.

In a stability study, the data in Table 7.6 were available for
analysis. The equation representing the degradation process is

$$C = C_o e^{-kt} \qquad (7.24)$$

The concentration values are known to be normal with the variance
constant at each value of time. Therefore, the usual least squares
analysis will *not* be used to estimate the parameters C_o and k after
the simple linearizing transformation:

$$\ln C = \ln C_0 - kt$$

The estimate of the parameters using nonlinear regression as
demonstrated here uses the first terms of Taylor's expansion,
which approximates the function and results in a linear equation.

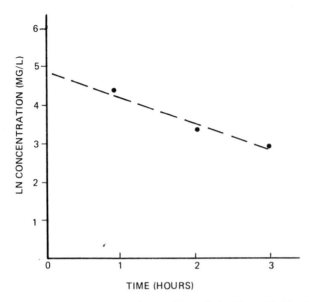

Figure 7.13   Plot of stability data from Table 7.6.

It is important to obtain good initial estimates of the parameters,
which may be obtained graphically. In the present example, a plot
of ln C vs. time (Fig. 7.13) results in initial estimates of 104 for C_0
and -0.53 for k. The process then estimates a change in C_0 and
a change in k that will improve the equation based on the comparison
of the fitted data to the original data. Typical of least squares procedures, the fit is measured by the sum of the squares of the
deviations of the observed values from the fitted values. The best
fit results from an iterative procedure. The new estimates result in
a better fit to the data. The procedure is repeated using the new
estimates, which results in a better fit than that observed in the
previous iteration. When the fit, as measured by the sum of the
squares of deviations, is negligibly improved, the procedure is
stopped. Computer programs are available to carry out these
tedious calculations.

The Taylor expansion requires taking partial derivatives of the
function with respect to C_0 and k. For the equation, $C = C_0 e^{-kt}$,
the resulting expression is:

$$dC = dC_0'(e^{-k't}) + dk' (C_0')(te^{-k't}) \qquad (7.25)$$

Table 7.7   Results of First Iteration

Time (t)	C	C'	dC'	X1	X2
1	63	61.2	1.8	0.5886	61.2149
2	34	36.0	−2.0	0.3465	72.0628
3	22	21.2	0.8	0.2039	63.6248

$$\Sigma \ dC'^2 \ = \ 7.88$$

In Eq. (7.25), dC is the change in C resulting from small changes in C_0 and k evaluated at the point, C_0' and k'. dC_0' is the change in the estimate of C_0, and dk' is the change in the estimate of k. $(e^{-k't})$ and C_0' $(te^{-k't})$ are the partial derivatives of Eq. (7.24) with respect to C_0 and k, respectively.

Equation (7.25) is linear in dC_0' and dk'. The coefficients of dC_0' and dk' are $(e^{-k't})$ and $(C_0')(te^{-k't})$, respectively. In the computations below, the coefficients are referred to as X1 and X2, respectively, for convenience. Because of the linearity, we can obtain the least squares estimates of dC_0' and dk' by the usual regression procedures.

The computations for two iterations are shown below. The solution to the least squares equation is usually accomplished using matrix manipulations. The solution for the coefficients can be proven to have the following form:

$$B \ = \ (X'X)^{-1} \ (X'Y)$$

The matrix B will contain the estimates of the coefficients. With two coefficients, this will be a 2 × 1 (2 rows and 1 column) matrix.

In Table 7.7, the values of X1 and X2 are $(e^{-k't})$ and (C_0') $(te^{-k't})$, respectively, using the initial estimates of $C_0' = 104$ and $k' = -0.53$ (Fig. 7.13). Note that the fit is measured by the $\Sigma \ dC'^2 = 7.88$.

The solution of $(X'X)^{-1}$ $(X'Y)$ gives the estimates of the parameters, dC_o' and k':

$$
| X'X |^{-1} \qquad\qquad | X'Y |
$$

$$
\begin{vmatrix} 4.82778 & -0.023239 \\ -0.023239 & 0.00018886 \end{vmatrix}
\begin{vmatrix} 0.5296 \\ 16.9611 \end{vmatrix}
=
\begin{vmatrix} 2.1 \\ -0.009 \end{vmatrix}
$$

Table 7.8   Results of Second Iteration

Time (t)	C	C'	dC'	X1	X2
1	63	61.9	1.1	0.5833	61.8915
2	34	36.2	−2.2	0.3403	72.2064
3	22	21.1	0.9	0.1985	63.1804

$$\Sigma \ dC'^2 \ = \ 6.86$$

The new estimates of C_o and k are:

$$C_o' \ = \ 104 + 2.1 \ = \ 106.1$$

$$k' \ = \ -0.53 - 0.009 \ = \ -0.539$$

With these estimates, new values of C' are calculated in Table 7.8.

Note that the $\Sigma \ dC'^2$ is 6.86, which is reduced from 7.88, from the initial iteration.

The solution of $(X'X)^{-1} \ (X'Y)$ is:

$$\begin{vmatrix} 11.85390 & -0.06656 \\ -0.06656 & 0.0004504 \end{vmatrix} \begin{vmatrix} 0.0716 \\ -33.911 \end{vmatrix} = \begin{vmatrix} 3.1 \\ -0.02 \end{vmatrix}$$

Therefore, the new estimates of C_o and k are

$$C_o' \ = \ 106.1 + 3.1 \ = \ 109.2$$

$$k \ = \ -0.539 - 0.02 \ = \ -0.559$$

The reader can verify that the new value of dC'^2 is now 5.81. The process is repeated until dC'^2 becomes stable.

Another way of expressing the decomposition is:

$$C \ = \ e^{\ln C_o - kt}$$

or

$$\ln C \ = \ \ln C_o - kt$$

The ambitious reader may wish to try a few iterations using this approach. Note that the partial derivatives of C with respect to C_0 and k are $(1/C_0)$ $(e^{\ln C_0 - kt})$ and $-t(e^{\ln C_0 - kt})$, respectively.

7.10   CORRELATION

Correlation methods are used to measure the "association" of two or more variables. Here we will be concerned with two observations for each sampling unit. We are interested in determining if the two values are related, in the sense that one variable may be predicted from a knowledge of the other. The better the prediction, the better the correlation. For example, if we could predict the dissolution of a tablet based on tablet hardness, we say that dissolution and hardness are *correlated*. Correlation analysis assumes a linear or *straight-line relationship* between the two variables.

Correlation is usually applied to the relationship of continuous variables, and is best visualized as a *scatter plot* or correlation diagram. Figure 7.14A shows a scatter plot for two variables, tablet weight and tablet potency. Tablets were individually weighed and than assayed. Each point in Fig. 7.14A represents a single tablet (X = weight, Y = potency). Inspection of this diagram suggests that weight and potency are *positively* correlated, as is indicated by the positive slope, or trend. Low-weight tablets are associated with low potencies, and vice versa. This positive relationship would probably be expected on intuitive grounds. If the tablet granulation is homogeneous, a larger weight of material in a tablet would contain larger amounts of drug. Figure 7.14B shows the correlation of tablet weights and dissolution rate. Smaller tablet weights are related to higher dissolution rates, a *negative* correlation (negative trend).

Inspection of Fig. 7.14A and B reveals what appears to be an obvious relationship. Given a tablet weight, we can make a good "ball-park" estimate of the dissolution rate and potency. However, the relationship between variables is not always as apparent as in these examples. The relationship may be partially obscured by variability, or the variables may not be related at all. The relationship between a patient's blood pressure reduction after treatment with an antihypertensive agent and serum potassium levels is not as obvious (Fig. 7.14C). There seems to be a trend toward higher blood pressure reductions associated with higher potassium levels — or is this just an illusion? The data plotted in Fig. 7.14D, illustrating the correlation of blood pressure and age, show little or no correlation.

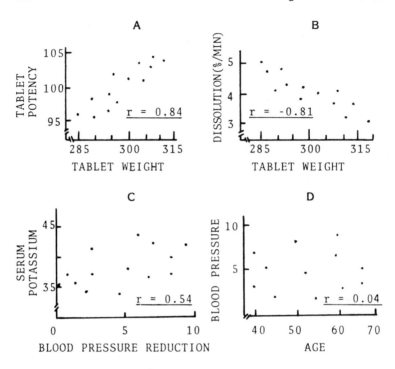

Figure 7.14 Examples of various correlation diagrams or scatter plots. The correlation coefficient, r, is defined in Sec. 7.10.1.

The various scatter diagrams illustrated in Fig. 7.14 should give the reader an intuitive feeling for the concept of correlation. There are many experimental situations where a researcher would be interested in relationships among two or more variables. Similar to applications of regression analysis, correlation relationships may allow for prediction and interpretation of experimental mechanisms. Unfortunately, the concept of correlation is often misused, and more is made of it than is deserved. For example, the presence of a strong correlation between two variables does not necessarily imply a causal relationship. Consider data that show a positive relationship between cancer rate and consumption of fluoridated water. Regardless of the possible validity of such a relationship, such an observed correlation does not necessarily imply a causal effect. One would have to investigate further other factors in the environment occurring concurrently with the implementation of fluoridation, which may be responsible for the cancer rate increase. Have other industries appeared and grown during this period, exposing the population to potential carcinogens? Have the population characteristics (e.g., racial, age, sex, economic factors) changed during this period? Such questions may be resolved by examining the cancer rates in control areas where fluoridation was not enforced.

The correlation coefficient is a measure of the "degree" of correlation, which is often *erroneously* interpreted as a measure of "linearity." That is, a strong correlation is sometimes interpreted as meaning that the relationship between X and Y is a straight line. As we shall see further in this discussion, this interpretation of correlation is not necessarily correct.

7.10.1 Correlation Coefficient

The correlation coefficient is a quantative measure of the relationship or correlation between two variables.

$$\text{Correlation coefficient} = r = \frac{\Sigma\ (X - \overline{X})(y - \overline{y})}{\sqrt{\Sigma\ (X - \overline{X})^2\ \Sigma\ (y - \overline{y})^2}}$$

(7.26)

A shortcut computing formula is

$$r = \frac{N\ \Sigma\ Xy - \Sigma\ X\ \Sigma\ y}{\sqrt{[N\ \Sigma\ X^2 - (\Sigma\ X)^2][N\ \Sigma\ y^2 - (\Sigma\ y)^2]}}$$

(7.27)

where N is the number of X, y pairs.

The correlation coefficient, r, may be better understood by its relationship to $S_{Y.x}^2$, the variance calculated from regression line fitting procedures. r^2 represents the relative reduction in the sum of squares of the variable y resulting from the fitting of the X, y line. For example, the sum of squares $[\Sigma\ (y - \overline{y})^2]$ for the y values 0, 1, and 5 is equal to 14 [see Eq. (1.4)].

$$\Sigma\ (y - \overline{y})^2 = 0^2 + 1^2 + 5^2 - \frac{(0 + 1 + 5)^2}{3} = 14$$

If these same y values were associated with X values, the sum of squares of y from the regression of y and X will be *equal to or less*

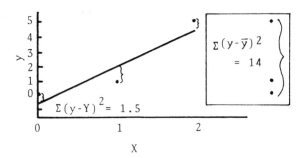

Figure 7.15   Reduction in sum of squares due to regression.

than $\Sigma\ (y - \bar{y})^2$, or 14 in this example. Suppose that X and y values are as follows (see Fig. 7.15):

	X	y	Xy	
	0	0	0	$\Sigma\ (X - \bar{X})^2 = 2$
	1	1	1	
	2	5	10	$\Sigma\ (y - \bar{y})^2 = 14$
Sum	3	6	11	

According to Eq. (7.9), the sum of squares due to deviations of the y values from the regression line is

$$\Sigma\ (y - \bar{y})^2 - b^2\ \Sigma\ (X - \bar{X})^2 \qquad\qquad (7.28)$$

where b is the slope of the regression line (y on X). The term $b^2\ \Sigma\ (X - \bar{X})^2$ is the reduction in the sum of squares due to the straight-line regression fit. Applying Eq. (7.28), the sum of squares is

$$14 - (2.5)^2(2)\ =\ 14 - 12.5\ =\ 1.5\ \text{ (the slope, b, is 2.5)}$$

r^2 is the relative reduction of the sum of squares:

$$\frac{14 - 1.5}{14}\ =\ 0.893 \qquad\qquad r\ =\ \sqrt{0.893}\ =\ 0.945$$

The usual calculation of r, according to Eq. (7.27), follows:

$$\frac{3(11) - (3)(6)}{\sqrt{[3(5) - (3)^2][3(26) - (36)]}} = \frac{15}{\sqrt{6(42)}} = 0.945$$

Thus, according to this notion, r can be interpreted as the relative degree of scatter about the regression line. If X and y values lie exactly on a straight line (a perfect fit), $S_{y.x}^2$ is 0, and r is equal to ±1; +1 for a line of positive slope and −1 for a line of negative slope. For a correlation coefficient equal to 0.5, $r^2 = 0.25$. The sum of squares for y is reduced 25%. A correlation coefficient of 0 means that the X, y pairs are not correlated (see Fig. 7.14D).

Although there are no assumptions necessary to calculate the correlation coefficient, statistical analysis of r is based on the notion of a bivariate normal distribution of X and y. We will not delve into the details of this complex probability distribution here. However, there are two interesting aspects of this distribution which deserve some attention with regard to correlation analysis.

1. In typical correlation problems, *both X and y are variable.* This is in contrast to the linear regression case, where X is considered *fixed*, chosen, a priori, by the investigator.
2. In a bivariate normal distribution, X and y are linearly related. The regression of both X and y and y on X is a straight line.* Thus, when statistically testing correlation coefficients, we are not testing for linearity. As described below, the statistical test of a correlation coefficient is a test of correlation or independence. According to Snedecor and Cochran, the correlation coefficient "estimates the degree of *closeness* of a linear relationship between two variables, Y and X, and the meaning of this concept is not easy to grasp" [8].

---

*The regression of y on X means that X is assumed to be the fixed variable when calculating the line. This line is different from that calculated when Y is considered the fixed variable (unless the correlation coefficient is 1, when both lines are identical). The slope of the line is rS_y/S_x for the regression of y on X and rS_x/S_y for x on Y.

7.10.2   Test of Zero Correlation

The correlation coefficient is a rough measure of the degree of association of two variables. The degree of association may be measured by how well one variable can be predicted from another; the closer the correlation coefficient is to $+1$ or -1, the better the correlation, the better the predictive power of the relationship. A question of particular importance from a statistical point of view is whether or not an observed correlation coefficient is "real" or due to chance. If two variables from a bivariate normal distribution are uncorrelated (independent), the correlation coefficient is 0. Even in these cases, in actual experiments, random variation will result in a correlation coefficient different from zero. Thus, it is of interest to test an observed correlation coefficient, r, versus a hypothetical value of 0. This test is based on an assumption that y is a normal variable [8]. The test is a t test with $(N - 2)$ degrees of freedom, as follows:

$$H_0: \quad \rho = 0 \qquad H_a: \quad \rho \neq 0$$

where ρ is the true correlation coefficient, estimated by r.

$$t_{N-2} = \frac{|r\sqrt{N-2}|}{\sqrt{1 - r^2}} \qquad\qquad (7.29)$$

The value of t is referred to a t distribution with $(N - 2)$ d.f., where N is the sample size (i.e., the number of pairs). Interestingly, this test is identical to the test of the slope of the least squares fit, $Y = a + bX$ [Eq. (7.13). In this context, one can think of the test of the correlation coefficient as a test of the significance of the slope versus 0.

   To illustrate the application of Eq. (7.29), Table 7.9 shows data of diastolic blood pressure and cholesterol levels of 10 randomly selected men. The data are plotted in Fig. 7.16. r is calculated from Eq. (7.27):

$$r = \frac{N \, \Sigma \, Xy - \Sigma \, X \, \Sigma \, y}{\sqrt{[N \, \Sigma \, X^2 - (\Sigma \, X)^2][N \, \Sigma \, y^2 - (\Sigma \, y)^2]}} \qquad\qquad (7.27)$$

$$= \frac{10(260,653) - (825)(3111)}{\sqrt{[10(69,279) - 825^2][10(987,893) - 3111^2]}} = 0.809$$

r is tested for significance using Eq. (7.29).

Table 7.9 Diastolic Blood Pressure and Serum Cholesterol
of 10 Persons

Person	Diastolic blood pressure (DBP), y	Cholesterol (C), X	Xy
1	80	307	24,560
2	75	259	19,425
3	90	341	30,690
4	74	317	23,458
5	75	274	20,550
6	110	416	45,760
7	70	267	18,690
8	85	320	27,200
9	88	274	24,112
10	78	336	26,208

$$\Sigma \text{ y} = 825 \qquad \Sigma \text{ X} = 3,111 \qquad \Sigma \text{ Xy} = 260,653$$

$$\Sigma \text{ y}^2 = 69,279 \qquad \Sigma \text{ X}^2 = 987,893$$

Source: Ref. 9.

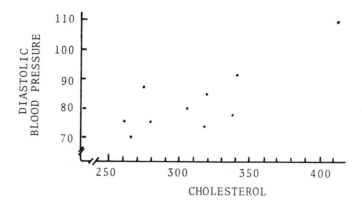

Figure 7.16 Plot of data from Table 7.8.

$$t_8 = \frac{|\, 0.809 \,\sqrt{8}\,|}{\sqrt{1 - (0.809)^2}} = 3.89$$

A value of t equal to 2.31 is needed for significance at the 5% level
(see Table IV.4). Therefore, the correlation between diastolic blood
pressure and cholesterol is significant. The correlation is apparent
from inspection of Fig. 7.16.

Significance tests for the correlation coefficient versus values
other than 0 are not very common. However, for these tests, the t
test described above [Eq. (7.29)] should not be used. An approximate test is available to test for correlation coefficients other than 0
(e.g., H_0: $\rho = 0.5$). Since applications of this test occur infrequently in pharmaceutical experiments, the procedure will not be
presented here. The statistical test is an approximation to the normal distribution, and the approximation can also be used to place
confidence intervals on the correlation coefficient. A description of
these applications is presented in Ref. 8.

7.10.3   Miscellaneous Comments

Before leaving the topic of correlation, the reader should once more
be warned about the potential misuses of interpretations of correlation and the correlation coefficient. In particular, the association
of high correlation coefficients with a "cause and effect" and
"linearity" is not necessarily valid. Strong correlation *may* imply a
direct causal relationship, but the nature of the measurements should
be well understood before firm statements can be made about cause
and effect. One should be keenly aware of the common occurrence
of spurious correlations due to indirect causes or remote mechanisms.

The correlation coefficient does not test the linearity of two
variables. If anything, it is more related to the slope of the line
relating the variables. Linearity is assumed for the routine statistical test of the correlation coefficient. As has been noted above,
the correlation coefficient measures the degree of correlation, a
measure of the variability of a predictive relationship. A proper
test for linearity (i.e., do the data represent a straight-line relationship between X and Y?) is described in App. II and requires
replicate measurements in the regression model. Usually, correlation
problems deal with cases where both variables, X and y, are variable in contrast to the regression model where X is considered
fixed. In correlation problems, the question of linearity is usually
not of primary interest. We are more interested in the degree of
association of the variables. Two examples will show that a high
correlation coefficient does not necessarily imply "linearity" and

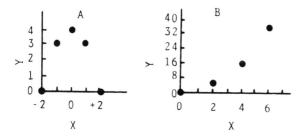

Figure 7.17 Plot of data in Table 7.10 showing problems with interpretation of the correlation coefficient.

that a small correlation coefficient does not necessarily imply lack of correlation (if the relationship is nonlinear).

Table 7.10 shows two sets of data which are plotted in Fig. 7.17. Both data sets A and B show perfect (but nonlinear) relationships between X and y. Set A is defined by $Y = 4 - X^2$. Set B is defined by $Y = X^2$. Yet the correlation coefficient for set A is 0, an implication of no correlation, and set B has a correlation coefficient of 0.96, very strong correlation (*but not linearity!*). These examples should emphasize the care needed in the interpretation of the correlation coefficient, particularly in nonlinear systems.

Table 7.10 Two Data Sets Illustrating
Some Problems of Interpreting
Correlation Coefficients

Set A		Set B	
X	y	X	y
−2	0	0	0
−1	3	2	4
0	4	4	16
+1	3	6	36
+2	0		

Table 7.11   Data to Illustrate a Problem
that Can Result in Misinterpretation of
the Correlation Coefficient

pH	Stability, $t_{1/2}$ (weeks)
2.0	48
2.1	50
1.9	50
2.0	46
2.1	47
5.5	12

Another example of data for which the correlation coefficient can
be misleading is shown in Table 7.11 and Fig. 2.18.   In this example, drug stability is plotted versus pH.   Five experiments were
performed at low pH and one at high pH.   The correlation coefficient
is 0.994, a highly significant result (P < 0.01).   Can this be interpreted that the data in Fig. 7.18 are a good fit to a straight line?
Without some other source of information, it would take a great deal
of imagination to assume that the relationship between pH and $t_{1/2}$
is linear over the range of pH equal to 2.0 to 5.5.   Even if the
relationship were linear, had data been available for points in between pH 2.0 and 5.5, the fit may not be as good as that implied

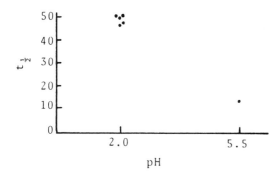

Figure 7.18   Plot of data from Table 7.10.

by the large value of r in this example. This situation can occur when one value is far from the cluster of the main body of data. One should be cautious in "over-interpreting" the correlation coefficient in these cases. When relationships between variables are to be quantified for predictive or theoretical reasons, regression procedures, if applicable, are recommended. Correlation, per se, is not as versatile or informative as regression analysis for describing the relationship between variables.

7.11 COMPARISON OF VARIANCES IN RELATED SAMPLES

In Sec. 5.3, a test was presented to compare variances from two independent samples. If the samples are related, the simple F test for two independent samples is not valid [8]. Related, or paired-sample tests arise, for example, in situations where the same subject tests two treatments, such as in clinical or bioavailability studies. To test for the equality of variances in related samples, we must first calculate the correlation coefficient and the F ratio of the variances. The test statistic is calculated as follows:

$$r_{ds} = \frac{F - 1}{\sqrt{(F + 1)^2 - 4r^2 F}} \tag{7.30}$$

where F is the ratio of the variances in the two samples and r is the correlation coefficient.

The ratio in Eq. (7.30), r_{ds}, can be tested for significance in the same manner as the test for the ordinary correlation coefficient, with $(N - 2)$ d.f., where N is the number of pairs [Eq. (7.29)]. As is the case for tests of the correlation coefficient, we assume a bivariate normal distribution for the related data. The following example demonstrates the calculations.

In a bioavailability study, 10 subjects were given each of two formulations of a drug substance on two occasions, with the results for AUC (area under the blood level versus time curve) given in Table 7.12.

The correlation coefficient is calculated according to Eq. (7.27).

$$r = \frac{(64,421)(10) - (781)(815)}{\sqrt{[(62,821)(10) - (781)^2][(67,087)(10) - (815)^2]}} = 0.699$$

Table 7.12   AUC Results of the
Bioavailability Study (A versus B)

	Formulation	
Subject	A	B
1	88	88
2	64	73
3	69	86
4	94	89
5	77	80
6	85	71
7	60	70
8	105	96
9	68	84
10	73	78
Mean	78.1	81.5
s^2	202.8	73.8

The ratio of the variances (Table 7.12), F, is

$$\frac{202.8}{73.8} = 2.75$$

[Note: The ratio of the variances may also be calculated as
73.8/202.8 = 0.36, with the same conclusions based on Eq. (7.30).]
    The test statistic, r_{ds}, is calculated from Eq. (7.30).

$$r_{ds} = \frac{2.75 - 1}{\sqrt{(2.75 + 1)^2 - 4(0.699)^2(2.75)}} = 0.593$$

r_{ds} is tested for significance using Eq. (7.29).

$$t_8 = \frac{|0.593 \sqrt{8}|}{\sqrt{1 - 0.593^2}} = 2.08$$

Referring to the t table (Table IV.4, 8 d.f.), a value of 2.31 is
needed for significance at the 5% level.   Therefore, we cannot
reject the null hypothesis of equal variances in this example.

Formulation A appears to be more variable, but more data would be needed to substantiate such a claim.

KEY TERMS

Best-fitting line	Nonlinear regression
Bivariate normal distribution	Nonlinearity
Confidence band for line	One-sided confidence interval
Confidence interval for X and Y	Prediction interval
Correlation	Reduction of sum of squares
Correlation coefficient	Regression
Correlation diagram	Regression analysis
Dependent variable	Residuals
Fixed value (X)	Scatter plot
Independence	Simple linear regression
Independent variable	Slope
Intercept	$S_{Y.x}^2$
Inverse prediction	
Lack of fit	Trend
Linear regression	Variance of correlated samples
Line through the origin	Weighted regression

EXERCISES

1. A drug seems to decompose in a manner such that appearance of degradation products is linear with time (i.e., $C_d = kt$).

t	C_d
1	3
2	9
3	12
4	17
5	19

   (a) Calculate the slope (k) and intercept from the least squares line.
   (b) Test the significance of the slope (test versus 0) at the 5% level.
   (c) Test the slope versus 5 (H_0: B = 5) at the 5% level.
   (d) Put 95% confidence limits on C_d at t = 3 and t = 5.
   (e) Predict the value of C_d at t = 20. Place a 95% prediction interval on C_d at t = 20.
   (f) If it is known that $C_d = 0$ at t = 0, calculate the slope.

2. A Beer's law plot is constructed by plotting ultraviolet absorb-
    ance versus concentration, with the following results:

Concentration, X	Absorbance, y	Xy
1	0.10	0.10
2	0.36	0.72
3	0.57	1.71
5	1.09	5.45
10	2.05	20.50

(a) Calculate the slope and intercept.
(b) Test to see if the intercept is different from 0 (5% level).
    How would you interpret a significant intercept with re-
    gard to the actual physical nature of the analytical method?
**(c) An unknown has an absorbance of 1.65. What is the con-
    centration? Put confidence limits on the concentration (95%).

3. Five tablets were weighed and then assayed with the following
    results:

Weight (mg)	Potency (mg)
205	103
200	100
202	101
198	98
197	98

(a) Plot potency versus weight (weight = X). Calculate the
    least squares line.
(b) Predict the potency for a 200-mg tablet.
(c) Put 95% confidence limits on the potency for a 200-mg tab-
    let.

4. Tablets were weighed and assayed with the following results:

Weight	Assay	Weight	Assay
200	10.0	198	9.9
205	10.1	200	10.0
203	10.0	190	9.6
201	10.1	205	10.2
195	9.9	207	10.2
203	10.1	210	10.3

  (a) Calculate the correlation coefficient.
  (b) Test the correlation coefficient versus 0 (5% level).
  (c) Plot the data in the table (scatter plot).
5. Tablet dissolution was measured in vitro for 10 generic formulations. These products were also tested in vivo. Results of these studies showed the following time to 80% dissolution and time to peak (in vivo).

Formulation	Time to 80% dissolution (min)	T_p (hr)
1	17	0.8
2	25	1.0
3	15	1.2
4	30	1.5
5	60	1.4
6	24	1.0
7	10	0.8
8	20	0.7
9	45	2.5
10	28	1.1

Calculate r and test for significance (versus 0)(5% level). Plot the data.
6. Shah et al. [10] measured the percent of product dissolved in vitro and the time to peak (in vivo) of nine phenytoin sodium products, with approximately the following results:

Product	Time to peak (hr)	Percentage dissolved in 30 min
1	6	20
2	4	60
3	2.5	100
4	4.5	80
5	5.1	35
6	5.7	35
7	3.5	80
8	5.7	38
9	3.8	85

Plot the data. Calculate the correlation coefficient and test to see if it is significantly different from 0 (5% level). (Why is the correlation coefficient negative?)

7. In a study to compare the effects of two pain-relieving drugs
    (A and B), 10 patients took each drug in a paired design
    with the following results (drug effectiveness based on a
    rating scale).

Patient	Drug A	Drug B
1	8	6
2	5	4
3	5	6
4	2	5
5	4	5
6	7	4
7	9	6
8	3	7
9	5	5
10	1	4

Are the drug effects equally variable?

8. Compute the intercept and slope of the least squares line for
    the data of Table 7.4 after a ln transformation of both X and
    Y. Calculate the residuals and compare to the data in
    Table 7.5.

9. In a drug stability study, the following data were obtained:

Time (months)	Concentration (mg)
0	2.56
1	2.55
3	2.50
9	2.44
12	2.40
18	2.31
24	2.25
36	2.13

(a) Fit a least squares line to the data.

(b) Predict the time to decompose to 90% of label claim
    (2.25 mg).

(c) Based on a two-sided 95% confidence interval, what ex-
    piration date should be applied to this formulation?

(d) Based on a one-sided 95% confidence interval, what
    expiration date should be applied to this formulation?

**10. Fit the following data to the exponential $y = e^{ax}$. Use nonlinear least squares.

x	y
1	1.62
2	2.93
3	4.21
4	7.86

REFERENCES

1. Draper, N. R. and Smith, H., *Applied Regression Analysis*, 2nd ed., Wiley, New York, 1981.
2. Youden, W. J., *Statistical Methods for Chemists*, Wiley, New York, 1964.
3. Current Good Manufacturing Practices (CGMP) 21 CFR, 210–229, Commissioner of the Food and Drug Administration, Washington, D.C.
4. Davies, O. L. and Hudson, H. E., Stability of Drugs: Accelerated Storage Tests, in *Statistics in the Pharmaceutical Industry*, C. R. Buncher and J.-Y. Tsay, Eds., Marcel Dekker, New York, 1981.
5. Tootill, J. P. R., *J. Pharm. Pharmacol.*, *13*, Suppl., 75T–86T, 1961.
6. Davis, J., *The Dating Game*, Food and Drug Administration, Washington, D.C., 1978.
7. Norwood, T. E., *Drug Dev. and Ind. Pharm.*, *12*, 553–560, 1986.
8. Snedecor, G. W. and Cochran, W. G., *Statistical Methods*, 7th ed., Iowa State University Press, Ames, Iowa, 1980.
9. Dixon, W. J. and Massey, F. J., Jr., *Introduction to Statistical Analysis*, 3rd ed., McGraw-Hill, New York, 1969.
10. Shah, V. P. et al., *J. Pharm. Sci.*, *72*, 306, 1983.
11. Weisberg, S., *Applied Linear Regression*, Wiley, New York, 1980.
12. duToit, S. H. C., Steyn, A. G. W., and Stumpf, R. H., *Graphical Exploratory Data Analysis*, Springer-Verlag, New York, 1986.

8
Analysis of Variance

Analysis of variance, also known as *ANOVA*, is perhaps the most powerful statistical tool. ANOVA is a general method of analyzing data from designed experiments, whose objective is to *compare two or more group means*. The t test is a special case of ANOVA in which only two means are compared. By *designed experiments*, we mean experiments with a particular structure. Well-designed experiments are usually optimal with respect to meeting study objectives. The statistical analysis depends on the design, and the discussion of ANOVA therefore includes common statistical designs used in pharmaceutical research. Analysis of variance designs can be more or less complex. The designs can be very simple, as in the case of the t-test procedures presented in Chap. 5. Other designs can be quite complex, sometimes depending on computers for their solution and analysis. As a rule of thumb, one should use the simplest design that will achieve the experimental objectives. This is particularly applicable to experiments otherwise difficult to implement, such as is the case in clinical trials.

8.1 ONE-WAY ANALYSIS OF VARIANCE

An elementary approach to ANOVA may be taken using the two-independent-groups t test as an example. This is an example of one-way analysis of variance, also known as a "completely randomized" design. (Certain simple "parallel-groups" designs in clinical trials correspond to the one-way analysis of variance design.) In the t test, the two treatments are assigned at random to different independent experimental units. In a clinical study, the t test is appropriate when two treatments are randomly assigned to different patients. This results in two groups, each group representing one of the two treatments. One-way ANOVA is used when we wish to test the equality of treatment means in experiments where two or more treatments are randomly assigned to different, independent experimental units. The typical null hypothesis is H_0: $\mu_1 = \mu_2 = \mu_3 = \cdots$ where μ_1 refers to treatment 1, and so on.

Suppose that 15 tablets are available for the comparison of three assay methods, five tablets for each assay. The one-way ANOVA design would result from a random assignment of the tablets to the three groups. In this example, five tablets are assigned to each group. Although this allocation (five tablets per group) is optimal with regard to the precision of the comparison of the three assay methods, it is not a necessary condition for this design. The number of tablets analyzed by each analytical procedure need not be equal for purposes of comparing the mean results. However, one can say, in general, that symmetry is a desirable feature in the design of experiments. This will become more apparent as we discuss various designs. In the one-way ANOVA, symmetry can be defined as an equal number of experimental units in each treatment group.

We will pursue the example above to illustrate the ANOVA procedure. Five replicate tablets are analyzed in each of the three assay method groups, one assay per tablet. Thus we assay the 15 tablets, five tablets by each method, as shown in Table 8.1. If only two assay methods were to be compared, we could use a t test to compare the means statistically. If more than two assay methods are to be compared, the correct statistical procedure to compare the means is the one-way analysis of variance (ANOVA).

Analysis of variance is a technique of separating the total variability in a set of data into component parts, represented by a statistical model. In the simple case of the one-way ANOVA, the model is represented as

Table 8.1 Results of Assays Comparing Three Analytical Methods

	Method A	Method B	Method C
	102	99	103
	101	100	100
	101	99	99
	100	101	104
	102	98	102
$\overline{X}$	101.2	99.4	101.6
s.d.	0.84	1.14	2.07

$$Y_{ij} = \mu + T_i + e_{ij} \tag{8.1}$$

where

Y_{ij} = jth response in treatment group i (e.g., 1 = 3, j = 2, second tablet in third group)

T_i = deviation of the ith treatment mean from the overall mean, μ

e_{ij} = random error in the experiment (measurement error, biological variability, etc.) assumed to be normal with mean 0 and variance σ^2

The model says that the response is a function of the true treatment mean ($\mu + T_i$) and a random error that is normally distributed, with mean zero and variance σ^2. In the case of a clinical study, $T_i + \mu$ is the true average of treatment i. If a patient is treated with an antihypertensive drug whose true mean effect is a 10-mmHg reduction in blood pressure, then $Y_{ij} = 10 + e_{ij}$, where Y_{ij} is the jth observation among patients taking the drug i. (Note that if treatments are identical, T_i is the same for all treatments.) The error, e_{ij}, is a normally distributed variable, identically distributed for all observations. It is composed of many factors, including interindividual variation and measurement error. Thus the observed experimental values will be different for different people, a consequence of the nature of the assigned treatment and the random error, e_{ij} (e.g., biological variation).

In addition to the assumption that the error is normal with mean 0 and variance σ^2, the errors must be independent. This is a very important assumption in the analysis of variance model. The fact that the error has mean 0 means that some people will show positive deviations from the treatment mean, and others will show negative deviations; but on the average, the deviation is zero.

As in the t test, statistical analysis and interpretation of the ANOVA is based on the following assumptions.

1. The errors are normal with constant variance.
2. The errors (or observations) are independent.

As will be discussed below, ANOVA separates the variability of the data into parts, comparing that due to treatments to that due to error.

8.1.1 Computations and Procedure for One-Way Analysis of Variance

Analysis of variance for a one-way design separates the variance into two parts, that due to *treatment differences* and that due to

Table 8.2 Sample Data to Illustrate Eq. (8.2)

Group I (Y_{1j})	Group II (Y_{2j})	Group III (Y_{3j})
0	2	6
2	4	10
$\overline{Y}_i$ 1	3	8

$\overline{Y} = (1 + 3 + 8)/3 = (0 + 2 + 2 + 4 + 6 + 10)/6$

$\quad = 4$

error. It can be proven that the *total sum of squares* (the squared deviations of each value from the overall mean)

$$\Sigma \, (Y_{ij} - \overline{Y})^2$$

is equal to

$$\Sigma \, (Y_{ij} - \overline{Y}_i)^2 + \Sigma \, N_i (\overline{Y}_i - \overline{Y})^2 \qquad (8.2)$$

where $\overline{Y}$ is the overall mean and $\overline{Y}_i$ is the mean of the ith group. N_i is the number of observations in treatment group i. The first term in expression (8.2) is called the *within* sum of squares, and the second term is called the *between* sum of squares.

A simple example to demonstrate the equality in Eq. (8.2) is shown below, using the data of Table 8.2.

$$\Sigma \, (Y_{ij} - \overline{Y})^2 = \Sigma \, Y^2 - \frac{(\Sigma \, Y)^2}{N} = 160 - \frac{(24)^2}{6} = 64$$

$$\Sigma \, (Y_{ij} - \overline{Y}_i)^2 = (0 - 1)^2 + (2 - 1)^2 + (2 - 3)^2 + (4 - 3)^2 + (6 - 8)^2$$

$$= (10 - 8)^2 = 2 + 2 + 8 = 12$$

$$\Sigma \, N_i (\overline{Y}_i - \overline{Y})^2 = 2(1 - 4)^2 + 2(3 - 4)^2 + 2(8 - 4)^2 = 52$$

Thus, according to Eq. (8.2), 64 = 12 + 52.

The calculations for the analysis make use of simple arithmetic with shortcut formulas for the computations similar to that used in the t-test procedures. Computer programs are available for the analysis of all kinds of analysis of variance designs from the most simple to the most complex. In the latter cases, the calculations can be very extensive and tedious, and use of computers may be almost mandatory. For the one-way design, the calculations pose no difficulty. In many cases, use of a pocket calculator will result in a quicker answer than can be obtained using a less accessible computer. A description of the calculations, with examples, are presented below.

The computational process consists first of obtaining the *sum of squares* (SS) for all of the data.

$$\text{Total sum of squares (SS)} = \Sigma \, (Y_{ij} - \overline{Y})^2 \tag{8.3}$$

The *total sum of squares* is divided into two parts: (a) the SS due to treatment differences (*between-treatment sum of squares*), and (b) the error term derived from the *within-treatment sum of squares*. The within-treatment sum of squares (within SS) divided by the appropriate degrees of freedom is the *pooled variance*, the same as that obtained in the t test for the comparison of two treatment groups. The ratio of the between-treatment mean square to the within-treatment mean square is a measure of treatment differences (see below).

To illustrate the computations, we will use the data from Table 8.1, a comparison of three analytical methods with five replicates per method. Remember that the objective of this experiment is to compare the average results of the three methods. We might think of method A as the standard, accepted method, and methods B and C as modifications of the method, meant to replace method A. As in the other tests of hypotheses described in Chap. 5, we first state the null and alternative hypotheses as well as the significance level, prior to the experiment. For example, in the present case,

$$H_0: \quad \mu_A = \mu_B = \mu_C \qquad H_a: \quad \mu_i \neq \mu_j \qquad \text{for any two means*}$$

1. First, calculate the *total sum of squares* (total SS or TSS). Calculate $\Sigma \, (Y_{ij} - \overline{Y})^2$ [Eq. (8.3)] using all of the data, ignoring the treatment grouping. This is most easily calculated using the shortcut formula

---

*Alternatives to H_0 may also include more complicated comparisons than $\mu_i \neq \mu_j$; see, for example, Sec. 8.2.1.

$$\Sigma \ Y^2 - \frac{(\Sigma \ Y)^2}{N} \tag{1.4}$$

$(\Sigma \ Y)^2$ is the grand total of all of the observations squared, divided by the total number of observations N, and is known as the *correction term*, *C.T.* As mentioned in Chap. 1, the correction term is commonly used in statistical calculations, and is important in the calculation of the sum of squares in the ANOVA.

$$\text{Total sum of squares} \ = \ \Sigma \ Y^2 - \frac{(\Sigma \ Y)^2}{N} \tag{8.4}$$

$$= \ (102^2 + 101^2 + \cdots + 103^2 + \cdots$$

$$+ \ 102^2) - \frac{(1511)^2}{15}$$

$$= \ 152,247 - 152,208.07 \ = \ 38.93$$

2. The *between-treatment sum of squares* (between SS or BSS) is calculated as follows:

$$\text{Between-treatment sum of squares} \ = \ \Sigma \ \frac{T_i^2}{N_i} - C.T. \tag{8.5}$$

T_i is the sum of observations in treatment group i and N_i is the number of observations in treatment group i. N_i need not be the same for each group. In our example, the BSS is equal to

$$\left(\frac{506^2}{5} + \frac{497^2}{5} + \frac{508^2}{5} \right) - 152,208.07 \ = \ 13.73$$

As previously noted, the *treatment* sum of squares is a measure of treatment differences. A large sum of squares means that the treatment differences are large. If the treatment means are identical, the treatment sum of squares will be exactly equal to zero (0).

3. The *within-treatment sum of squares* (WSS) is equal to the difference between the TSS and BSS; that is, TSS = BMS + WMS. The WSS can also be calculated, as in the t test, by calculating $\Sigma \ (Y_{ij} - \overline{Y}_i)^2$ within each group, and pooling the results.

Table 8.3   Analysis of Variance for the Data Shown in
Table 8.1:   Comparison of Three Analytical Methods

Source	d.f.	SS	MS	F
Between methods	2	13.73	6.87	$F = 3.27^*$
Within methods	<u>12</u>	<u>25.20</u>	2.10	
Total	14	38.93		

*P < 0.10.

$$\text{Within-treatment sum of squares} = \text{total SS} - \text{between SS}$$
$$= 38.93 - 13.73$$
$$= 25.20 \qquad\qquad (8.6)$$

Having performed the calculations above, the sum of squares for
each "source" is set out in an "analysis of variance" table, as
shown in Table 8.3.   The ANOVA table includes the *source, degrees
of freedom, sum of squares* (SS), *mean square* (MS) and the *probability* based on the statistical test (F ratio).

The degrees of freedom, noted in Table 8.3, are calculated as
$N_t - 1$ *for the total* (N_t is the total number of observations); *number of treatments minus one for the treatments*; and for the *within
error, subtract d.f. for treatments from the total degrees of freedom*.   In our example,

Total degrees of freedom $= 15 - 1 = 14$

Between-treatment degrees of freedom $= 3 - 1 = 2$

Within-treatment degrees of freedom $= 14 - 2 = 12$

Note that for the within degrees of freedom, we have 4 d.f. from
each of the three groups.   Thus there are 12 d.f. for the within
error term.   The *mean squares* are equal to the sum of squares
divided by the degrees of freedom.

Before discussing the statistical test, the reader is reminded of
the assumptions underlying the analysis of variance model: *independence of errors, equality of variance,* and *normally distributed
errors.*

Testing the Hypothesis of Equal Treatment Means

The *mean squares are variance estimates*. One can demonstrate that the variance estimated by the treatment mean square is a sum of the within variance plus a term that is dependent on treatment differences. If the treatments are identical, the term due to treatment differences is zero, and the between mean square (BMS) will be approximately equal to the within mean square (WMS) on the average. In any given experiment, the presence of random variation will result in nonequality of the BMS and WMS terms, even though the treatments may be identical. If the null hypothesis of equal treatment means is true, the distribution of the BMS/WMS ratio is described by the *F distribution*. Note that under the null hypothesis, both WMS and BMS are estimates of σ^2, the within-group variance.

The F distribution is defined by two parameters, degrees of freedom in the numerator and denominator of the F ratio:

$$F = \frac{BMS \ (2 \ d.f.)}{WMS \ (12 \ d.f.)} = \frac{6.87}{2.10} = 3.27$$

In our example, we have an F with 2 d.f. in the numerator and 12 d.f. in the denominator. A test of significance is made by comparing the observed F ratio to a table of the F distribution with appropriate d.f. at the specified level of significance. The F distribution is an asymmetric distribution with a long tail at large values of F, as shown in Fig. 8.1. (See also Secs. 3.5 and 5.3.) To tabulate all the probability points of all F distributions would not be possible. Tables of F, similar to the t table, usually tabulate points at commonly used α levels. The cutoff points ($\alpha = 0.01, 0.05$) for F with n_1 and n_2 d.f. (numerator and denominator) are given in Table IV.6. The probabilities in this table (1% and 5%) are in the upper tail, usually reserved for one-sided tests. This table is used to determine statistical "significance" for the analysis of variance. Although the alternative hypothesis in ANOVA (H_a: at least two treatment means not equal) is two-sided, the ANOVA F test (BMS/WMS) uses the upper tail of the F distribution because, theoretically, the BMS cannot be smaller than the WMS.* (Thus the F ratio will be less than 1 only due to chance variability.) The BMS (between mean square) is composed of the WMS *plus* a possible

---

*This may be clearer if one thinks of the null and alternative hypotheses in ANOVA as H_0: $\sigma_B^2 = \sigma_W^2$; H_a: $\sigma_B^2 > \sigma_W^2$.

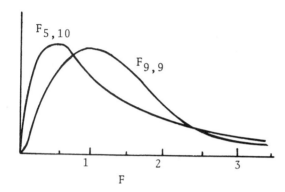

Figure 8.1   Some F distributions.

"treatment" term.   Only large values of the F ratio are considered to be significant.   In our example, Table 8.3 shows the F ratio to be equal to 3.27.   Referring to Table IV.6, the value of F needed for significance at the 5% level is 3.89 (2 d.f. in the numerator and 12 d.f. in the denominator).   Therefore, we cannot reject the hypothesis that all means are equal: method A = method B = method C ($\mu_A = \mu_B = \mu_C$).

8.1.2   Summary of Procedure for One-Way ANOVA

1.   Choose experimental design and state the null hypothesis.
2.   Define the α level.
3.   Choose samples, perform the experiment, and obtain data.
4.   Calculate the total sum of squares and between sum of squares.
5.   Calculate the within sum of squares as the difference between the total SS and the between SS.
6.   Construct an analysis of variance table with mean squares.
7.   Calculate the F statistic (BMS/WMS).
8.   Refer the F ratio statistic to Table IV.6 (n_1 and n_2 d.f., where n_1 is the d.f. for the BMS and n_2 is the d.f. for the WMS).
9.   If the calculated F is equal to or greater than the table value for F at the specified α level of significance, at least two of the treatments can be said to differ.

8.1.3 A Common but Incorrect Analysis of the Comparison of Means from More Than Two Groups

In the example in Sec. 8.1.1, if more than two assay methods are to be compared, the correct statistical procedure is a one-way ANOVA. A common error made by those persons not familiar with ANOVA is to perform three separate t tests on such data: comparing method A to method B, method A to method C, and method B to method C. This would require three analyses and "decisions," which can result in apparent contradictions. For example, decision statements based on three separate analyses could read:

Method A gives higher results than method B ($P < 0.05$).
Method A is not significantly different from method C ($P > 0.05$).
Method B is not significantly different from method C ($P > 0.05$).

These are the conclusions one would arrive at if separate t tests were performed on the data in Table 8.1 (see Exercise Problem 1). One may correctly question: If A is larger than B, and C is slightly larger than A, how can C not be larger than B? The reasons for such apparent contradictions are (a) the use of different variances for the different comparisons, and (b) performing three tests of significance on the same set of data. Analysis of variance obviates such ambiguities by using a common variance for the single test of significance (the F test).* The question of multiple comparisons (i.e., multiple tests of significance) is addressed in the following section.

8.2 PLANNED VERSUS A POSTERIORI (UNPLANNED) COMPARISONS IN ANOVA

Often, in an experiment involving more than two treatments, more specific hypotheses than the global hypothesis, $\mu_1 = \mu_2 = \mu_3 = \cdots$, are proposed in advance of the experiment. These are known as *a priori* or *planned comparisons*. For example, in our example of

---

*We have assumed in the previous discussion that the variances in the different treatment groups are the same. If the number of observations in each group are equal, the ANOVA will be close to correct in the case of moderate variance heterogeneity. If in doubt, a test to compare variances may be performed; see Sec. 5.3.

the three analytical methods, if method A is the standard method, we may have been interested in a comparison of each of the two new methods, B and C, with A (i.e., H_0: $\mu_A = \mu_C$ and $\mu_A = \mu_B$). We may proceed to make these comparisons at the conclusion of the experiment using the usual t-test procedure with the following proviso: *The estimate of the variance is obtained from the ANOVA, the pooled within mean square term.* This estimate comes from all the groups, not only the two groups being compared. ANOVA procedures, like the t test, assume that the variances are equal in the groups being tested.* Therefore, the *within mean square* is the best estimate of the common variance. In addition, the increased d.f. resulting from this estimate results in increased precision and power (Chap. 7) of the comparisons. A smaller value of t is needed to show "significance" compared to the t test, which uses only the data from a specific comparison, in general. Tests of only those comparisons planned a priori should be made using this procedure. This means that the α level (e.g., 5%) applies to each comparison.

Indiscriminate comparisons made after the data has been collected, such as looking for the largest differences as suggested by the data, will always result in more significant differences than those suggested by the stated level of significance. We shall see in Sec. 8.2.1 that a posteriori tests (i.e., unplanned tests made after data have been collected) can be made. However, a "penalty" is imposed which makes it more difficult to find "significant" differences. This keeps the "experiment-wise" α level at the stated value (e.g., 5%). (For a further explanation, see Sec. 8.2.1.) The statistical tests for the two planned comparisons as described above are performed as follows (a two-independent-groups t test with WMS equal to error, the pooled variance):

Method A vs. method B:

$$\frac{|\,101.2 - 99.4\,|}{\sqrt{2.1(1/5 + 1/5)}} = 1.96$$

Method A vs. method C:

$$\frac{|\,101.2 - 101.6\,|}{\sqrt{2.1(1/5 + 1/5)}} = 0.44$$

---

*We have assumed in the previous discussion that the variances in the different treatment groups are the same. If the number of observations in each group are equal, the ANOVA will be close to correct in the case of moderate variance heterogeneity. If in doubt, a test to compare variances may be performed; see Sec. 5.3.

Since the t value needed for significance at the 5% level ($d.f. = 12$) is 2.18 (Table IV.4), neither of the comparisons noted previously is significant. However, when reporting such results, a researcher should be sure to include the actual averages. A confidence interval for the difference may also be appropriate. The confidence interval is calculated as described previously [Eq. (5.2)]; but remember to use the WMS for the variance estimate (12 d.f.). Also, the fact that methods A and B are not significantly different does not mean that they are the same. If one were looking to replace method A, other things being equal, method C would be the most likely choice.

If the comparison of methods B and C had been planned in advance, the t test would show a significant difference at the 5% level (see Exercise Problem 3). However, it would be unfair to decide to make such a comparison using the t-test procedure described above only after having seen the results. Now, it should be more clear why the analysis of variance results in different conclusions from that resulting from the comparison of all pairs of treatments using separate t tests:

1. *The variance is pooled from all of the treatments.* Thus it is the pooled variance from all treatments which is used as the error estimate. When performing separate t tests, the variance estimate differs depending on which pair of treatments is being compared. The pooled variance for the ordinary t test uses only the data from the specific two groups that are being compared. The estimates of the variance for each separate t test differ due to chance variability. That is, although an assumption in ANOVA procedures is that the variance is the same in all treatment groups, the *observed* sample variances will be different in different treatment groups because of the variable nature of the observations. This is what we have observed in our example. By chance, the variability for methods A and B was smaller than that for method C. Therefore, when performing individual t tests, a smaller difference of means is necessary to obtain significance when comparing methods A and B than that needed for the comparison of methods A and C, or methods B and C. Also, the degrees of freedom for the t tests are 8 for the separate tests, compared to 12 when the pooled variance from the ANOVA is used. In conclusion, we obtain different results because we used different variance estimates for the different tests, which can result in ambiguous and conflicting conclusions.

2. The F test in the ANOVA takes into account the number of treatments being compared. An α level of 5% means that if all treatments are identical, 1 in 20 experiments (on the average) will show a significant F ratio. That is, the risk of erroneously observing a significant F is 1 in 20. If separate t tests are performed, each at the 5% level, for each pair of treatments (three in our example), the

chances of finding at least one pair of treatments different in a given experiment will be greater than 5%, when the treatments are, in fact, identical. *We should differentiate between the two situations* (a) where we plan, a priori, specific comparisons of interest, and (b) where we make tests a posteriori suggested by the data. In case (a), each test is done at the α level, and each test has an α percent chance of being rejected if treatments are the same. In case (b), having seen the data we are apt to choose only those differences that are large. In this case, experiments will reveal differences where none truly exist much more than α percent of the time.

Multiple testing of data from the same experiment results in a higher significance level than the stated α level *on an experiment-wise basis*. This concept may be made more clear if we consider an experiment in which five assay methods are compared. If we perform a significance (t) test comparing each pair of treatments, there will be 10 tests, $(n)(n - 1)/2$, where n is the number of treatments: $5(4)/2 = 10$ in this example. To construct and calculate 10 t tests is a rather tedious procedure. If treatments are identical and each t test is performed at the 5% level, the probability of finding at least one significant difference in an experiment will be much more than 5%. Thus the probability is very high that at the completion of such an experiment, this testing will lead to the conclusion that *at least* two methods are different. If we perform 10 separate t tests, the α level, on an experiment-wise basis, would be approximately 29%; that is, 29% of experiments analyzed in this way would show at least one significant difference, when none truly exists [2].

The Bonferroni method is often used to control the alpha level for multiple comparisons. For an overall level of alpha, the level is set at α/k for each test, where k is the number of comparisons planned. For the data of Table 8.1, for a test of 2 planned comparisons at an overall level of 0.05, each would be performed at the $0.05/2 = 0.025$ level. If the tests consisted of comparisons of the means (A vs. C) and (A vs. B), t tests could be performed. A more detailed t table than IV.4 would be needed to identify the critical value of t for a two-sided test at the 0.025 level with 12 d.f. This value lies between the tabled values for the 0.05 and 0.01 level and is equal to 2.56. The difference needed for significance at the 0.025 level is

$$2.56 \times \sqrt{2.1 \times 2/5} = 2.35$$

Since the absolute differences for the two comparisons (A vs. C) and (A vs. B) are 0.4 and 1.8, respectively, neither difference is statistically significant.

In the case of preplanned comparisons, significance may be found even if the F test in the ANOVA is not significant. This procedure is considered acceptable by many statisticians. Comparisons made after seeing the data which were not preplanned fall into the category of *a posteriori multiple* comparisons. Many such procedures have been recommended and are commonly used. Several frequently used methods are presented in the following section.

8.2.1 Multiple Comparisons in Analysis of Variance

The discussion above presented compelling reasons to avoid the practice of using many separate t tests when analyzing data where more than two treatments are compared. On the other hand, for the null hypothesis of no treatment differences, a significant F in the ANOVA does not immediately reveal which of the multiple treatments tested differ. Sometimes, with a small number of treatments, inspection of the treatment means is sufficient to show obvious differences. Often, differences are not obvious. Table 8.4 shows the average results and ANOVA table for four drugs with regard to their effect on the reduction of pain, where the data are derived from subjective pain scores (see also Fig. 8.2). The null hypothesis is H_0: $\mu_A = \mu_B = \mu_C = \mu_D$. The alternative hypothesis here is that at least two treatment means differ. The α level is set at 5%. Ten patients were assigned to each of the four treatment groups. The F test with 3 and

Table 8.4 Average Results and ANOVA for Four Analgesic Drugs

	Reduction in pain with drugs			
	A	B	C	D
$\overline{X}$	4.5	5.7	7.1	6.3
S^2	3.0	4.0	4.5	3.8
S	1.73	2.0	2.12	1.95
N	10	10	10	10

ANOVA

Source	d.f.	SS	MS	F
Between drugs	3	36	12	$F_{3,36} = 3.14*$
Within drugs	36	137.7	3.83	
Total	39	173.7		

*P < 0.05.

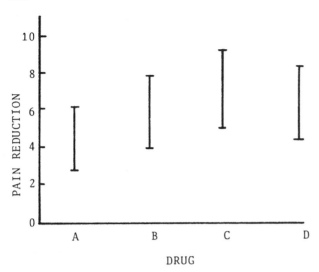

Figure 8.2   Result of pain reduction (± standard deviation) for four drugs with 10 patients per treatment group.

36 d.f. is significant at the 5% level.   An important question that we wish to address here is: Which treatments are different?   Are all treatments different from one another, or are some treatments not significantly different?   This problem may be solved using "multiple comparison" procedures.   The many proposals that address this question result in similar but not identical solutions.   Each method has its merits and deficiencies.   We will present some approaches commonly used for performing a posteriori comparisons. Using these methods, we can test differences specified by the alternative hypothesis, as well as differences suggested by the final experimental data.   These methods will be discussed with regard to comparing individual treatment means.   Some of these methods can be used to compare any linear combination of the treatment means, such as the mean of drug A versus the average of the means for drugs B, C, and D [$\overline{A}$ versus ($\overline{B}$ + $\overline{C}$ + $\overline{D}$)/3].   For a further discussion of this problem, see the Scheffé method below.

Least Significant Difference

The method of "least significant difference" (LSD) proposed by R. A. Fisher, is the simplest approach to a posteriori comparisons. This test is a simple t test comparing all possible pairs of treatment means.   (Note that this approach is not based on preplanned comparisons, discussed in the previous section.) However, the LSD method results in more significant differences than would be expected according to the α level. Because of this, many statisticians do not recommend its use. The LSD test differs from the indiscriminate use of multiple t tests in that one proceeds (a) *only if the F test in the ANOVA is significant,* and (b) *the pooled (within MS) variance is used as the variance estimate in* the t test procedure. The least significant difference (LSD) approach is illustrated using the data from Table 8.4.

Since $t = (\overline{X}_1 - \overline{X}_2)/ \sqrt{S^2(1/N_1 + 1/N_2)}$,

$$LSD = (\overline{X}_1 - \overline{X}_2) = t \sqrt{S^2\left(\frac{1}{N_1} + \frac{1}{N_2}\right)} \tag{8.7}$$

If the sample sizes are equal in each group ($N_1 = N_2 = N$),

$$LSD = t \sqrt{\frac{2S^2}{N}} \tag{8.8}$$

where S^2 is the within mean square variance and t is the tabulated value of t at the α level, with appropriate degrees of freedom (d.f. = the number of degrees of freedom from the WMS of the ANOVA table). Any difference of two means that is equal to or exceeds the LSD is significant at the α level. From Table IV.4, the value of t at the 5% level with 36 d.f. is 2.03. The variance (from the ANOVA in Table 8.4 is 3.83. Therefore, the LSD is

$$LSD = 2.03 \sqrt{\frac{2(3.83)}{10}} = 1.78$$

The average pain reductions for drugs C and D are significantly greater than that for drug A ($\overline{C} - \overline{A} = 2.6$; $\overline{D} - \overline{A} = 1.8$).

Note that in the example shown in Table 8.1 (ANOVA table in Table 8.3), the F test is *not* significant. Therefore, one would not use the LSD procedure to compare the methods, after seeing the experimental results. If a comparison had been planned a priori, the LSD test could be correctly applied to the comparison.

Tukey's Multiple Range Test

Tukey's multiple range test is a commonly used multiple comparison test based on keeping the error rate at α (e.g., 5%) from an "experiment-wise" viewpoint. By "experiment-wise" we mean that if no treatment differences exist, the probability of finding at least one significant difference for a posteriori tests in a given experiment is α (e.g., 5%). This test is more conservative than the LSD test. This means that a larger difference between treatments is needed for significance in the Tukey test than in the LSD test. On the other hand, although the experiment-wise error is underestimated using the LSD test, the LSD test is apt to find real differences more often than will the Tukey multiple range test. (The LSD test has greater power.) Note that a trade-off exists. The easier it is to obtain significance, the greater the chance of mistakenly calling treatments different (α error), but the less chance of missing real differences (β error). The balance between these risks depends on the costs of errors in each individual situation. (See Chap. 6 for a further discussion of these risks.)

In the multiple range test, treatments can be compared without the need for a prior significant F test. However, the analysis of variance should always be carried out. The error term for the treatment comparisons comes from the ANOVA, the within mean square in the one-way ANOVA. Similar to the LSD procedure, a least significant difference can be calculated. Any difference of treatment means exceeding

$$Q \sqrt{\frac{S^2}{N}} \tag{8.9}$$

is significant. S^2 *is the "error" variance from the ANOVA* (within mean square for the one-way ANOVA) *and N is the sample size.* This test is based on equal sample sizes in each group. If the sample sizes are not equal in the two groups to be compared, an approximate method may be used with N replaced by $2N_1 N_2/(N_1 + N_2)$, where N_1 and N_2 are the sample sizes of the two groups. Q is the value of the "studentized range" found in Table IV.7, a short table of Q at the 5% level. More extensive tables of Q may be found in Ref. 1 (Table A-18a). The value of Q depends on the *number of means being tested* (the number of treatments in the ANOVA design) and the *degrees of freedom for error* (again, the within mean square d.f. in the one-way ANOVA). In the example of Table 8.4, the number of treatments is 4, and the d.f. for error is 36. From Table IV.7, the value of Q is approximately 3.81. Any difference of means greater than

$$3.81 \sqrt{\frac{1.83}{10}} = 2.36$$

is significant at the 5% level. Therefore, this test finds only drugs A and C to be significantly different.

This test is more conservative than the LSD test. However, one must understand that the multiple range test tries to keep the error rate at α on an experiment-wise basis. In the LSD test, the error rate is greater than α for each experiment.

Scheffé Method

The Tukey method should be used if we are only interested in the comparison of treatment means (after having seen the data). However, for more complicated comparisons (also known as *contrasts*) for a large number of treatments, the Scheffé method will often result in shorter intervals needed for significance. As in the Tukey method, the Scheffé method is meant to keep the α error rate at 5%, for example, on an experiment-wise basis. For the comparison of two means, the following statistic is computed:

$$\sqrt{S^2(k - 1)F\left(\frac{1}{N_1} + \frac{1}{N_2}\right)} \qquad (8.10)$$

S^2 is the appropriate variance estimate (WMS for the one-way ANOVA), k is the number of treatments in the ANOVA design, and N_1 and N_2 are the sample sizes of the two groups being compared. F is the table value of F (at the appropriate level) with d.f. of $(k - 1)$ in the numerator, and d.f. in the denominator equal to that of the error term in the ANOVA. Any difference of means equal to or greater than the value computed from expression (8.10) is significant at the α level. Applying this method to the data of Table 8.4 results in the following [$S^2 = 3.83$, $k = 4$, $F(3, 36 \text{ d.f.}) = 2.86$, $N_1 = N_2 = 10$]:

$$\sqrt{3.83(3)(2.86)\left(\frac{1}{10} + \frac{1}{10}\right)} = 2.56$$

Using this method, treatments A and C are significantly different. This conclusion is the same as that obtained using the Tukey method. However, treatments A and C barely make the 5% level; the difference needed for significance in the Scheffé method is greater than that needed for the Tukey method for this simple comparison of means. However, one should appreciate that the Scheffé method can be applied to more complicated contrasts with suitable modification of Eq. (8.10).

Suppose that drug A is a control or standard drug, and drugs B and C are homologous experimental drugs. Conceivably, one may be interested in comparing the results of the average of drugs B and C to drug A. From Table 8.4, the average of the means of drugs B and C is

$$\frac{5.7 + 7.1}{2} = 6.4$$

For tests of significance of comparisons (contrasts) for the general case, Eq. (8.10) may be written as

$$\sqrt{(k - 1)FV(\text{contrast})} \qquad\qquad\qquad (8.11)$$

where $(k - 1)$ and (F) are the same as in Eq. (8.10), and V(contrast) is the variance estimate of the contrast. Here the contrast is

$$\frac{\overline{X}_B + \overline{X}_C}{2} - \overline{X}_A$$

The variance of this contrast is (see also App. I)

$$\frac{s^2/N_B + s^2/N_C}{4} + \frac{s^2}{N_A} = s^2\left(\frac{1}{20} + \frac{1}{10}\right) = \frac{3s^2}{20}$$

(Note that $N_A = N_B = N_C = 10$ in this example.)   From Eq. (8.11), a difference of $(\overline{X}_B + \overline{X}_C)/2 - \overline{X}_A$ exceeding

$$\sqrt{3(2.86)(3.83)\,\frac{3}{20}} = 2.22$$

will be significant at the 5% level.   The observed difference is

$$6.4 - 4.5 = 1.9$$

Since the observed difference does not exceed 2.22, the difference between the average results of drugs B and C versus drug A is not significant $(P > 0.05)$.   For a further discussion of this more advanced topic, the reader is referred to Ref. 3.

Newman-Keuls Test

The Newman-Keuls test uses the multiple range factor Q (see Tukey's Multiple Range Test) in a sequential fashion.   In this test, the means to be compared are first arranged in order of magnitude.   For the data of Table 8.4, the means are 4.5, 5.7, 6.3, and 7.1 for treatments A, B, D, and C, respectively.

To apply the test, compute the difference needed for significance for the comparison of 2, 3 . . . n means (where n is the total number of treatment means).   In this example, the experiment consists of 4 treatments.   Therefore, we will obtain differences needed for significance for 2, 3, and 4 means.

Initially, consider the first two means using the Q test:

$$Q \sqrt{S^2/N} \qquad\qquad (8.12)$$

From Table IV.7, with 2 treatments and 36 d.f. for error, Q = approximately 2.87. From Eq. (8.12),

$$Q \sqrt{S^2N} = 2.87 \sqrt{3.83/10} = 1.78$$

For 3 means, find Q from Table IV.7 for $k = 3$.

$$3.45 \sqrt{3.83/10} = 2.14$$

For 4 means, find Q from Table IV.7 for $k = 4$

$$3.81 \sqrt{3.83/10} = 2.36$$

Note that the last value, 2.36, is the same value as that obtained for the Tukey test.

Thus, the differences needed for 2, 3, and 4 means to be considered significantly different are 1.78, 2.14, and 2.36. This can be represented as follows:

Number of treatments	2	3	4
Critical difference	1.78	2.14	2.36

The 4 ordered means are

A	B	D	C
4.5	5.7	6.3	7.1

The above notation is standard. Any two means connected by the same underscored line are not significantly different. Two means not connected by the underscored line are significantly different. Examination of the two underscored lines in this example shows that the only two means not connected are 4.5 and 7.1, corresponding to treatments A and C, respectively.

The determination of significant and nonsignificant differences follows. The difference between treatments A and C, covering 4 means, is equal to 2.6, which exceeds 2.36, resulting in a significant difference. The difference between treatments A and D is 1.8, which is less than the critical value of 2.14 for 3 means. This is described by the first underscore. (Note that we need not compare A and B or B and D since these will not be considered different based on the first underscore.) Treatments B, D, and C are considered to be not significantly different because the difference between B and C, encompassing 3 treatment means, is 1.4, which is less than 2.14. Therefore, a second underscore includes treatments B, D, and C.

Dunnett's Test

Sometimes experiments are designed to compare several treatments against a control but not among each other. For the data of Table 8.4, treatment A may have been a placebo treatment, whereas treatments B, C, and D are 3 different active treatments. The comparisons of interest are A vs. B, A vs. C, and A vs. D. Dunnett [4,5] devised a multiple comparison procedure for treatments vs. a control. The critical difference for a 2-sided test for any of the comparisons vs. control, D', is defined as:

$$D' = t' \sqrt{s^2(1/N_1 + 1/N_2)}$$

where t' is obtained from Table IV.7A.

In the present example, p, the number of treatments, is equal to 3, and d.f. = 36. For a 2-sided test at the 0.05 level, the value of t' is 2.48 from Table IV.7A. Therefore the critical difference is:

$$2.48 \sqrt{3.83(1/10 + 1/10)} = 2.17$$

Again, the only treatment with a difference from treatment A greater than 2.17 is treatment C. Therefore, only treatment C can be shown to be significantly different from treatment A, the control.

Those readers interested in further pursuing the topic of multiple comparisons are referred to Ref. 4.

8.3 ANOTHER EXAMPLE OF ONE-WAY ANALYSIS OF VARIANCE: UNEQUAL SAMPLE SIZE AND THE FIXED AND RANDOM MODELS

Before leaving the topic of one-way ANOVA, we will describe an example in which the sample sizes of the treatment groups are not equal. We will also introduce the notion of "fixed" and "random" models in analysis of variance.

Table 8.5 shows the results of an experiment comparing tablet dissolution as performed by five laboratories. Each laboratory determined the dissolution of tablets from the same batch of a standard product. Because of a misunderstanding, one laboratory (D) tested 12 tablets, whereas the other four laboratories tested six tablets. The null hypothesis is

Table 8.5 Percent Dissolution After 15 Min for Tablets
from a Single Batch Tested in Five Laboratories

	Laboratory				
	A	B	C	D	E
	68	55	78	75	65
	78	62	63	60	60
	63	67	78	66	66
	56	60	65	69	75
	61	67	70	58	75
	69	73	74	64	70
				71	
				71	
				65	
				77	
				60	
				63	
Total	395	384	428	799	411
$\overline{X}$	65.8	64.0	71.3	66.6	68.5
s.d.	7.6	6.3	6.4	6.1	6.0

$$H_0: \quad \mu_a = \mu_B = \mu_C = \mu_D = \mu_E$$

and

$$H_a: \quad \mu_i \neq \mu_j \quad \text{for at least two means}$$

The analysis of variance calculations are performed in an identical manner to that shown in the previous example (Sec. 8.1.1). The analysis of variance table is shown in Table 8.6. The F test for laboratories (4, 31 d.f.) is 1.15, which is *not* significant at the 5% level (Table IV.6). Therefore, the null hypothesis that the laboratories obtain the same average result for dissolution cannot be rejected.

$$\Sigma X = 2417 \qquad \Sigma X^2 = 163,747 \qquad N = 36$$

$$\text{Total SS} = \Sigma X^2 - \frac{(\Sigma X)^2}{N} = 1472.306$$

Table 8.6   Analysis of Variance Table for the Data in
Table 8.5 for Tablet Dissolution

Source	d.f.	SS	MS	F
Between labs	4	189.726	47.43	$F_{4,31} = 1.15$
Within labs	31	1282.58	41.37	
Total	35	1472.306		

$$\text{Between lab SS} = \frac{(395)^2}{6} + \frac{(384)^2}{6} + \frac{(428)^2}{6} + \frac{(799)^2}{12}$$

$$+ \frac{(411)^2}{6} - \frac{(2417)^2}{36} = 189.726$$

Within lab SS = TSS − BSS = 1472.306 − 189.726 = 1282.58

One should always question the validity of ANOVA assumptions.
In particular, the assumption of independence may be suspect in
this example.   Are tablets tested in sets of six, or is each tablet
tested separately?   If tablets are tested one at a time in separate
runs, the results are probably independent.   However, if six tablets
are tested at one time, it is possible that the dissolution times may
be related due to particular conditions which exist during the experiment.   For example, variable temperature setting and mixing speed
would affect all six tablets in the same (or similar) way.   A knowledge of the particular experimental system and apparatus, and/or
experimental investigation, are needed to assess possible dependence
in such experiments.   The assumption of equality of variance seems
to be no problem in this experiment (see the standard deviations in
Table 8.5).

Fixed and Random Models

In this example, the interpretation (and possible further analysis)
of the experimental results depends on the nature of the laboratories
participating in the experiment.   The laboratories can be considered to be:

1.   The only laboratories of interest with respect to dissolution
     testing; for example, perhaps the laboratories include only
     those which have had trouble performing the procedure.

2. A random sampling of five laboratories, selected to determine the reproducibility (variability) of the method when performed at different locations.

The former situation is known as a *fixed model*. Inferences based on the results apply only to those laboratories included in the experiment. The latter situation is known as a *random model*. The random selection of laboratories suggests that the five laboratories are a sample chosen among many possible laboratories. Thus inferences based on these results can be applied to all laboratories in the population of laboratories being sampled.

One way of differentiating a fixed and random model is to consider which treatment groups (laboratories) would be included if the experiment were to be run again. If the same groups would always be chosen in these perhaps hypothetical subsequent experiments, then the groups are fixed. If the new experiment includes different groups, the groups are random.

The statistical test of the hypothesis of equal means among the five laboratories is the same for both situations, *fixed* and *random*. However, in the random case, one may also be interested in estimating the variance. The estimates of the *within-laboratory* and *between-laboratory* variance are important in defining the reproducibility of the method. This concept is discussed further in Sec. 12.4.1.

8.4 TWO-WAY ANALYSIS OF VARIANCE (RANDOMIZED BLOCKS)

As the one-way ANOVA is an extension of the two-independent-groups t test when an experiment contains more than two treatments, *two-way ANOVA* is an extension of the paired t test to more than two treatments. The two-way design, which we will consider here, is known as a randomized block design (the nomenclature in statistical designs is often a carryover based on the original application of statistical designs in agricultural experiments). In this design, treatments are assigned at random to each experimental unit or "block." (In clinical trials, where a patient represents a block, each patient receives each of the two or more treatments to be tested in random order.)

The randomized block design is advantageous when the level of response of the different experimental units are very different. The statistical analysis separates these differences from the experimental error, resulting in a more precise (sensitive) experiment. For example, in the paired t test, taking differences of the two

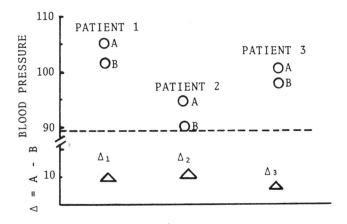

Figure 8.3   Increased precision in two-way designs.

treatments should result in increased precision if the experimental
units receiving the treatments are very different from each other,
but they differentiate the treatments similarly.   In Fig. 8.3, the
three patients are very different in their levels of response (blood
pressure).   However, each patient shows a similar difference between
drugs A and B (A > B).   In a two-independent-groups design
(parallel groups), the experimental error is estimated from differences among experimental units within treatments.   This is usually
larger than the experimental error in a corresponding two-way
design.
        Another example of a two-way (randomized block) design is the
comparison of analytical methods using product from different
batches.   The design is depicted in Table 8.7.   If the batches have
a variable potency, a rational approach is to run each assay method
on material from each batch.   The statistical analysis will separate
the variation due to different batches from the other random error.
The experimental error is free of batch differences, and will be
smaller than that obtained from a one-way design using the same
experimental material.   In the latter case, material would be assigned
to each analytical method at random.
        A popular type of two-way design which deserves mention is
that which consists of pretreatment or baseline readings.   These
designs, called *repeated measures* designs, often consist of pretreatment readings followed by treatment and posttreatment readings observed over time.   Repeated measure designs are discussed
further in Chap. 11.   In these designs, order (order is *time* in
these examples) cannot be randomized.   One should be careful to

Table 8.7 Two-Way Layout for Analytical
Procedures Applied to Different Batches of
Material

	Analytical method			
Batch	A	B	C	•••
1				
2				
3				
•				
•				
•				

avoid bias in situations where a concomitant control is not part of
these experiments. For example, suppose that it is of interest to
determine if a drug causes a change in a clinical effect. One possible approach is to observe pretreatment (baseline) and posttreatment measurements, and to perform a statistical test (a paired t
test) on the "change from baseline." Such an experiment lacks an
adequate control group and interpretation of the results may be
difficult. For example, any observed change or lack of change
could be dependent on the time of observation, when different environmental conditions exist, in addition to any possible drug effect.
A better experiment would include a *parallel* group taking a control
product: a placebo or an active drug (positive control). The difference between change from baseline in the placebo group and test
drug would be an unbiased estimate of the drug effect.

8.4.1 A Comparison of Dissolution of Various Tablet Formulations: Random and Fixed Models in Two-Way ANOVA

Eight laboratories were requested to participate in an experiment
whose objective was to compare the dissolution rates of two generic
products and a standard drug product. The purpose of the experiment was to determine (a) if the products had different rates of
dissolution, and (b) to estimate the laboratory variability (differences) and/or test for significant differences among laboratories.
If the laboratory differences are large, the residual or error sum
of squares will be substantially reduced compared to the corresponding

Table 8.8   Tablet Dissolution After 30 Min for Three Products
(Percent Dissolution)

Laboratory	Generic A	Generic B	Standard	Row total
1	89	83	94	266
2	93	75	78	246
3	87	75	89	251
4	80	76	85	241
5	80	77	84	241
6	87	73	84	244
7	82	80	75	237
8	68	77	75	220
Column total	666	616	664	1946
$\overline{X}$	83.25	77.0	83.0	

$\Sigma\ X^2 = 158,786$

error in the one-way design. The laboratory sum of squares and
the product sum of squares in the analysis of variance are computed
in a manner similar to the calculations in the one-way design. The
residual sum of squares is calculated as the total sum of squares
minus the laboratory and product sum of squares. (The laboratory
and product sum of squares are also denoted as the row and column
sum of squares, respectively.) The *error* or *residual* sum of squares
squares, that part of the total sum of squares remaining after subtracting out that due to rows and columns, is also often denoted as
the *interaction* (C × R) sum of squares.

The hypothesis of interest is

$$H_0: \quad \mu_A = \mu_B = \mu_C$$

That is, the average dissolution rates of the three products are
equal. The level of significance is set at 5%. The experimental results are shown in Table 8.8.

The analysis proceeds as follows:

Total sum of squares (TSS)

$$= \Sigma\ X^2 - C.T. = 89^2 + 93^2 + \cdots + 75^2 + 75^2 - \frac{(1946)^2}{24}$$

$$= 158,786 - 157,788.2 = 997.8$$

Column sum of squares (CSS) or product SS

$$= \frac{\Sigma C_j^2}{R} - C.T. = \frac{(666^2 + 616^2 + 664^2)}{8} - 157,788.2$$

$= 200.3$ (C_j is the total of column j, R is the number of rows

Row sum of squares (RSS) or laboratory SS

$$= \frac{\Sigma R_i^2}{C} - C.T. = \frac{(266^2 + 246^2 + \cdots + 220^2)}{3} - 157,788.2$$

$= 391.8$ (R_i is the total of row i, C is the number of columns

Residual (C × R) sum of squares (ESS) = TSS − CSS − RSS

$= 997.8 - 200.3 - 391.8 = 405.7$

The ANOVA table is shown in Table 8.9. The *degrees of freedom* are calculated as follows:

Total $= N_t - 1$ N_t = total number of observations

Column $= C - 1$ C = number of columns

Row $= R - 1$ R = number of rows

Residual (C × R) $= (C - 1)(R - 1)$

Tests of Significance

To test for differences among *products* (H_0: $\mu_A = \mu_B = \mu_C$), an F ratio is formed:

$$\frac{\text{drug product MS}}{\text{residual MS}} = \frac{100.2}{29} = 3.5$$

The F distribution has 2 and 14 d.f. According to Table IV.6, an F of 3.74 is needed for significance at the 5% level. Therefore, the products are not significantly different at the 5% level. However, had the a priori comparisons of each generic product versus the standard been planned, one could perform a t test for each of the two comparisons (using 29.0 as the error from the ANOVA), *generic A versus standard* and *generic B versus standard*. Generic

Table 8.9   Analysis of Variance Table for the Data
(Dissolution) from Table 8.8

Source	d.f.	SS	MS	F[a]
Drug products	2	200.3	100.2	$F_{2,14} = 3.5$
Laboratories	7	391.8	56.0	$F_{7,14} = 1.9$
Residual (C × R)	14	405.7	29.0	
Total	23	997.8		

[a]See the text for a discussion of proper F tests.

A is clearly not different from the standard.   The t test for
generic B versus the standard is

$$t = \frac{|\overline{X}_B - \overline{X}_S|}{\sqrt{29(1/8 + 1/8)}} = \frac{6}{2.69} = 2.23$$

This is significant at the 5% level (see Table IV.4, t with 14 d.f. =
2.14).   Also, one could apply one of the multiple comparisons tests,
such as the Tukey test described in Sec. 8.2.1.   According to Eq.
(8.9), any difference exceeding $Q\sqrt{S^2(1/N)}$ will be significant.
From Table IV.7, Q for three treatments and 14 d.f. for error is
3.70 at the 5% level.   Therefore, the difference needed for significance for any pair of treatments for a posteriori tests is

$$3.70 \sqrt{29 \frac{1}{8}} = 7.04$$

Since none of the means differ by more than 7.04, individual comparisons decided upon after seeing the data would show no significance in this experiment.
    The test for laboratory differences is (laboratory MS)/(residual
MS), which is an F test with 7 and 14 d.f.   According to Table
IV.6, this ratio is not significant at the 5% level.   (A value of 2.77
is needed for significance.)   As discussed further below, if *drug
products* is a fixed effect, this test is valid only if interaction
(drug product × laboratories) is absent.   Under these conditions,
the laboratories are not sufficiently different to show a significant
F value at the 5% level.

**Fixed and Random Effects in the Two-Way Model

The proper test of significance in the two-way design depends on the model and the presence of *interaction*. The notion of interaction will be discussed further in the presentation of factorial designs (Chap. 9). In the previous example, the presence of *interaction* means that the three products are ranked differently with regard to dissolution rate by at least some of the eight laboratories. For example, laboratory 2 shows that generic A dissolves fastest among the three products, with generic B and the standard being similar. On the other hand, laboratory 8 shows that generic A is the slowest-dissolving product. Interaction is conveniently shown graphically as in Fig. 8.4. "Parallel curves" indicate no interaction.

Of course, in the presence of error (variability), it is not obvious if the apparent lack of parallelism is real or is due to the inherent variability of the system. An experiment in which a lab makes a single observation on each product, such as is the case in the present experiment, usually contains insufficient information to make decisions concerning the presence or absence of interaction. To test for interaction, an additional error term is needed to test for the significance of the C × R residual term. In this case, the experiment should be designed to have replicates (at least duplicate determinations). In the absence of replication, it is best (usually) to assume that interaction is present. This is a conservative point of view. A knowledge of the presence or absence of interaction is

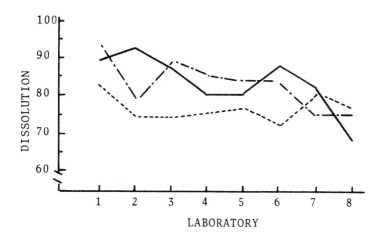

Figure 8.4   Average results of dissolution for eight laboratories.
— · — · — standard; ———— generic A; — — — — generic B.

important in order that one may choose the proper error term for statistical testing (the term in the denominator of the F test) as described below.

The concept of fixed and random effects was introduced under the topic of one-way ANOVA. A "fixed" category includes all the treatments of interest. In the present example, it is apparent that the columns, drug products, are fixed. We are only interested in comparing the two generic products with the standard. Otherwise, we would have included other products of interest in the experiment. On the other hand, the nature of the rows, laboratories, is not obvious. Depending on the context, laboratories may be either *random* or *fixed*. If the laboratories were selected as a random sample among many laboratories that perform such dissolution tests, then "laboratories" is a random factor. In the present situation, the laboratories are chosen as a means of replication in order to compare the dissolution of the three products. Then, inferences based on the result of the experiment are applied to the population of laboratories from which this sample of eight was drawn. We might also be interested in estimating the variance among laboratories in order to have some estimate of the difference to be expected when two or more laboratories perform the same test (see Sec. 12.4.1). If the laboratories chosen were the only laboratories of interest, and inferences based on the experimental results apply only to these eight laboratories, then laboratories are considered to be fixed. Table 8.10 shows when the F tests in the two-way ANOVA are valid depending on the model and the presence of interaction.

Table 8.10   Tests in the Two-Way Analysis of Variance (One Observation per Cell)

Columns	Rows	Interaction	Error term for the F test[a]
Fixed	Fixed	None	Residual (C × R) or within
Fixed	Random	None	Residual (C × R) or within
Random	Random	None	Residual (C × R) or within
Fixed	Fixed	Present	Within
Fixed	Random	Present	Residual (C × R) for fixed effect; use within for random effect
Random	Random	Present	Residual (CR)

[a]*Residual* is the usual residual mean square and includes (C × R), column × row interaction. *Within* is the within mean square calculated from replicate determinations and will be called "error" in future discussions.

In the usual situation, columns are fixed (e.g., drug treatments, formulations) and rows are random (patients, batches, laboratories). In these cases, in the absence of replication, the proper test for columns is (column mean square)/(residual mean square).

Usually, the test for rows is not pertinent if rows are "random." For example, in a clinical study, in which two or more treatments are to be compared, the rows are "patients." The statistical test of interest in such situations is a comparison of the treatments; one does not usually test for patient differences. However, in many laboratory experiments, both column and row effects are of interest. In these cases, if significance testing is to be performed for *both row* and *column* effects (where either or both are fixed), it is a good good idea to include proper replication (see Table 8.10). *Duplicate assays* on the same sample such as may be performed in a dissolution experiment are not adequate to estimate the relevant variability. Replication in this example would consist of repeat runs, using different tablets for each run. An example of a two-way analysis in which replication is included is described in the following section.

8.4.2   Two-Way Analysis of Variance with Replication

Before discussing an example of the analysis of two-way designs with replications, two points should be addressed regarding the implementation of such experiments.

1. It is best to have equal number of replications for each cell of the two-way design. In the dissolution example, this means that each lab replicates each formulation an equal number of times. If the number of replicates is very different for each cell, the analysis and interpretation of the experimental results can be very complicated and difficult.
2. The experimenter should be sure that the experiment is *properly* replicated. As noted above, merely replicating assays on the same tablet is not proper replication in the dissolution example. Replication is an independently run sample in most cases. Each particular experiment has its own problems and definitions regarding replication. If there is any doubt about what constitutes a proper replicate, a statistician should be consulted.

As an example of a replicated, two-way experiment, we will consider the dissolution data of Table 8.8. Suppose that the data presented in Table 8.8 are the average of two determinations (either *two* tablets or *two averages of six tablets each* — a total of 12 tablets). The actual duplicate determinations are shown in Table 8.11. We will consider "products" fixed and "laboratories" random.

Table 8.11   Replicate Tablet Dissolution Data for Eight
Laboratories Testing Three Products (Percent Distribution)

| | Generic | | | |
Laboratory	A	B	Standard	Row total
1	87, 91	81, 85	93, 95	532
2	90, 96	74, 76	74, 82	492
3	84, 90	72, 78	84, 94	502
4	75, 85	73, 79	81, 89	482
5	77, 83	76, 78	80, 88	482
6	85, 89	70, 76	80, 88	488
7	79, 85	74, 86	71, 79	474
8	65, 71	73, 81	70, 80	440
Total	1332	1232	1328	3892
Average	83.25	77.0	83.0	

The analysis of these data results in one new term in the
ANOVA, that due to the *within cell sum of squares*. The *within
cell SS* represents the variability or error due to replicate determinations, and is the pooled SS from within the cells. In the example
shown previously, the SS is calculated for each cell, $\Sigma \, (X - \overline{X})^2$.
For example, for the first cell (generic A in laboratory 1),
$\Sigma \, (X - \overline{X})^2 = (87 - 89)^2 + (91 - 89)^2 = (87 - 91)^2/2 = 8$. The sum
of squares is equal to 8. The within sum of squares is the total of
the sum of squares for the 24 (8 × 3) cells. The residual or inter-
ation SS is calculated as the difference between the total SS and the
sum of the column SS, row SS, and within-cell SS. The calculations
for Table 8.11 are shown below.

$$\text{Total sum of squares} = \Sigma \, X^2 - \text{C.T.}$$

$$= 87^2 + 91^2 + 90^2 + \cdots + 71^2 + 79^2 + 70^2 + 80^2 - \frac{3892^2}{48}$$

$$= 318,160 - 315,576.3 = 2583.7$$

Product sum of squares $= \dfrac{\Sigma \ C_j^2}{Rr} - C.T.$

$$= \frac{1332^2 + 1232^2 + 1328^2}{16} - \frac{3892^2}{48} = 315,977 - 315,576.3$$

$$= 400.7$$

C_j = sum of observations in column j

R = number of rows

r = number of replicates per cell

Laboratory sum of squares $= \dfrac{\Sigma \ R_i^2}{Cr} - C.T.$

$$= \frac{532^2 + 492^2 + \cdots + 440^2}{6} - \frac{3892^2}{48} = 316,360 - 315,576.3$$

$$= 783.7$$

R_i = sum of observations in row i

C = number of columns

r = number of replicates per cell

Within-cell sum of squares*

$$= \Sigma \ (X - \overline{X})^2 \text{ where the sum extends over all cells}$$

$$= \frac{(87 - 91)^2}{2} + \frac{(90 - 96)^2}{2} + \frac{(84 - 90)^2}{2} + \cdots + \frac{(70 - 80)^2}{2}$$

$$= 588$$

$C \times R$ sum of squares $= TSS - PSS - LSS - WSS$

$$= 2583.7 - 400.7 - 783.7 - 588$$

$$= 811.3$$

The ANOVA table is shown in Table 8.12. Note that the F test for drug products is identical to the previous test, where the averages

---

*For duplicate determinations, $\Sigma \ (X - \overline{X})^2 = (X_1 - X_2)^2/2$.

Table 8.12   ANOVA Table for the Replicated Dissolution Data
Shown in Table 8.11

Source	d.f.	SS	MS	F^a
Drug products	2	400.7	200.4	$F_{2,14} = 3.5$
Laboratories	7	783.7	112	$F_{7,24} = 4.6*$
C × R (residual)	14	811.3	58.0	$F_{14,24} = 2.37*$
Within cells (error)	24^b	588	24.5	

[a] Assume drug products fixed, laboratories random.

[b] d.f. for within cells is the pooled d.f., one d.f. for each of 24
cells in general, d.f. = R × C (n − 1), where n is the number of
replicates.
*P < 0.05.

of duplicate determinations were analyzed. However, the laboratory
MS is compared to the within MS to test for laboratory differences.
This test is correct if laboratories are considered either to be fixed
(all FDA laboratories, for example), or random, when drug products
are fixed (see Table 8.10). For significance, $F_{7,24}$ must exceed
2.43 at the 5% level (Table IV.6). The significant result for laboratories suggests that at least some of the laboratories may be considered to give different levels of response. For example, compare
the results for laboratory 1 versus laboratory 8.

Another statistical test, not previously discussed, is available
in this analysis. The F test (C × R MS/within MS) is a test of
interaction. In the absence of interaction (laboratory × drug product), the C × R mean square would equal the within mean square
on the average. A value of the ratio sufficiently larger than 1 is
an indication of interaction. In the present example, the F ratio is
2.37, 58.0/24.5. This is significant at the 5% level (see Table
IV.6, $F_{14,24} = 2.13$ at the 5% level). The presence of a laboratory ×
drug product interaction in this experiment suggests that laboratories
are not similar in their ability to distinguish the three products
(see Fig. 8.4).

****8.4.3   Another Worked Example of Two-Way
Analysis of Variance**

Before leaving the subject of the basic analysis of variance designs,
we will present one further example of a two-way experiment. The

design is a form of a factorial experiment, discussed further in Chap. 9. In this experiment, three drug treatments are compared at three clinical sites. The treatments consist of two doses of an experimental drug (low and high dose) and a control drug. Eight patients were observed for each treatment at each site. The data represent increased performance in an exercise test in asthmatic patients. The results are shown in Table 8.13. In order to follow the computations, the following table of totals (and definitions) should be useful.

$$C.T. = \frac{(371.5)^2}{72} = 1916.84$$

R = number of rows = 3

C = number of columns = 3

r = number of replicates = 8

R_i = total of row i (row 1 = 108.9, row 2 = 140.7, row 3 = 121.9)

C_j = total of column j (column 1 = 69.7, column 2 = 156.1, column 3 = 145.7)

The cell totals are shown below:

	A	B	C	Total
I	27.8	29.4	51.7	108.9
Site II	25	63.8	51.9	140.7
III	16.9	62.9	42.1	121.9
Total	69.7	156.1	145.7	371.5

The computations for the statistical analysis proceed as described in the previous example. The *within-cell mean square* is the pooled variance over the nine cells with 63 degrees of freedom (7 d.f. from each cell). In this example (equal number of observations in each cell), the within-cell mean square is the average of the nine variances calculated from within-cell replication (eight values per cell). The computations are detailed below.

$$\text{Total sum of squares} = \Sigma X^2 - C.T.$$

$$= 4.0^2 + 2.3^2 + 2.1^2 + \cdots + 6.8^2 + 5.2^2 - \frac{(371.5)^2}{72}$$

$$= 2416.77 - 1916.84 = 499.93$$

Table 8.13 Increase in Exercise Time for Three Treatments (Antiasthmatic) at Three Clinical Sites (Eight Patients per Cell)

Site	Treatment			Cell means (standard deviation)		
	A (low dose)	B (high dose)	C (control)	A	B	C
I	4.0, 2.3, 2.1, 3.0, 1.6, 6.4, 1.4, 7.0	3.6, 2.6, 5.5, 6.0, 2.5, 6.0, 0.1, 3.1	5.1, 6.6, 5.1, 6.3, 5.9, 6.2, 6.3, 10.2	3.475 (2.16)	3.675 (2.06)	6.463 (1.61)
II	2.4, 5.4, 3.7, 4.0, 3.3, 0.8, 4.6, 0.8	6.6, 6.4, 6.8, 8.3, 6.9, 9.0, 12.0, 7.8	5.6, 6.4, 8.2, 6.5, 4.2, 5.6, 6.4, 9.0	3.475 (2.16)	3.675 (2.06)	6.463 (1.61)
III	1.0, 1.3, 0.0, 5.1, 0.2, 2.4, 4.5, 2.4	6.0, 8.1, 10.2, 6.6, 7.3, 8.0, 6.8, 9.9	5.8, 4.1, 6.3, 7.4, 4.5, 2.0, 6.8, 5.2	2.113 (1.88)	7.863 (1.52)	5.263 (1.73)

Column sum of squares (treatment SS)

$$= \frac{\Sigma C_j^2}{Rr} - C.T. = \frac{69.7^2 + 156.1^2 + 145.7^2}{3 \times 8} - 1916.84$$

$$= 185.40$$

Row sum of squares (site SS)

$$= \frac{\Sigma R_i^2}{Cr} - C.T. = \frac{108.9^2 + 140.7^2 + 121.9^2}{3 \times 8} - 1916.84$$

$$= 21.30$$

Within cell mean square = pooled sum of squares from the nine cells

$$= \Sigma X^2 - \frac{\Sigma (\text{cell total})^2}{r} = 2416.7 -$$

$$- \frac{27.8^2 + 29.4^2 + 51.7^2 + \cdots + 42.1^2}{8} = 2416.77 - 2214.2$$

$$= 202.57$$

C × R sum of squares (treatment × site interaction SS)

$$= \text{total SS} - \text{treatment SS} - \text{site SS} - \text{within SS}$$

$$= 499.93 - 185.40 - 21.30 - 202.57$$

$$= 90.66$$

Note the shortcut calculation for within SS using the squares of the cell totals. Also note that the C × R SS is a measure of *interaction* of sites and treatments. Before interpreting the results of the experiment from a statistical point of view, both the ANOVA table (Table 8.14) and a plot of the average results should be constructed (Fig. 8.5). The figure helps as a means of interpretation of the ANOVA as well as a means of presenting the experimental results to the "client" (e.g., management).

Conclusions of the Experiment Comparing Three Treatments at Three Sites: Interpretation of the ANOVA Table

The comparisons of most interest come from the treatment and treatment × site terms. The *treatment MS* measures differences among the three treatments. The *treatment × site MS* is a measure of how

Table 8.14 Analysis of Variance Table for the Data of Table 8.13 (Treatments and Sites Fixed)

Source	d.f.	SS	MS	F
Treatments	2	185.4	92.7	$F_{2,63} = 28.8$**
Sites	2	21.3	10.7	$F_{2,63} = 3.31$*
Treatment × site	4	90.66	22.7	$F_{4,63} = 7.05$**
Within	63	202.57	3.215	
Total	71	499.93		

*$P < 0.05$.
**$P < 0.01$.

the three sites differentiate the three treatments. As is usually the case, interactions are most easily visualized by means of a plot (Fig. 8.5). The lack of "parallelism" is most easily seen as a difference between site I and the other two sites. Site I shows that treatment C has the greatest increase in exercise time, whereas the other two sites find treatment B most efficacious. Of course, the

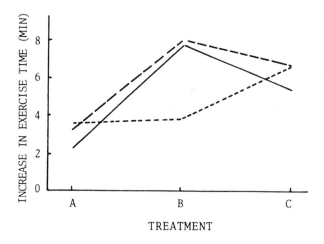

Figure 8.5 Plot of average results from data of Table 8.13.
———— site III; — — — site II; -------- site I.

apparent differences, as noted in Fig. 8.5, may be due to experimental variability. However, the treatment × site interaction term (Table 8.14) is highly significant ($F_{4,63} = 7.05$). Therefore, this interaction can be considered to be real. The presence of interaction has important consequences on the interpretation of the results. The lack of consistency makes it difficult to decide if treatment B or treatment C is the better drug. Certainly, the decision would have been easier had all sites found the same drug best. The final statistical decision depends on whether one considers sites fixed or random. In this example treatments are fixed.

Case 1: Sites fixed. If both treatments and sites are fixed, the proper error term for treatments and sites is the within MS. As shown in Table 8.14, both treatments and sites (as well as interaction) are significant. Inspection of the data suggests that treatments B and C are not significantly different, but that both of these treatments are significantly greater than treatment A (see Exercise Problem 11 for an a posteriori test). Although not of primary interest in such studies, the significant difference among sites may be attributed to the difference between site II and site I, site II showing greater average exercise times (due to higher results for treatment B). However, this difference is of less importance than the interaction of sites and treatments which exists in this study. Thus, although treatments B and C do not differ, on the average, in the fixed site case, site I is different from the other sites in the comparison of treatments B and C. One may wish to investigate further to determine the cause of such differences (e.g., different kinds of patients, different exercise equipment, etc.). If the difference between the results for treatments B and C were dependent on the type of patient treated, this would be an important parameter in drug therapy. In most multiclinic drug trials, clinical sites are selected at random, although it is impractical, if not impossible, to choose clinical sites in a truly random fashion (see also Sec. 11.5). Nevertheless, the interpretation of the data is different if sites are considered to be a random effect.

Case 2: Sites random. If sites are random, and interaction exists, the correct error term for treatments is the treatment × site (interaction) mean square. In this case the F test ($F_{2,4} = 4.09$) shows a lack of significance at the 5% level. The apparently "obvious" difference between treatment A and treatments B and C is not sufficiently large to result in significance because of the paucity of degrees of freedom (4 d.f.). The disparity of the interpretation here compared to the fixed sites case is due to the large interaction. The data suggest that differences among treatments are dependent on the site at which the drugs are tested. If the three sites are random selection from among many possible sites, this very small

Table 8.15   Tests for Treatment Differences in Two-Way
ANOVA with Replicate Observations (Treatments Fixed)

Rows	Interaction	Proper error term
Fixed	Present	Within MS
Fixed	Absent	Within MS or C × R MS
Random	Present	C × R (interaction) MS
Random	Absent	Within MS (conservative test: use C × R MS; pool C × R and within MS — see the text)

sample of sites does not give a reliable estimate of the population averages.

Table 8.15, abstracted from Table 8.10, shows the proper error terms for testing treatment differences, depending on whether sites (rows) are random or fixed. The testing also depends on whether or not there is interaction in the model. Ordinarily, it is not possible to predict the presence (or absence) of interaction in advance of the study. The conservative approach for statistical tests is to assume interaction exists. In this example, if sites are random, the C × R (interaction) mean square is the proper error term for treatments. Often, however, the interaction mean square has few degrees of freedom. This can considerably reduce the power of the test, as is the case in this example. In these situations, if the interaction mean square is not significant, the *interaction* and *within* mean squares may be pooled. This gives a pooled error term with more degrees of freedom than either term alone. This is a controversial procedure, but can be considered acceptable if interaction is clearly not present.

KEY TERMS

Alpha level	Block
ANOVA	Bonferroni test
ANOVA table	Completely randomized design
A posteriori comparisons	Components of variance
A priori comparisons	Contrasts
Assumptions	Control
Between-treatment sum of	Correction term
squares or mean square	Degrees of freedom
(BSS or BMS)	Designed experiments

Dunnett's test	Precision
Error	Randomized block design
Error sum of squares or mean square (ESS or EMS)	Random model
	Repeated measures design
Experimental error	Replicates
Experimental units	Residual
F distribution	Scheffé method for multiple comparisons
Fixed model	
Independence	Shortcut computing formulas
Interaction	Source
LSD procedure for multiple comparisons mean square	Sum of squares
	Symmetry
Model	Total sum of squares (TSS)
Multiple comparisons	Treatments
Newman-Keuls' test	Treatment sum of squares or mean square
One-way analysis of variance	
Parallel groups	T tests
Parallelism	Tukey's multiple range test
Placebo	Two-way analysis of variance
Pooled variance	Within sum of squares or mean square (WSS or WMS)
Positive control	
Power	

EXERCISES

1. Perform three separate t tests to compare method A to method B, method A to method C, and method B to method C in Table 8.1. Compare the results to that obtained from the ANOVA (Table 8.3).

2. Treatments A, B, and C are applied to six experimental subjects with the following results:

A	B	C
1	3	4
5	2	1

Perform an ANOVA and interpret the between-treatment mean square.

3. Repeat the t tests from Exercise Problem 1, but use the "pooled" error term for the tests. Explain why the results are different from those calculated in Problem 1. When is it appropriate to perform separate t tests?

4. It is suspected that four analysts in a laboratory are not performing accurately. A known sample is given to each analyst and replicate assays performed by each with the following results:

	Analyst		
I	II	III	IV
10	9	8	9
11	10	9	9
10	11	8	8

(a) State the null and alternative hypotheses.
(b) Is this a fixed or a random model?
(c) Perform an ANOVA. Use the LSD procedure to show which analysts differ if the "analyst" mean square is significant at the 5% level.
(d) Use Tukey's and Scheffé's multiple comparison procedures to test for treatment (analyst) differences. Compare the results to those in part (c).

5. Physicians from seven clinics in the United States were each asked to test a new drug on three patients. These physicians are considered to be among those who are expert in the disease being tested. The seventh physician tested the drug on only two patients. The physicians had a meeting prior to the experiment to standardize the procedure so that all measurements were uniform in the seven sites. The results were as follows:

			Clinic			
1	2	3	4	5	6	7
9	11	6	10	5	7	12
8	9	9	10	3	7	10
7	13	9	7	4	7	—

(a) Perform an ANOVA
(b) Are the results at the different clinics significantly different at the 5% level?
(c) If the answer to part (b) is yes, which clinics are different? Which multiple comparison test did you use?

**6. Are the following examples random or fixed? Explain.
    (a) Blood pressure readings of rats are taken after the administration of four different drugs.
    (b) A manufacturing plant contains five tablet machines. The same product is made on all machines, and a random sample of 100 tablets is chosen from each machine and weighed individually. The problem is to see if the machines differ with respect to the weight of tablets produced.
    (c) Five formulations of the same product are compared. After 6 months, each formula is assayed in triplicate to compare stability.
    (d) Same as part (b) except that the plant has 20 machines. Five machines are selected at random for the comparison.
    (e) Ten bottles of 100 tablets are selected at random in clusters 10 times during the packaging of tablets (a total of 10,000 tablets). The number of defects in each bottle are counted. Thus we have 10 groups, each with 10 readings. We want to compare the average number of defects in each cluster.

7. Dissolution is compared for three experimental batches with the following results (each point is the time in minutes for 50% dissolution for a single tablet).

Batch 1: 15, 18, 19, 21, 23, 26
Batch 2: 17, 18, 24, 20
Batch 3: 13, 10, 16, 11, 9

    (a) Is there a significant difference among batches?
    (b) Which batch is different?
    (c) Is this a fixed or a random model?

8. In a clinical trial, the following data were obtained comparing placebo and two drugs:

	Placebo		Drug 1		Drug 2	
Patient	Predrug	Postdrug	Predrug	Postdrug	Predrug	Postdrug
1	180	176	170	161	172	165
2	140	142	143	140	140	141
3	175	174	180	176	182	175
4	120	128	115	120	122	122
5	165	165	176	170	171	166
6	190	183	200	195	192	185

(a) Test for treatment differences, using only postdrug values.

(b) Test for treatment differences by testing the change from baseline (predrug).

(c) For problem 8(b), perform a posteriori multiple comparison tests (1) comparing all pairs of treatments using Tukey's multiple range rest and the Newman-Keuls' test and (2) comparing drug 1 and drug 2 to control using Dunnett's test.

9. Tablets were made on six different tablet presses during the course of a run (batch). Five tablets were assayed during the 5-hour run, one tablet during each hour. The results are as follows:

Hour	Press					
	1	2	3	4	5	6
1	47	49	46	49	47	50
2	48	48	48	47	50	50
3	52	50	51	53	51	52
4	50	47	50	48	51	50
5	49	46	50	49	47	49

(a) Are presses and hours fixed or random?

(b) Do the presses give different results (5% level)?

(c) Are the assay results different at the different hours (5% level)?

(d) What assumptions are made about the presence of interaction?

(e) If the assay results are significantly different at different hours, which hour(s) is different from the others?

**10. Duplicate tablets were assayed at hours 1, 3, and 5 for the data in Problem 9, using only presses 2, 4, and 6, with the following results:

Hour	Press		
	2	4	6
1	49,52	49,50	50,53
3	50,48	53,51	52,55
5	46,47	49,52	49,53

If presses and hours are fixed, test for the significance of presses and hours at the 5% level. Is there significant interaction? Explain in words what is meant by interaction in this example.

11. Use Tukey's multiple range test to compare all three treatments (a posteriori test) for the data of Tables 8.13 and 8.14.

REFERENCES

1. Dixon, W. J. and Massey, F. J., Jr., *Introduction to Statistical Analysis*, 3rd ed., McGraw-Hill, New York, 1969.
2. Snedecor, G. W. and Cochran, W. G., *Statistical Methods*, 7th ed., Iowa State University Press, Ames, Iowa, 1980.
3. Scheffe, H., *The Analysis of Variance*, Wiley, New York, 1964.
4. Dunnett, C. and Goldsmith, C., in *Statistics in the Pharmaceutical Industry*, C. R. Buncher and J.-Y. Tsay, Eds., Marcel Dekker, New York, 1981.
5. Steel, R. G. D. and Torrie, J. H., *Principles and Procedure of Statistics*, McGraw-Hill, New York, 1960.

9

**Factorial Designs

Factorial designs are used in experiments where the effects of different factors, or conditions, on experimental results are to be elucidated. Some practical examples where factorial designs are optimal are experiments to determine the effect of pressure and lubricant on the hardness of a tablet formulation, to determine the effect of disintegrant and lubricant concentration on tablet dissolution, or to determine the efficacy of a combination of two active ingredients in an over-the-counter cough preparation. Factorial designs are the designs of choice for simultaneous determination of the effects of several factors and their interactions. This chapter introduces some elementary concepts of the design and analysis of factorial designs.

9.1 DEFINITIONS (VOCABULARY)

9.1.1 Factor

A *factor* is an *assigned variable* such as concentration, temperature, lubricating agent, drug treatment, or diet. The choice of factors to be included in an experiment depends on experimental objectives and is predetermined by the experimenter. A factor can be qualitative or quantitative. A *quantitative factor* has a numerical value assigned to it. For example, the factor "concentration" may be given the values 1%, 2%, and 3%. Some examples of *qualitative factors* are treatment, diets, batches of material, laboratories, analysts, and tablet diluent. Qualitative factors are assigned names rather than numbers. Although factorial designs may have one or many factors, only experiments with two factors will be considered in this chapter. Single-factor designs fit the category of one-way

ANOVA designs. For example, an experiment designed to compare three drug substances using different patients in each drug group is a one-way design with the single factor "drugs."

9.1.2 Levels

The *levels* of a factor are the values or designations assigned to the factor. Examples of levels are 30° and 50° for the factor "temperature," 0.1 molar and 0.3 molar for the factor "concentration," and "drug" and "placebo" for the factor "drug treatment."

The *runs* or *trials* that comprise factorial experiments consist of all combinations of all levels of all factors. As an example, a two-factor experiment would be appropriate for the investigation of the effects of drug concentration and lubricant concentration on dissolution time of a tablet. If both factors were at two levels (two concentrations for each factor), four runs (dissolution determinations for four formulations) would be required, as follows:

Symbol	Formulation
(1)	Low drug and low lubricant concentration
a	Low drug and high lubricant concentration
b	High drug and low lubricant concentration
ab	High drug and high lubricant concentration

"Low" and "high" refer to the low and high concentrations preselected for the drug and lubricant. (Of course, the actual values selected for the low and high concentrations of drug will probably be different from those chosen for the lubricant.) The notation (symbol) for the various combinations of the factors, (1), a, b, ab, is standard. When both factors are at their low levels, we denote the combination as (1). When factor A is at its high level and factor B is at its low level, the combination is called a. b means that only factor B is at the high level, and ab means that both factors A and B are at their high levels.

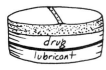 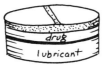 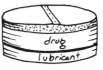 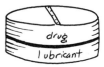

(1)   a   b   ab

9.1.3 Effects

The *effect* of a factor is the change in response caused by varying
the level(s) of the factor. The *main effect* is the *effect* of a factor
averaged over all levels of the other factors. In the previous example, a two-factor experiment with two levels each of drug and
lubricant, the main effect due to drug would be the difference between the average response when drug is at the high level (runs b
and ab) and the average response when drug is at the low level
[runs (1) and a]. For this example the main effect can be characterized as a linear response, since the effect is the difference between the two points shown in Fig. 9.1.

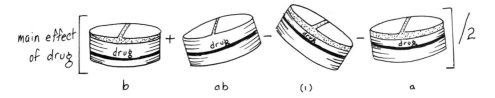

More than two points would be needed to define more clearly the
nature of the response as a function of the factor drug concentration. For example, if the response plotted against the levels of a
quantitative factor is not linear, the definition of the main effect is
less clear. Figure 9.2 shows an example of a curved (quadratic)
response based on experimental results with a factor at three levels.
In many cases, an important objective of a factorial experiment is to

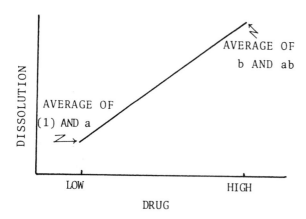

Figure 9.1   Linear effect of drug.   a = lubricant; b = drug.

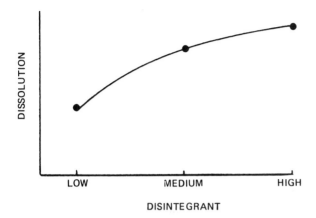

Figure 9.2 Nonlinear (quadratic) effect.

characterize the effect of changing levels of a factor or combinations of factors on the response variable.

9.1.4 Interaction

Interaction may be thought of as a lack of "additivity of factor effects." For example, in a two-factor experiment, if factor A has an effect equal to 5 and factor B has an effect of 10, additivity would be evident if an effect of 15 (5 + 10) were observed when both A and B are at their high levels (in a two-level experiment). (It is well worth the extra effort to examine and understand this concept as illustrated in Fig. 9.3.)

If the effect is greater than 15 when both factors are at their high levels, the result is *synergistic* (in biological notation) with respect to the two factors. If the effect is less than 15 when A and B are at their high levels, an *antagonistic* effect is said to exist. In statistical terminology, the lack of additivity is known as *interaction*. In the example above (two factors each at two levels), interaction can be described as the difference between the effects of drug concentration at the two lubricant levels. Equivalently, interaction is also the difference between the effects of lubricant at the two drug levels. More specifically, this means that the drug effect measured when the lubricant is at the low level [a − (1)] is *different* from the drug effect measured when the lubricant is at the high level (ab − b). If the drug effects are the same in the presence of both high and low levels of lubricant, the system is additive, and no interaction exists. Interaction is conveniently

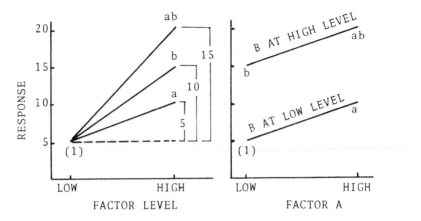

Figure 9.3   Additivity of effects: Lack of interaction.

shown graphically as depicted in Fig. 9.4.   If the lines representing the effect of drug concentration at each level of lubricant are
"parallel," there is no interaction.   Lack of parallelism, as shown in
Fig. 9.4B, suggests interaction.   Examination of the lines in Fig.
9.4B reveals that the effect of drug concentration on dissolution is
dependent on the concentration of lubricant.   The effects of drug
and lubricant are not additive.

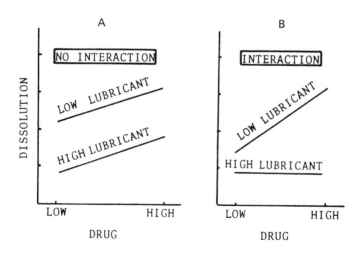

Figure 9.4   Illustration of interaction.

Factorial designs have many advantages [1].

1. In the absence of interaction, factorial designs have maximum efficiency in estimating main effects.

2. If interactions exist, factorial designs are necessary to reveal and identify the interactions.

3. Since factor effects are measured over varying levels of other factors, conclusions apply to a wide range of conditions.

4. Maximum use is made of the data since all main effects and interactions are calculated from all of the data (as will be demonstrated below).

5. Factorial designs are orthogonal; all estimated effects and interactions are independent of effects of other factors. Independence, in this context, means that when we estimate a main effect, for example, the result we obtain is due only to the main effect of interest, and is not influenced by other factors in the experiment. In nonorthogonal designs (as is the case in many multiple-regression-type "fits" — see App. III), effects are not independent. *Confounding* is a result of lack of independence. When an effect is confounded, one cannot assess how much of the observed effect is due to the factor under consideration. The effect is influenced by other factors in a manner that often cannot be easily unraveled, if at all. Suppose, for example, that two drugs are to be compared, with patients from a New York clinic taking drug A and patients from a Los Angeles clinic taking drug B. Clearly, the difference observed between the two drugs is confounded with the different locations. The two locations reflect differences in patients, methods of treatment, and disease state, which can affect the observed difference in therapeutic effects of the two drugs. A simple factorial design where both drugs are tested in both locations will result in an "unconfounded," clear estimate of the drug effect if designed correctly, e.g., equal or proportional number of patients in each treatment group at each treatment site.

9.2 TWO SIMPLE HYPOTHETICAL EXPERIMENTS TO ILLUSTRATE THE ADVANTAGES OF FACTORIAL DESIGNS

The following hypothetical experiment illustrates the advantage of the factorial approach to experimentation when the effects of multiple factors are to be assessed. The problem is to determine the effects of a special diet and a drug on serum cholesterol levels. To this end, an experiment was conducted in which cholesterol changes were measured in three groups of patients. Group A received the drug, group B received the diet, and group C received both the diet and drug. The results are shown below. The

experimenter concluded that there was no interaction between drug
and diet (i.e., their effects are additive).

Drug alone: decrease of 10 mg %
Diet alone: decrease of 20 mg %
Diet + drug: decrease of 30 mg %

However, suppose that patients given *neither* drug nor diet would
have shown a decrease of serum cholesterol of 10 mg % had they
been included in the experiment. (Such a result could occur because of "psychological effects" or seasonal changes, for example.)
Under these circumstances, we would conclude that drug alone has
no effect, that diet results in a cholesterol lowering of 10 mg %, and
that the combination of drug and diet is synergistic. The combination of drug and diet results in a decrease of cholesterol equal to
20 mg %. This concept is shown in Fig. 9.5.

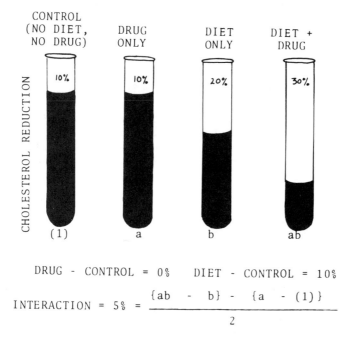

Figure 9.5   Synergism in cholesterol lowering as a result of drug
and diet.

Thus, without a fourth group, the control group (low level of diet and drug), we have no way of assessing the presence of interaction. This example illustrates how estimates of effects can be incorrect when pieces of the design are missing. Inclusion of a control control group would have completed the factorial design, two factors at two levels. Drug and diet are the factors, each at two levels, either present or absent. The complete factorial design consists of the following four groups:

(1) Group on normal diet without drug (drug and special diet at low level)
 a   Group on drug only (high level of drug, low level of diet)
 b   Group on diet only (high level of diet, low level of drug)
 ab Group on diet and drug (high level of drug and high level of diet)

The effects and interaction can be clearly calculated based on the results of these four groups (see Fig. 9.5).

Incomplete factorial designs such as those described above are known as the *one-at-a-time* approach to experimentation. Such an approach is usually very *inefficient*. By performing the entire factorial, we usually have to do *less work*, and we get *more* information. This is a consequence of an important attribute of factorial designs: effects are measured with maximum precision. To demonstrate this property of factorial designs, consider the following hypothetical example. The objective of this experiment is to weigh two objects on an insensitive balance. Because of the lack of reproducibility, we will weigh the items in duplicate. The balance is in such poor condition that the zero point (balance reading with no weights) is in doubt. A typical one-at-a-time experiment is to weigh each object separately (in duplicate) in addition to a duplicate reading with no weights on the balance. The weight of item A is taken as the average of the readings with A on the balance minus the average of the readings with the pans empty. Under the assumption that the variance is the same for all weighings, regardless of the amount of material being weighed, the variance of the weight of A is the sum of the variances of the average weight of A and the average weight with the pans empty (see App. I):

$$\frac{\sigma^2}{2} + \frac{\sigma^2}{2} = \sigma^2 \tag{9.1}$$

Note that the variance of the *difference* of the average of two weighings is the *sum of the variances* of each weighing. (The variance of the average of *two* weighings is $\sigma^2/2$.) Similarly, the variance of the weight of B is $\sigma^2 = \sigma^2/2 + \sigma^2/2$. Thus, based on six readings (two weighings each with the balance empty, with A on the balance and with B on the balance), we have estimated the weights of A and B with variance equal to σ^2, where σ^2 is the variance of a single weighing.

In a factorial design, an extra reading(s) would be made, a reading with both A and B on the balance. In the following example, using a full factorial design, we can estimate the weight of A with the same precision as above using only 4 weighings (instead of 6). In this case the weighings are made without replication. That is, four weighings are made as follows:

(1)	Reading with balance empty	0.5 kg
a	Reading with item A on balance	38.6 kg
b	Reading with item B on balance	42.1 kg
ab	Reading with both items A and B on balance	80.5 kg

With a full factorial design, as illustrated above, the *weight of A* is estimated as (the main effect of A)

$$\frac{a - (1) + ab - b}{2} \tag{9.2}$$

Expression (9.2) says that the estimate of the weight of A is the average of the weight of A alone minus the reading of the empty balance [a − (1)] and the weight of both items A and B minus the weight of B. According to the weights recorded above, the weight of A would be estimated as

$$\frac{38.6 - 0.5 + 80.5 - 42.1}{2} = 38.25 \text{ kg}$$

Similarly, the weight of B is estimated as

$$\frac{42.1 - 0.5 + 80.5 - 38.6}{2} = 41.75 \text{ kg}$$

Note how we use *all the data* to estimate the weights of A and B; the weight of B alone is used to help estimate the weight of A, and vice versa!

Interaction is measured as the average difference of the weights of A in the presence and absence of B as follows:

$$\frac{(ab - b) - [a - (1)]}{2} \tag{9.3}$$

We can assume that there is no interaction, a very reasonable assumption in the present example. (The weights of the combined items should be the sum of the individual weights.) The estimate of interaction in this example is

$$\frac{(80.5 - 42.1) - (38.6 - 0.5)}{2} = 0.3$$

The estimate of interaction is not zero because of the presence of random errors made on this insensitive balance.

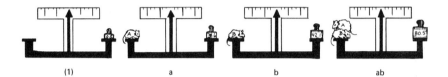

(1)	a	b	ab

In this example, we have made *four* weighings. The variance of the main effects (i.e., the average weights of A and B) is σ^2, *exactly the same variance as was obtained using six weightings in the one-at-a-time experiment!** We obtain the same precision with two-thirds of the work: four readings instead of six. In addition to the advantage of greater precision, if interaction were present, we would have had the opportunity to estimate the interaction effect in the full factorial design. *It is not possible to estimate interaction in the one-at-a-time experiment.*

9.3 PERFORMING FACTORIAL EXPERIMENTS: RECOMMENDATIONS AND NOTATION

The simplest factorial experiment, as illustrated above, consists of four trials, two factors each at two levels. If three factors, A, B, and C, each at two levels, are to be investigated, eight trials are necessary for a full factorial design, as shown in Table 9.1. This is also called a 2^3 experiment, three factors each at two levels.

As shown in Table 9.1, in experiments with factors at two levels, the low and high levels of factors in a particular run are

---

*The main effect of A, for example, is $[a - (1) + ab - b]/2$. The variance of the main effect is $(\sigma_a^2 + \sigma_{(1)}^2 + \sigma_{ab}^2 + \sigma_b^2)/4 = \sigma^2$. σ^2 is the same for all weighings (App. I).

Table 9.1   Eight Experiments for a 2^3
Factorial Design[a]

Combination	A	B	C
(1)	−	−	−
a	+	−	−
b	−	+	−
ab	+	+	−
c	−	−	+
ac	+	−	+
bc	−	+	+
abc	+	+	+

[a]−, factor at low level; +, factor at
high level.

denoted by the absence or presence of the letter, respectively. For
example, if all factors are at their low levels, the run is denoted as
(1). If factor A is at its high level, and B and C are at their low
levels, we use the notation a. If factors A and B are at their high
levels, and C is at its low level, we use the notation ab; and so on.

Before implementing a factorial experiment, the researcher should
carefully consider the experimental objectives vis-à-vis the appropriateness of the design. The results of a factorial experiment may
be used (a) to help interpret the mechanism of an experimental system; (b) to recommend of implement a practical procedure or set of
conditions in an industrial manufacturing situation; or (c) as guid-
ance for further experimentation. In most situations where one is
interested in the effect of various factors or conditions on some experimental outcome, factorial designs will be optimal.

The choice of factors to be included in the experimental design
should be considered carefully. Those factors not relevant to the
experiment, but which could influence the results, should be carefully controlled or kept constant. For example, if the use of different technicians, different pieces of equipment, or different excipients can affect experimental outcomes, but are not variables of
interest, they should not be allowed to vary randomly, if possible.
Consider an example of the comparison of two analytical methods.
We may wish to have a single analyst perform both methods on the
same spectrophotometer to reduce the variability that would be present if different analysts used different instruments. However, there
will be circumstances where the effects due to different analysts and
different spectrophotometers are of interest. In these cases,

different analysts and instruments may be designed into the experiment as additional factors.

On the other hand, we may be interested in the effect of a particular factor, but because of time limitations, cost, or other problems, the factor is held constant, retaining the option of further investigation of the factor at some future time. In the example above, one may wish to look into possible differences among analysts with regard to the comparison of the two methods (an analyst × method interaction). However, time and cost limitations may restrict the extent of the experiment. One analyst may be used for the experiment, but testing may continue at some other time using more analysts to confirm the results.

The more extraneous variables that can be controlled, the smaller with be the residual variation. The residual variation is the random error remaining after the ANOVA removes the variability due to factors and their interactions. If factors known to influence the experimental results, but of no interest in the experiment, are allowed to vary "willy-nilly," the effects caused by the random variation of these factors will become part of the residual error. Suppose the temperature influences the analytical results in the example above. If the temperature is not controlled, the experimental error will be greater than if the experiment is carried out under constant-temperature conditions. The smaller the residual error, the more sensitive the experiment will be in detecting effects or changes in response due to the factors under investigation.

The choice of levels is usually well defined if factors are qualitative. For example, in an experiment where a product supplied by several manufacturers is under investigation, the levels of the factor "product" could be denoted by the name of the manufacturer: company X, company Y, and so on. If factors are quantitative, we can choose two or more levels, the choice being dependent on the size of the experiment (the number of trials and the amount of replication) and the nature of the anticipated response. If a response is known to be a linear function of a factor, two levels would be sufficient to define the response. If the response is "curved" (a quadratic response for example*), at least three levels of the quantitative factor would be needed to characterize the response. Two levels are often used for the sake of economy, but a third level or more can be used to meet experimental objectives as noted above. A rule of thumb used for the choice of levels in two-level experiments is to divide extreme ranges of a factor into four equal parts and take the one-fourth (1/4) and three-fourths (3/4) values as the

---

*A quadratic response is of the form $Y = A + BX + CX^2$, where Y is the response and X is the factor level.

choice of levels [1]. For example, if the minimum and maximum concentrations for a factor are 1% and 5%, respectively, the choice of levels would be 2% and 4% according to this empirical rule.

The trials comprising the factorial experiment should be done in random order if at all possible. This helps ensure that the results will be unbiased (as is true for many statistical procedures). The fact that all effects are averaged over all runs in the analysis of factorial experiments is also a protection against bias.

9.4   A WORKED EXAMPLE OF A FACTORIAL EXPERIMENT

The data in Table 9.2 were obtained from an experiment with three factors each at two levels. There is no replication in this experiment. Replication would consist of repeating each of the eight runs one or more times. The results in Table 9.2 are presented in standard order. Recording the results in this order is useful when analyzing the data by hand (see below) or for input into computers where software packages require data to be entered in a specified or standard order. The standard order for a 2^2 experiment consists of the first four factor combinations in Table 9.2. For experiments with more than three factors, see Davies for tables and an explanation of the ordering [1].

The experiment that we will analyze is designed to investigate the effects of three components (factors) — stearate, drug, and starch — on the thickness of a tablet formulation. In this example,

Table 9.2   Results of 2^3 Factorial Experiment: Effect of Stearate, Drug, and Starch Concentration on Tablet Thickness[a]

Factor combination	Stearate	Drug	Starch	Response (thickness) (cm × 10^3)
(1)	−	−	−	475
a	+	−	−	487
b	−	+	−	421
ab	+	+	−	426
c	−	−	+	525
ac	+	−	+	546
bc	−	+	+	472
abc	+	+	+	522

[a] −, factor at low level; +, factor at high level.

two levels were chosen for each factor. Because of budgetary constraints, use of more than two levels would result in too large an experiment. For example, if one of the three factors were to be studied at three levels, 12 formulations would have to be tested for a 2 × 2 × 3 factorial design. Because only two levels are being investigated, nonlinear responses cannot be elucidated. However, the pharmaceutical scientist felt that the information from this two-level experiment would be sufficient to identify effects that would be helpful in designing and formulating the final product. The levels of the factors in this experiment were as follows:

Factor	Low level (mg)	High level (mg)
A: Stearate	0.5	1.5
B: Drug	60.0	120.0
C: Starch	30.0	50.0

The computation of the main effects and interactions as well as the ANOVA may be done by hand in simple designs such as this one. Readily available computer programs are usually used for more complex analyses. (For n factors, an n-way analysis of variance is appropriate. In typical factorial designs, the factors are usually considered to be fixed.)

For two-level experiments, the effects can be calculated by applying the signs (+ or −) arithmetically for each of the eight responses as shown in Table 9.3. This table is constructed by placing a + or − in columns A, B, and C depending on whether or not the appropriate factor is at the high or low level in the particular run. If the letter appears in the factor combination, a + appears in the column corresponding to that letter. For example, for the product combination ab, a + appears in columns A and B, and a − appears in column C. Thus for column A, runs a, ab, ac, and abc have a + because in these runs, A is at the high level. Similarly, for runs (1), b, c, and bc, a − appears in column A since these runs have A at the low level.

Columns denoted by AB, AC, BC, and ABC in Table 9.3 represent the indicated interactions (i.e., AB is the interaction of factors A and B, etc.). The signs in these columns are obtained by multiplying the signs of the individual components. For example, to obtain the signs in column AB we refer to the signs in column A and column B. For run (1), the + sign in column AB is obtained by multiplying the − sign in column A times the − sign in column B. For run a, the − sign in column AB is obtained by multiplying the

Table 9.3   Signs to Calculate Effects in a 2^3 Factorial Experiment[a]

Factor combination	Level of factor in experiment			Interaction[b]			
	A	B	C	AB	AC	BC	ABC
(1)	−	−	−	+	+	+	−
a	+	−	−	−	−	+	+
b	−	+	−	−	+	−	+
ab	+	+	−	+	−	−	−
c	−	−	+	+	−	−	+
ac	+	−	+	−	+	−	−
bc	−	+	+	−	−	+	−
abc	+	+	+	+	+	+	+

[a] −, factor at low level; +, factor at high level.
[b] Multiply signs of factors to obtain signs for interaction terms in combination [e.g., AB at (1) = (−) × (−) = (+)].

sign in column A (+) times the sign in column B (−). Similarly, for column ABC, we multiply the signs in columns A, B, and C to obtain the appropriate sign. Thus run ab has a − sign in column ABC as a result of multiplying the three signs in columns A, B, and C: (+) × (+) × (−).

The average effects can be calculated using these signs as follows. To obtain the average effect, multiply the response times the sign for each of the eight runs in a column, and divide the result by 2^{n-1}, where n is the number of factors (for three factors, 2^{n-1} is equal to 4). This will be illustrated for the calculation of the main effect of A (stearate). The main effect for factor A is

$$\frac{[-(1) + a - b + ab - c + ac - bc + abc] \times 10^{-3}}{4} \qquad (9.4)$$

Note that the main effect of A is the average of all results at the high level of A minus the average of all results at the low level of A. This is more easily seen if formula (9.4) is rewritten as follows:

$$\text{Main effect of A} = \frac{a + ab + ac + abc}{4} - \frac{(1) + b + c + bc}{4} \qquad (9.5)$$

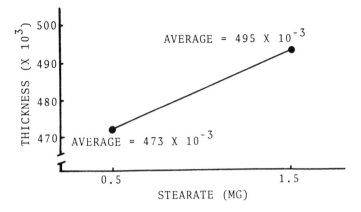

Figure 9.6 Main effect of the factor "stearate."

"Plugging in" the results of the experiment for each of the eight runs in Eq. (9.5), we obtain

$$\frac{[487 + 426 + 456 + 522 - (475 + 421 + 525 + 472)] \times 10^{-3}}{4} = 0.022 \text{ cm}$$

The *main effect of A is interpreted* to mean that the net effect of increasing the stearate concentration from the low to the high level (averaged over all other factor levels) is to increase the tablet thickness by 0.022 cm. This result is illustrated in Fig. 9.6.

The interaction effects are estimated in a manner similar to the estimation of the main effects. The signs in the column representing the interaction (e.g., AC) are applied to the eight responses, and as before the total divided by 2^{n-1}, where n is the number of factors. The interaction AC, for example, is defined as one-half the difference between the effect of A when C is at the high level and the effect of A when C is at the low level (see Fig. 9.7). Applying the signs as noted above, the AC interaction is estimated as

$$\text{AC interaction} = \frac{1}{4} \left\{ (abc + ac - bc - c) - [ab + a - b - (1)] \right\}$$

$$(9.6)$$

The interaction is shown in Fig. 9.7. With starch (factor C) at the high level, 50 mg, increasing the stearate concentration from the low to the high level (from 0.5 mg to 1.5 mg) results in an increased thickness of 0.0355 cm.* At the low level of starch, 30 mg,

---

*(1/2)(abc + ac − bc − c).

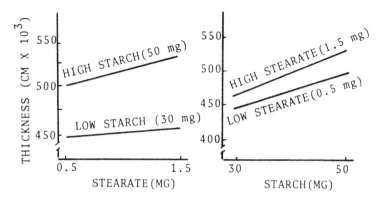

Figure 9.7   Starch × stearate interaction.

increasing stearate concentration from 0.5 mg to 1.5 mg results in
an increased thickness of 0.0085 cm. Thus stearate has a greater
effect at the higher starch concentration, a possible starch × stearate interaction.

Lack of interaction would be evidenced by the same effect of
stearate at both low and high starch concentrations. In a real experiment, the effect of stearate would not be identical at both levels
of starch concentration in the absence of interaction because of the
presence of experimental error. The statistical tests described below show how to determine the significance of observed nonzero
effects.

The description of interaction is "symmetrical." The AC interaction can be described in two equivalent ways: (a) the effect of
stearate is greater at high starch concentrations, or (b) the effect
of starch concentration is greater at the high stearate concentration (1.5 mg) compared to its effect at low stearate concentration
(0.5 mg). The effect of starch at low stearate concentration is
0.051. The effect of starch at high stearate concentration is 0.078.
(Also see Fig. 9.7.)

9.4.1   Data Analysis

Method of Yates

Computers are usually used to analyze factorial experiments. However, hand analysis of simple experiments can give insight into the
properties of this important class of experimental designs. A method devised by Yates for systematically analyzing data from 2^n factorial experiments (n factors each at two levels) is demonstrated in
Table 9.4. The data are first tabulated in standard order (see

Table 9.4 Yates Analysis of the Factorial Tableting Experiment for Analysis Variance

Combination	Thickness (× 10³)	(1)	(2)	(3)	Effect (× 10³) (3)/4	Mean square (× 10⁶) (3)²/8
(1)	475	962	1809	3874	—	—
a	487	847	2065	88	22.0	968
b	421	1071	17	-192	-48.0	4608
ab	426	994	71	22	5.5	60.5
c	525	12	-115	256	64.0	8192
ac	546	5	-77	54	13.5	364.5
bc	472	21	-7	38	9.5	180.5
abc	522	50	29	36	9.0	162

Ref. 1 for experiments with more than three factors). The data are
first added in pairs, followed by taking differences in pairs as
shown in column (1) in Table 9.4.

$$475 + 487 = 962$$
$$421 + 426 = 847$$
$$525 + 546 = 1071$$
$$472 + 522 = 994$$

$$487 - 475 = 12$$
$$426 - 421 = 5$$
$$546 - 525 = 21$$
$$522 - 472 = 50$$

This addition and subtraction process is repeated sequentially on
the n columns. (Remember that n is the number of factors, three
columns for three factors.) Thus the process is repeated in column
(2), operating on the results in column (1) of Table 9.4. Note, for
example, that 1809 in column (2) is 962 + 847 from column (1).
Finally, the process is repeated, operating on column (2) to form
column (3). Column (3) is divided by 2^{n-1} ($2^{n-1} = 4$ for 3 factors)
to obtain the average effect. The mean squares for the ANOVA
(described below) are obtained by dividing the square of column (n)
by 2^n. For example, the mean square attributable to factor A is

$$\text{Mean square for A} = \frac{(88)^2}{8} = 968$$

The mean squares are presented in an ANOVA table, as discussed
below.

Analysis of Variance

The results of a factorial experiment are typically presented in an
ANOVA table, as shown in Table 9.5. In a 2^n factorial, each effect
and interaction has 1 degree of freedom. The error mean square
for statistical tests and estimation) can be estimated in several ways
for a factorial experiment. Running the experiment with replicates
is best. Duplicates are usually sufficient. However, replication
may result in an inordinately large number of runs. Remember that
replicates do not usually consist of replicate analyses or observations on the same run. A true replicate usually is obtained by repeating the run, from "scratch." For example, in the 2^3 experiment described above, determining the thickness of several tablets
from a single run [e.g., the run denoted by a (A at the high
level)] would probably not be sufficient to estimate the experimental
error in this system. The proper replicate would be obtained by

Table 9.5 Analysis of Variance for the Factorial Tableting Experiment

Factor	Source	d.f.	Mean square $(\times 10^6)$	F^a
A	Stearate	1	968	7.2*
B	Drug	1	4608	34.3**
C	Starch	1	8192	61.0**
AB	Stearate × drug	1	60.5	
AC	Stearate × starch	1	364.5	2.7
BC	Drug × starch	1	180.5	
ABC	Stearate × drug × starch	1	162	

[a]Error mean square based on AB, BC, and ABC interactions, 3 d.f.
*P < 0.1.
**P < 0.01.

preparing a new mix with the same ingredients, retableting, and measuring the thickness of tablets in this new batch.* In the absence of replication, experimental error may be estimated from prior experience in systems similar to that used in the factorial experiment. To obtain the error estimate from the experiment itself is always most desirable. Environmental conditions in prior experiments are apt to be different from those in the current experiment. In a large experiment, the experimental error can be estimated without replication by pooling the mean squares from higher-order interactions (e.g., three-way and higher-order interactions) as well as other interactions known to be absent, a priori. For example, in the tableting experiment, we might average the mean squares corresponding to the two-way interactions, AB and BC, and the three-way ABC interaction, if these interactions were known to be zero from prior considerations. The error estimated from the average of the AB, BC, and ABC interactions is

---

*If the tableting procedure in the different runs were identical in all respects (with the exception of tablet ingredients), replicates within each run would be a proper estimate of error.

$$(60.5 + 180.5 + 162) \times \frac{10^{-6}}{3} = 134.2 \times 10^{-6}$$

with 3 degrees of freedom (assuming that these interactions do not exist).

Interpretation

In the absence of interaction, the main effect of a factor describes the change in response when going from one level of a factor to another. If a large interaction exists, the main effects corresponding to the interaction do not have much meaning as such. Specifically, an AC interaction suggests that the effect of A depends on the level of C and a description of the results should specify the change due to A at each level of C. Based on the mean squares in Table 9.5, the effects which are of interest are A, B, C, and AC. Although not statistically significant, stearate and starch interact to a small extent, and examination of the data is necessary to describe this effect (see Fig. 9.7). Since B does not interact with A or C, it is sufficient to calculate the effect of drug (B), averaged over all levels of A and C, to explain its effect. The effect of drug is to *decrease* the thickness 0.048 mm when the drug concentration is raised from 60 mg to 120 mg [Table 9.4, column (3)/4].

9.5   FRACTIONAL FACTORIAL DESIGNS

In an experiment with a large number of factors and/or a large number of levels for the factors, the number of experiments needed to complete a factorial design may be inordinately large. For example, a factorial design with 5 factors each at 2 levels requires 32 experiments; a 3-factor experiment each at 3 levels requires 27 experiments. If the cost and time considerations make the implementation of a full factorial design impractical, fractional factorial experiments can be used in which a fraction (e.g., 1/2, 1/4, etc.) of the original number of experiments can be run. Of course, something must be sacrificed for the reduced work. If the experiments are judiciously chosen, it may be possible to design an experiment so that effects which we believe are negligible are confounded with important effects. (The word "confounded" has been noted before in this chapter.) In fractional factorial designs, the negligible and important effects are indistinguishable, and thus confounded. This will become clearer in the first example.

    To illustrate some of the principles of fractional factorial designs, we will discuss and present an example of a fractional design based on a factorial design where each of 3 factors is at 2 levels, a 2^3 design. Table 9.3 shows the 8 experiments required for the

Table 9.6 2^2 Factorial Design

Experiment	A level	B level	AB
(1)	−	−	+
a	+	−	−
b	−	+	−
ab	+	+	+

full design. With the full factorial design, we can estimate 7 effects from the 8 experiments, the 3 main effects (A, B, and C), and the 4 interactions (AB, AC, BC, and ABC). In a 1/2 replicate fractional design, we perform 4 experiments, but we can only estimate 3 effects. With 3 factors, a 1/2 replicate can be used to estimate the main effects, A, B, and C. The following procedure is used to choose the 4 experiments.

Table 9.6 shows the 4 experiments that define a 2^2 factorial design using the notation described in Sec. 9.3.

To construct the 1/2 replicate with 3 factors, we equate one of the effects to the third factor. In the 2^2 factorial, the interaction, AB is equated to the third factor, C. Table 9.7 describes the 1/2 replicate design for 3 factors. The 4 experiments consist of (1) c at the high level (a, b at the low level); (2) a at the high level (b, c at the low level); (3) b at the high level (a, c at the low level); and (4) a, b, c all at the high level.

From Table 9.7, we can define the confounded effects, also known as aliases. An effect is defined by the signs in the columns of Table 9.7. For example, the effect of A is

$$(a + abc) - (c + b)$$

Note that the effect of A is exactly equal to BC. Therefore, BC and A are confounded (they are aliases). Also note that C = AB

Table 9.7 One-Half Replicate of 2^3 Factorial Design

Experiment	A level	B level	C = AB	AC	BC
c	−	−	+	−	−
a	+	−	−	−	+
b	−	+	−	+	−
abc	+	+	+	+	+

(by definition) and B = AC. Thus, in this design the main effects are confounded with the two factor interactions. This means that the main effects cannot be clearly interpreted if interactions are not absent or negligible. If interactions are negligible, this design will give fair estimates of the main effects. If interactions are significant, this design is not recommended.

Example 1: Davies [1] gives an excellent example of weighing 3 objects on a balance with a zero error in a 1/2 replicate of a 2^3 design. This illustration is used because interactions are zero when weighing two or more objects together (i.e., the weight of two or more objects is the sum of the individual weights). The three objects are denoted as A, B, and C; the high level is the presence of the object to be weighed and the low level is the absence of the object. From Table 9.7, we would perform 4 weighings: A alone, B alone, C alone, and A, B, and C together (call this ABC).

1. The weight of A is the [weight of A + the weight of ABC − the weight of B − weight of C]/2.
2. The weight of B is the [weight of B + the weight of ABC − the weight of A − weight of C]/2.
3. The weight of C is the [weight of C + the weight of ABC − the weight of A − weight of B]/2.

As noted by Davies, this illustration is not meant as a recommendation of how to weigh objects, but rather to show how the design works in the absence of interaction. (See Exercise Problem 5 as another way to weigh these objects using a 1/2 replicate fractional factorial design.)

Example 2. A 1/2 replicate of a 2^4 experiment: Chariot et al. [5] reported the results of a factorial experiment studying the effect of processing variables on extrusion-spheronization of wet powder masses. They identified 5 factors each at 2 levels, the full factorial requiring 32 experiments. Initially, they performed a 1/4 replicate, requiring 8 experiments. One of the factors, extrusion speed, was not significant. To simplify the discussion, we will ignore this factor for our example. The design and results are shown in Table 9.8. A = spheronization time, B = spheronization speed, C = spheronization load, and D = extrusion screen.

Note the confounding pattern shown in Table 9.8. The reader can verify these confounded effects (see Exercise Problem 6 at the end of this chapter). Table 9.8 was constructed by first setting up the standard 2^3 factorial (Table 9.3) and substituting D for the ABC interaction. For the estimated effects to have meaning, the

Table 9.8 One-Half Replicate of 2^4 Factorial Design (Extrusion-Spheronization of Wet Powder Masses)

Experiment	A (min)	B (rpm)	C (kg)	D (mm)	AB[a] = CD	AC = BD	AD = BC	Response
(1)	−	−	−	−	+	+	+	75.5
ab	+	+	−	−	+	−	−	55.5
ac	+	−	+	−	−	+	−	92.8
ad	+	−	−	+	−	−	+	45.4
bc	−	+	+	−	−	−	+	46.5
bd	−	+	−	+	−	+	−	19.7
cd	−	−	+	+	+	−	−	11.1
abcd	+	+	+	+	+	+	+	55.0

Parameter

[a]Illustrates confounding.

confounded effects should be small. For example, if BC and AD
were both significant, the interpretation of BC and/or AD would be
fuzzy.

To estimate the effects, we add the responses multiplied by the
signs in the appropriate column and divide by 4. For example, the
effect of AB is

$$[75.5 + 55.5 - 92.8 - 45.4 - 46.5 - 19.7 + 11.1 + 55.0]/4$$

$$= -1.825$$

Estimates of the other effects are (see Exercise Problem 7)

$$
\begin{aligned}
A &= +23.98 \\
B &= -12.03 \\
C &= +2.33 \\
D &= -34.78 \\
AB &= -1.83 \\
AC &= +21.13 \\
AD &= +10.83
\end{aligned}
$$

We cannot perform tests for the significance of these parameters
without an estimate of the error (variance). The variance can be
estimated from duplicate experiments, nonexistent interactions, or
experiments from previous studies, for example. Based on the
estimate above, factor A, D, and AC are the largest effects. To
help clarify the possible confounding effects, 8 more experiments
can be performed. For example, the large effect observed for the
interaction AC, spheronization time × spheronization load could be
exagerrated due to the presence of a BD interaction. Without other
insights, it is not possible to separate these 2 interactions (they
are aliases in this design). Therefore, this design would not be
desirable if the nature of these interactions are unknown. Data for
the 8 further experiments that complete the factorial design are
given in Exercise Problem 8.

The conclusions given by Chariot et al. are

1. Spheronization time (factor A) has a positive effect on the pro-
    duction of spheres.
2. There is a strong interaction between factors A and C (spheron-
    ization time × spheronization load). Note that the BD inter-
    action is considered to be small.
3. Spheronization speed (factor B) has a negative effect on yield.
4. The interaction between spheronization speed and spheronization
    load (BC) appears significant. The AD interaction is consid-
    ered to be small.

Table 9.9 Some Fractional Designs for Up to 5 Factors

Observations	Factors	Fraction of full factorial	Defining contrast	Confounding	Design
4	3	1/2	-ABC	Main effects confused with 2-way interactions	(1), ab, ac, bc
8	4	1/2	ABCD	Main effects and 3 2-way interactions are not confused	(1), ab, ac, bc, ad, bd, cd, abcd
8	5	1/4	-BCE -ADE	Main effects confused with 2-way interactions; see references note below	(1), ad, bc, abcd, abe, bde, ace, cde
16	5	1/2	ABCDE	Main effects and 2-factor interactions are not confused	(1), ab, ac, bc, ad, bd, cd, abcd, ae, be, ce, abce, de, abde, acde, bcde

See References 1 and 6 for more detailed discussion and other designs.

333

5. The interaction between spheronization speed and spheroniza-
    tion time (AB) appears significant. The CD interaction is con-
    sidered to be small.
6. Extrusion screen (D) has a very strong negative effect.

Table 9.9 presents some fractional designs with up to 8 observations. To find the aliases (confounded effects), multiply the defining contrast in the table by the effect under consideration. Any
letter that appears twice is considered to be equal to 1. The result is the confounded effect. For example, if the defining contrast
is $-ABC$ and we are interested in the alias of A, we multiply $-ABC$
by $A = -A^2BC = -BC$. Therefore, A is confounded with $-BC$.
Similarly, B is confounded with $-AC$ and C is confounded with $-AB$.

9.6   SOME GENERAL COMMENTS

As noted previously, experiments need not be limited to factors at
two levels, although the use of two levels is often necessary to keep
the experiment at a manageable size. Where factors are quantitative,
experiments at more than two levels may be desirable when curvature
of the response is anticipated. As the number of levels increase,
the size of the experiment increases rapidly and fractional designs
are recommended.

The theory of factorial designs is quite fascinating from a mathematical viewpoint. Particularly, the algebra and arithmetic lead to
very elegant concepts. For those readers interested in pursuing
this topic further, the book *The Design and Analysis of Industrial
Experiments*, edited by O. L. Davies, is indispensable [1]. This
topic is also discussed in some detail in Ref. 2. Applications of
factorial designs in pharmaceutical systems have appeared in the recent pharmaceutical literature. Plaizier-Vercammen and De Neve investigated the interaction of povidone with low-molecular-weight
organic molecules using a factorial design [3]. Bolton has shown
the application of factorial designs to drug stability studies [4].

KEY TERMS

Additivity	Half replicate
Aliases	Interaction
Confounding	Level
Effects	Main effect
Factor	One-at-a-time experiment
Fractional factorial designs	Replication

Residual variation 2^n factorials
Runs Yates analysis
Standard order

EXERCISES

1. A 2^2 factorial design was used to investigate the effects of stearate concentration and mixing time on the hardness of a tablet
   formulation. The results below are the averages of the hardness of 10 tablets. The variance of an average of 10 determinations was estimated from replicate determinations as 0.3 (d.f. =
   36). This is the error term for performing statistical tests of
   significance.

Mixing time (min)	Stearate	
	0.5%	1%
15	9.6 (1)	7.5 (a)
30	7.4 (b)	7.0 (ab)

   (a) Calculate the ANOVA and present the ANOVA table.
   (b) Test the main effects and interaction for significance.
   (c) Graph the data showing the possible AB interaction.

2. Show how to calculate the effect of increasing stearate concentration at low starch level for the data in Table 9.2. The
   answer is an increased thickness of 0.085 cm. Also, compute
   the drug × starch interaction.

3. The end point of a titration procedure is known to be affected
   by (1) temperature, (2) pH, and (3) concentration of indicator.
   A factorial experiment was conducted to estimate the effects of
   the factors. Before the experiment was conducted, all interactions were thought to be negligible except for a pH × indicator concentration interaction. The other interactions are to
   be pooled to form the error term for statistical tests. Use the
   Yates method to calculate the ANOVA based on the following
   assay results:

Factor combination	Recovery (%)	Factor combination	Recovery (%)
(1)	100.7	c	99.9
a	100.1	ac	99.6
b	102.0	bc	98.5
ab	101.0	abc	98.1

(a) Which factors are significant?

(b) Plot the data to show main effects and interactions which are significant.

(c) Describe, in words, the BC interaction.

4. A clinical study was performed to assess the effects of a combination of ingredients to support the claim that the combination product showed a synergistic effect compared to the effects of the two individual components. The study was designed as a factorial with each component at two levels.

Ingredient A: low level, 0; high level, 5 mg
Ingredient B: low level, 0; high level, 50 mg

Following is the analysis of variance table:

Source	d.f.	MS	F
Ingredient A	1	150	12.5
Ingredient B	1	486	40.5
A × B	1	6	0.5
Error	20	12	

The experiment consisted of observing six patients in each cell of the 2^2 experiment. One group took placebo with an average result of 21. A second group took ingredient A at a 5-mg dose with an average result of 25. The third group had ingredient B at a 50-mg dose with an average result of 29, and the fourth group took a combination of 5 mg of A and 50 mg of B with a result of 35. In view of the results and the ANOVA, discuss arguments for or against the claim of synergism.

5. The 3 objects in the weighing experiment described in Sec. 9.5, Example 1, may also be weighed using the other 4 combinations from the 2^3 design not included in the example. Describe how you would weigh the 3 objects using these new 4 weighings. (Note that these combinations comprise a 1/2 replicate of a fractional factorial with a different confounding pattern from that described in Sec. 9.5. [Hint: See Table 9.9.]

6. Verify that the effects (AB = CD, AC = BD, and AD = BC) shown in Table 9.8 are confounded.

7. Compute the effects for the data in Sec. 9.5, example 2 (Table 9.8).

**8. In example 2 in Sec. 9.5 (Table 9.8), eight more experiments were performed with the following results:

Experiment	Response
a	78.7
b	56.9
c	46.7
d	21.2
abc	67.0
abd	29.0
acd	34.9
bcd	1.2

Using the entire 16 experiments (the 8 given here plus the 8 in Table 9.8), analyze the data as a full 2^4 factorial design. Pool the 3-factor and 4-factor interactions (5 d.f.) to obtain an estimate of error. Test the other effects for significance at the 5% level. Explain and describe any significant interactions.

REFERENCES

1. Davies, O. L., *The Design and Analysis of Industrial Experiments*, Hafner, New York, 1963.
2. Box, G. E., Hunter, W. G., and Hunter, J. S., *Statistics for Experimenters*, Wiley, New York, 1978.
3. Plaizier-Vercammen, J. A. and De Neve, R. E., *J. Pharm. Sci.*, 70, 1252, 1981.
4. Bolton, S., *J. Pharm. Sci.*, 72, 362, 1983.
5. Chariot, M., Francès, G. A., Lewis, D., Mathieu, R., Phan Tan, L., and Stevens, N. H. E., *Drug Dev. and Ind. Pharm.*, 13(9−11), 1639−1649, 1987.
6. Beyer, W. H., Editor, *Handbook of Tables for Probability and Statistics*, The Chemical Rubber Co., Cleveland, 1966.

10
Transformations and Outliers

Critical examination of the data is an important step in statistical analyses. Often, we observe either what seem to be unusual observations (outliers) or observations that appear to violate the assumptions of the analysis. When such problems occur, several courses of action are available depending on the nature of the problem and statistical judgement. Most of the analyses described in previous chapters are appropriate for groups in which data are normally distributed with equal variance. As a result of the Central Limit theorem, these analyses perform well for data that are not normal provided the deviation from normality is not large and/or the data sets are not very small. (If necessary and appropriate, nonparametric analyses, Chap. 15, can be used in these instances.) However, lack of equality of variance (heteroscedascity) in t tests, analysis of variance and regression, for example, is more problematic. The Fisher-Behrens test is an example of a modified analysis that is used in the comparison of means from two independent groups with unequal variances in the two groups (Chap. 5). Often, variance heterogeneity and/or lack of normality can be corrected by a data transformation, such as the logarithmic or square root transformation. Transformations of data may also be appropriate to help linearize data. For example, a plot of log potency vs. time is linear for stability data showing first-order kinetics.

Variance heterogeneity may also be corrected using an analysis in which each observation is weighted appropriately, i.e., a weighted analysis. In regression analysis of kinetic data, if the variances at each time point differ, depending on the magnitude of drug concentration, for example, a weighted regression would be appropriate. For an example of the analysis of a regression problem requiring a weighted analysis for its solution, see Chap. 7.

Data resulting from gross errors in observations or overt mis-
takes such as recording errors should clearly be omitted from the
statistical treatment. However, upon examining experimental data,
we often find unusual values that are not easily explained. The
prudent experimenter will make every effort to find a cause for
such aberrant data and modify the data or analysis appropriately.
If no cause is found, one should be wary about discarding these
results. In such cases, a statistical test may be used to detect an
outlying value. An outlier may be defined as an observation that
is extreme and appears not to belong to the bulk of data. Many
tests to identify outliers have been proposed and several of these
are presented in this chapter.

10.1   TRANSFORMATIONS

A transformation applied to a variable changes each value of the
variable as described by the transformation. In a *logarithmic (log)
transformation*, each data point is changed to its logarithm prior to
the statistical analysis. Thus the value 10 is transformed to 1
(i.e., log 10 = 1). The log transformation may be in terms of logs
to the base 10 or logs to the base e (e = 2.718 . . .), known as
natural logs (ln). For example, using natural logs, 10 would be
transformed to 2.303 (ln 10 = 2.303). The *square-root* transformation would change the number 9 to 3.

Parametric analyses such as the t test and analysis of variance
are the methods of choice in most situations where experimental
data are continuous. For these methods to be valid, data is assumed to have a normal distribution with constant variance within
treatment groups. Under appropriate circumstances, a transformation can change a data distribution which is not normal into a distribution that is approximately normal and/or can transform data
with heterogeneous variance into a distribution with approximately
homogeneous variance.

Thus, data transformations can be used in cases where (1) the
variance in regression and analysis of variance is not constant
and/or (2) data are clearly not normally distributed (highly skewed
to the left or right).

Another application of transformations is to linearize relationships such as may occur when fitting a least squares line (not all
relationships can be linearized). Table 10.1 shows some examples
of such linearizing transformations. When making linearizing transformations, if statistical tests are to be made on the transformed
data, one should take care that the normality and variance homogeneity assumptions are not invalidated by the transformation.

Table 10.1   Some Transformations Used to Linearize
Relationships Between Two Variables, X and Y

Function	Transformation	Linear form
$Y = Ae^{-BX}$	Logarithm of Y	$\ln Y = \ln A - BX$
$Y = 1/(A + BX)$	Reciprocal of Y	$1/Y = A + BX$
$Y = X/(AX + B)$	Reciprocal of Y	$1/Y = A + B (1/X)$[a]

[a]A plot of $1/Y$ vs. $1/X$ is linear.

10.1.1   The Logarithmic Transformation

Probably the most common transformation used in scientific research
is the log transformation. Either logs to the base 10 ($\log_{10}$) or the
base e, $\log_e$ (ln) can be used. Data skewed to the right as shown
in Fig. 10.1 can often be shown to have an approximately lognormal
distribution. A lognormal distribution is a distribution that would
be normal following a log transformation, as illustrated in Fig. 10.2.
When statistically analyzing data with a distribution similar to that
shown in Fig. 10.1, a log transformation should be considered.
One should understand that a reasonably large data set or prior
knowledge is needed in order to know the form of the distribution.
Table 10.2 shows examples of two data sets, listed in ascending
order of magnitude. Data set A would be too small to conclude that
the underlying distribution is not normal in the absence of prior
information. Data set B, an approximately lognormal distribution,
is strongly suggestive of nonnormality. (See Exercise Problem 1.)

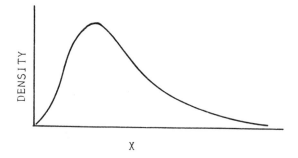

Figure 10.1   Lognormal distribution.

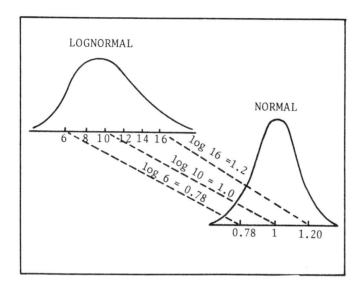

Figure 10.2 Transformation of a lognormal distribution to a normal distribution via the log transformation.

Two problems may arise as a consequence of using the log transformation.

1. Many people have trouble interpreting data reported in logarithmic form. Therefore, when reporting experimental results, such as means for example, a back transformation (the antilog) may be needed. For example, if the mean of the logarithms of a data set is 1.00, the antilog, 10, might be more meaningful in a formal report of the experimental results. The mean of a set of untransformed numbers is not, in general, equal to the antilog of the mean of the logs of these numbers. If the data are relatively nonvariable, the means calculated by these two methods will be close. The mean

Table 10.2 Two Data Sets that May be Considered Lognormal

Data set A: 2, 17, 23, 33, 43, 55, 125, 135

Data set B: 10, 13, 40, 44, 55, 63, 115, 145, 199, 218, 231, 370, 501, 790, 795, 980, 1260, 1312, 1500, 4520

Table 10.3 Illustration of Why the Antilog of the Mean of the
Logs Is Not Equal to the Mean of the Untransformed Values

	Case I			Case II	
	Original data	Log transform		Original data	Log transform
	5	0.699		4	0.603
	5	0.699		6	0.778
	5	0.699		8	0.903
	5	0.699		10	1.000
Mean	5		Mean	7	
	Antilog (0.699) = 5			Antilog (0.821) = 6.62	

of the logs and the log of the mean will be identical only if each
observation is the same, a highly unlikely circumstance. Table 10.3
illustrates this concept. Note that the antilog of the mean of a set
of log transformed variables is the geometric mean (see Chap. 1).
This lack of "equivalence" can raise questions when someone review-
ing the data is unaware of this divergence, "the nature of the
beast," so to speak.

    2. The second problem to be considered when making log trans-
formations is that the log transformation which "normalizes" lognormal data also changes the variance. If the variance is not very
large, the variance of the ln transformed values will have a variance
approximately equal to $S^2/\overline{X}^2$. That is, the standard deviation of the
data after the transformation will be approximately equal to the coefficient of variation (C.V.), $S/\overline{X}$. For example, consider the following data:

	X	ln X
	105	4.654
	102	4,625
	100	4.605
	110	4.700
	112	4.718
Mean	105.8	4.6606
s.d.	5.12	0.0483

The coefficient of variation of the original data is 5.12/105.8 = 0.0484. The standard deviation of the ln transformed values is 0.0483, very close to the C.V. of the untransformed data. This property of the transformed variance can be advantageous when working with data groups that are both *lognormal* and have a *constant coefficient of variation*. If the standard deviation within treatment groups, for example, is not homogeneous but is proportional to the magnitude of the measurement, the coefficient of variation (C.V.) will be constant. In analytical procedures, one often observes that the s.d. is proportional to the quantity of material being assayed. In these circumstances, the ln transformation will result in data with homogeneous s.d. equal to C.V. (The s.d. of the transformed data is approximately equal to C.V.*) This concept is illustrated in Example 1 which follows. Fortunately, in many situations, data that are approximately lognormal also have a constant C.V. In these cases, the log transformation results in normal data with approximately homogeneous variance. The transformed data can be analyzed using techniques that depend on normality and homogeneous variance for their validity (e.g., ANOVA).

Example 1: Experimental data were collected at three different levels of drug to show that an assay procedure is linear over a range of drug concentrations. "Linear" means that a plot of the *assay results*, or a suitable transformation of the results, versus the *known concentration* of drug is a straight line. In particular, we wish to plot the results such that a linear relationship is obtained, and calculate the least squares regression line to relate the assay results to the known amount of drug. The results of the experiment are shown in Table 10.4. In this example, the assay results are unusually variable. This large variability is intentionally presented in this example to illustrate the properties of the log transformation. The skewed nature of the data in Table 10.4 suggests a lognormal distribution, although there are not sufficient data to verify the exact nature of the distribution. Also in this example, the standard deviation increases with drug concentration. The standard deviation is approximately proportional to the mean assay, an approximately constant C.V. (10 − 12%). Note that the log transformation results in variance homogeneity and a more symmetric data distribution (Table 10.4). Thus, there is a strong indication for a log transformation.

The properties of this relatively variable analytical method can be evaluated by plotting the known amount of drug versus the

---

*The log transformation of data with constant C.V. results in data with variance approximately equal to C.V./2.303.

Table 10.4 Results of an Assay at Three Different Levels of Drug

	At 40 mg		At 60 mg		At 80 mg	
	Assay	Log assay	Assay	Log assay	Assay	Log assay
	37	1.568	63	1.799	82	1.914
	43	1.633	77	1.886	68	1.833
	42	1.623	56	1.748	75	1.875
	40	1.602	64	1.806	97	1.987
	30	1.477	66	1.820	71	1.851
	35	1.544	58	1.763	86	1.934
	38	1.580	67	1.826	71	1.851
	40	1.602	52	1.716	81	1.908
	39	1.591	55	1.740	91	1.959
	36	1.556	58	1.763	72	1.857
Average	38	1.578	61.6	1.787	79.4	1.897
s.d.	3.77	0.045	7.35	0.050	9.67	0.052
C.V.	0.10		0.12		0.12	

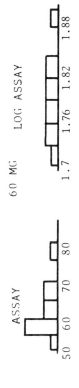

ASSAY
50   60   70   80

60 MG   LOG ASSAY
1.7   1.76   1.82   1.88

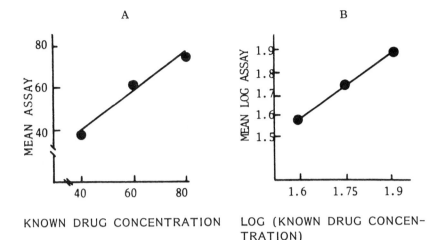

Figure 10.3   Plots of raw data means and log transformed means for data of Table 10.4.   (A) means of untransformed data; (B) log transformation.

amount recovered in the assay procedure.   Ideally, the relationship should be linear over the range of drug concentration being assayed. A plot of known drug concentration versus assay results is close to linear (Fig. 10.3A).   A plot of *log* drug concentration versus *log* assay is also approximately linear, as shown in Fig. 10.3B.   From a statistical viewpoint, the log plot has better properties because the data are more "normal" and the variance is approximately constant in the three drug concentration groups as noted above.   The line in Fig. 10.3B is the least squares line.   The details of the calculation are not shown here (see Exercise Problem 2 and Chap. 7 for further details of the statistical line fitting).

When performing the usual statistical tests in regression problems, the assumptions include:

1. The data at each X should be normal (i.e., the amount of drug recovered at a given amount added should be normally distributed).
2. The assays should have the same variance at each concentration.

The log transformation of the assay results (Y) helps to satisfy these assumptions.   In addition, in this example, the linear fit is improved as a result of the log transformation.

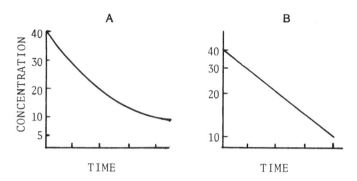

Figure 10.4   First-order plots.   (A) usual plot;   (B) semilog plot.

Example 2:   In the pharmaceutical sciences, the logarithmic
transformation has applications in kinetic studies, when ascertaining
stability and pharmacokinetic parameters.   First-order processes
are usually expressed in logarithmic form (see also Sec. 2.5):

$$\ln C = \ln C_0 - kt \tag{10.1}$$

Least squares procedures are typically used to fit concentration
versus time data in order to estimate the rate constant, k.   A plot
of concentration (C) versus time (t) is not linear for first-order
reactions (see Fig. 10.4A).   A plot of the log-transformed concentrations (the Y variable) versus time is linear for a first-order
process [Eq. (10.1)].   The plot of log C versus time is shown in
Fig. 10.4B, a semilog plot.

   Thus we may use linear regression procedures to fit a straight
line to log C versus time data for first-order reactions.   One should
recognize, as before, that if statistical tests are performed to test
the significance of the rate constant, for example, or when placing
confidence limits on the rate constant, the implicit assumption is
that log concentration is normal with constant variance at each value
of X (time).   These assumptions will hold, when linearizing such
concentration versus time relationships if the *untransformed* values
of "concentration" are *lognormal* with constant coefficient of variation.   In cases in which the assumptions necessary for statistical
inference are invalidated by the transformation, one may question
the validity of predictions based on least squares line fitting for
first-order processes.   For example, if the original, untransformed concentration values are normal with constant variance, the
log transformation will distort the distribution and upset the constant

variance condition. However, if the variance is small, and the concentrations measured are in a narrow range (as might occur in a short-term stability study to 10% decomposition), the log transformation will result in data that are close to normal with homogeneous variance. Predictions for stability during the short-term based on the least squares fit will be approximately correct under these conditions.

Analysis of Residuals

We have discussed the importance of carefully looking at and graphing data before performing transformations or statistical tests. The approach to examining data in this context is commonly known as Exploratory Data Analysis, EDA, introduced in Chap. 7. A significant aspect of EDA is the examination of residuals. Residuals are deviations of the observed data from the fit to the statistical model, the least squares line in this example. Figure 10.5 shows the residuals for the least squares fit of the data in Table 10.4, using the untransformed and transformed data analysis. Note that the residual plot vs. dose shows the dependency of the variance on dose. The log response vs. log dose shows a more uniform distribution of residuals.

Example 3: The log transformation may be used for data presented in the form of ratios. Ratios are often used to express the comparative absorption of drug from two formulations based on the area under the plasma level versus time curve from a bioavailability study. Another way of comparing the absorptions from the two formulations is to test statistically the *difference* in absorption $(AUC_1 - AUC_2)$, as illustrated in Sec. 5.2.3. However, reporting results of relative absorption using a *ratio*, rather than a difference, has great appeal. The ratio can be interpreted in a pragmatic sense. Stating that formulation A is absorbed *twice* as much as formulation B has more meaning than stating that formulation A has an AUC 525 µg·hr/ml more than formulation B. A statistical problem which is evident when performing statistical tests on ratios is that the ratios of random variables will probably not be normally distributed. In particular, if both A and B are normally distributed, the ratio A/B does not have a normal distribution. On the other hand, the test of the differences of AUC has statistical appeal because the difference of two normally distributed variables is also normally distributed. The practical appeal of the *ratio* and the statistical appeal of *differences* suggest the use of a log transformation, when ratios seem most appropriate for data analysis.

The differences of logs is analogous to ratios; the difference of the logs is the log of the ratio: log A − log B = log (A/B). The antilog of the average difference of the logs will be close to the

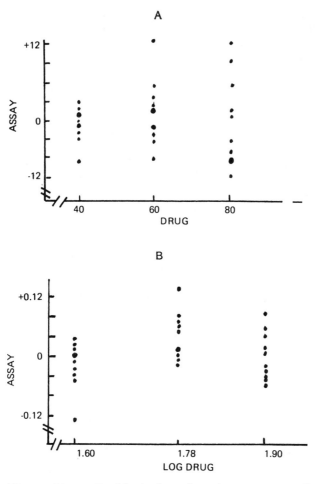

Figure 10.5   Residual plots from least squares line fitting of data from Table 10.4.

average of the ratios if the variability is not too large. The differences of the logs will also tend to be normally distributed. But
the normality assumption should not be a problem in these analyses
because we are testing *mean* differences (again, the central limit
theorem). After application of the log transformation, the data may
be analyzed by the usual t-test (or ANOVA) techniques which assess
treatment differences.

Table 10.5 shows AUC data for 10 subjects who participated in
a bioavailability study. The analysis (a paired t test in this example) is performed on both the difference of the *logarithms* and the
ratios. The t test for the ratios is a one-sample, two-sided test,
comparing the average ratio to 1 (H_0: R = 1), as shown in Sec.
5.2.1.

t test for ratios:

$$H_0: \quad R = 1$$

$$t = \frac{|1.025 - 1|}{0.378/\sqrt{10}} = 0.209$$

95% confidence interval:

$$1.025 \pm \frac{2.26(0.378)}{\sqrt{10}} = 1.025 \pm 0.27$$

t test for difference of logs:

$$H_0: \quad \log A - \log B = 0$$

$$t = \frac{|-0.01077|}{0.136/\sqrt{10}} = 0.250$$

95% confidence interval:

$$-0.01077 \pm \frac{2.26(0.136)}{\sqrt{10}} = -0.01077 \pm 0.0972$$

The confidence interval for the logs is -0.10797 to 0.08643. The
antilogs of these values are 0.78 to 1.22. The confidence interval
for the ratio is 0.75 to 1.30. Thus the conclusions using both
methods (ratio and difference of logs) are similar. Had the variability been smaller, the two methods would have been in better
agreement.

Table 10.5   Results of the Bioavailability Study: Areas Under the Plasma Level Versus Time Curve

Subject	Product A		Product B		Ratio AUCs: A/B	Log A - Log B
	AUC	Log AUC	AUC	Log AUC		
1	533	2.727	651	2.814	0.819	-0.087
2	461	2.664	547	2.738	0.843	-0.074
3	470	2.672	535	2.728	0.879	-0.056
4	624	2.795	326	2.513	1.914	0.282
5	490	2.690	386	2.587	1.269	0.104
6	476	2.678	640	2.806	0.744	-0.129
7	465	2.667	582	2.765	0.799	-0.097
8	365	2.562	420	2.623	0.869	-0.061
9	412	2.615	545	2.736	0.756	-0.121
10	380	2.580	280	2.447	1.357	0.133
Average					1.025	-0.01077
s.d.					0.378	0.136

t test		Confidence interval	
Ratio	Difference of logs	Ratio	Difference of logs
0.209	0.250	0.75—1.30	0.78—1.22

Another interesting result that recommends the analysis of differences of logs rather than the use of ratios is a consequence of the *symmetry* which is apparent with the former analysis. With the log transformation, the conclusion regarding the equivalence of the products will be the same whether we consider the difference as (log A − log B) or (log B − log A). However, when analyzing ratios, the analysis of A/B will be different from the analysis of B/A. The product in the numerator has the advantage (see Exercise Problem 3). In the example in Table 10.5 the average ratio of B/A is 1.066. B appears slightly better than A. When the ratios are calculated as A/B, A appeared somewhat better than B. Other authors have also recommended use of the log transformation for bioavailability parameters [2].

For data containing zeros, very small numbers (close to zero) or negative numbers, using ratios or logarithms is either not possible or not recommended. Clearly, if we have a ratio with a zero in the denominator or a mixture of positive and negative ratios, the analysis and interpretation is difficult or impossible. Logarithms of negative numbers and zero are undefined. Therefore, unless special adjustments are made, such data are not candidates for a log transformation.

10.1.2 The Arcsin Transformation for Proportions

Another commonly used transformation is the *arcsin* transformation for proportions. The arcsin is the inverse sine function, also denoted as $\sin^{-1}$. Thus, if sin 45° = 0.7, arcsin 0.7 = 45°. Many calculators have a sine and inverse sine function available.

The problem that arises when analyzing proportions, where the data consist of proportions of widely different magnitudes, is the lack of homogeneity of variance. The variance homogeneity problem is a result of the definition of the variance for proportions, pq/N. If the proportions under consideration vary from one observation to another, the variance will also vary. If the proportions to be analyzed are approximately normally distributed (Np and Nq $\geqslant$ 5; see Chap. 5), the arcsin transformation will equalize the variances. The arcsin values can then be analyzed using standard parametric techniques such as ANOVA. When using the arcsin transformation,

each proportion should be based on the same number of observations, N. If the number of observations is similar for each proportion, the analysis using arcsines will be close to correct. However,
if the numbers of observations are very different for the different
proportions, the use of the transformation is not appropriate. Also,
for very small or very large proportions (less than 0.03 or greater
than 0.97), a more accurate transformation is given by Mosteller
and Youtz [3]. The following example should clarify the concept
and calculations when applying the arcsin transformation.

Example 4: In preparation for a toxicological study for a new
drug entity, an estimate of the incidence of a particular adverse reaction in untreated mice was desired. Data were available from previous studies, as shown in Table 10.6. The arcsin transformation
is applied to the proportions as follows:

$$\text{Arcsin transformation} = \text{arcsin } \sqrt{p} \tag{10.2}$$

For example, in Table 10.6, the arcsin transformation of 10% (0.10)
is arcsin $\sqrt{0.10}$, which is equal to 18.43°.

The objective of this exercise is to estimate the incidence of the
adverse reaction in normal, untreated animals. To this end, we will
obtain the average proportion and construct a confidence interval
using the arcsin transformed data. The average arcsin is 26.197°.
The average proportions are not reported in terms of arcsines. As
in the case of the log transformation, one should back-transform
the average transformed value to the original terms. In this

Table 10.6   Incidence of an Adverse Reaction in
Untreated Mice from Six Studies

Proportion of mice showing adverse reaction	Arcsin P
5/50 = 0.10	18.43
12/50 = 0.24	29.33
8/50 = 0.16	23.58
15/50 = 0.30	33.21
13/50 = 0.26	30.66
7/50 = 0.14	21.97
Average 0.20	26.197°

example, we obtain the back-transform as sin $(\text{arcsin})^2$, or sin $(26.197)^2 = 0.195$. This is very close to the average of the un-transformed proportions, 20%. The *variance of a transformed proportion* can be shown to be equal to *820.7/N*, where N is the number of observations for each proportion [4]. Thus, in this example, the variance is 820.7/50 = 16.414.

A confidence interval for the average proportion is obtained by finding the confidence interval for the average arcsin and back-transforming to proportions. 95% confidence interval: $\overline{X} \pm$ 1.96 $\sqrt{\sigma^2/N}$ [Eq. (5.1)]:

$$26.197 \pm 1.96 \sqrt{\frac{16.414}{6}} = 26.197 \pm 3.242$$

The 95% confidence interval for the average arcsin is 22.955° to 29.439°. This interval corresponds to an interval for the proportion of 15.2 to 24.2% (0.152 to 0.242).*

10.1.3 Other Transformations

Two other transformations that are used to correct deviations from assumptions for statistical testing are the *square-root* and *reciprocal transformations*. As their names imply, these transformations change the data as follows:

Square-root transformation: $X \longrightarrow \sqrt{X}$

Reciprocal transformation: $X \longrightarrow 1/X$

The square-root transformation is useful in cases where the variance is proportional to the mean. The situation occurs often where the data consist of counts, such as may occur in blood and urine analyses or microbiological data. If some values are 0 or very small, the transformation, $\sqrt{X} + \sqrt{X + 1}$, has been recommended [5]. Different Poisson variables, whose variances equal their means, will have approximately equal variance after the square-root transformation (see Exercise Problem 6).

The reciprocal transformation may be used when the standard deviation is proportional to the square of the mean [6]. The transformation is also useful where time to a given response is being measured. For some objects (persons) the time to the response may

---

*sin $(22.955°)^2$ = 0.152 and sin $(29.439°)^2$ = 0.242.

Table 10.7   Summary of Some Common
Transformations

Transformation	When used
Logarithm (log X)	s.d. α $\overline{X}$
Arcsin ($\sin^{-1}$) $\sqrt{X}$	Proportions
Square root ($\sqrt{X}$ or $\sqrt{X}$ + $\sqrt{X + 1}$)	(s.d.)^2 α $\overline{X}$
Reciprocal (1/X)	s.d. α $\overline{X}^2$

be very long and a skewed distribution results.   The reciprocal
transformation helps make the data more symmetrical.

Table 10.7 summarizes the common transformations discussed in
this section.

10.2   OUTLIERS

Outliers, in statistics, refer to relatively small or large values which
are considered to be different from, and not belong to, the main

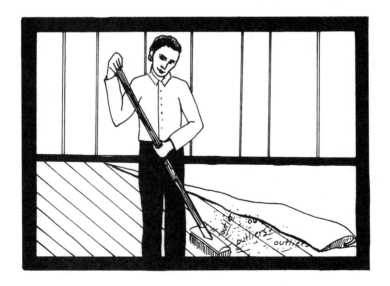

body of data. The problem of what to do with outliers is a constant dilemma facing research scientists. If the cause of an outlier is known, resulting from an obvious error, for example, the value can be omitted from the analysis and tabulation of the data. However, it is good practice to include the reason(s) for the omission of the aberrant value in the text of the report of the experimental results. For example, a container of urine, assayed for drug content in a pharmacokinetic study, results in too low a drug content because part of the urine was lost due to accidental spillage. This is just cause to discard the data from that sample. In most cases, extreme values are observed without obvious causes, and we are confronted with the problem of how to handle the apparent outliers. Do the outlying data really represent the experimental process that is being investigated? Can we expect such extreme values to occur routinely in such experiments? Or was the outlier due to an error of observation? Perhaps the observation came from a population different from the one being studied. In general, aberrant observations *should not be arbitrarily discarded* only because they look too large or too small, perhaps only for the reason of making the experimental data look "better." In fact, the presence of such observations may be a clue to an important process inherent in the experimental system. Therefore, the question of what to do with outliers is not an easy one to answer. The error of either incorrectly including or excluding outlying observations will distort the validity of interpretation and conclusions of the experiment.

Several statistical criteria for handling outlying observations will be presented here. These methods may be used if no obvious cause for the outlier can be found. If, for any reason, one or more outlying data are rejected, one has the option of (a) repeating the appropriate portion of the experiment to obtain a replacement value(s), (b) estimating the now "missing" value by statistical methods, or (c) analyzing the data without the discarded value(s). From a statistical point of view, the practice of looking at a set of data or replicates, and rejecting the value(s) that is most extreme (and possibly, rerunning the rejected point) is to be discouraged. Biases in the results are almost sure to occur. Certainly, the variance will be underestimated, since we are throwing out the extreme values, willy nilly. For example, when performing assays, some persons recommend doing the assay in triplicate and selecting the two best results (those two closest together). In other cases, two assays are performed and if they "disagree," a third assay is performed to make a decision as to which of the original two assays should be discarded. Arbitrary rules such as these often result in incorrect decisions about the validity of results [7]. Experimental scientists usually have a very good intuitive "feel" for their data, and this should be taken into account before coming to a final decision regarding the disposition of outlying values. However, in the absence of other information, the statistical criteria discussed below may be used to help make an objective decision. When in doubt, a useful approach is to analyze the data with and without the suspected value(s). If conclusions and decisions are the same with and without the extreme value(s), including the possible outlying observations would seem to be the most prudent action.

Statistical tests for the presence of outliers are usually based on an assumption that the data has a normal distribution. Thus, applying these tests to data that are known to be highly skewed, for example, would result too often in the rejection of legitimate data. If the national average income were to be estimated by an interview of 100 randomly selected persons, and 99 were found to have incomes of less than $100,000 while one person had an income of $1,000,000, it would be clearly incorrect to omit the latter figure, attributing it to a recording error or interviewer unreliability. The tests described below are based on statistics calculated from the observed data, which are then referred to tables to determine the level of significance. The significance level here has the same interpretation as that described for statistical tests of hypotheses (Chap. 5). At the 5% level, an outlying observation may be incorrectly rejected 1 time in 20.

10.2.1 Dixon's Test for Extreme Values

The data in Table 10.8 represent cholesterol values (ordered according to magnitude) for a group of healthy, normal persons. This example is presented particularly, because the problem that it represents has two facets. First, the possibility exists that the very low and very high values (165, 297) are the result of a recording or analytical error. Second, one may question the existence of such extreme values among *normal healthy* persons. Without the presence of an obvious error, one would probably be remiss if these two values (165, 297) were omitted from a report of "normal" cholesterol values in these normal subjects. However, with the knowledge that plasma cholesterol levels are approximately normally distributed,

Table 10.8   Ordered Values of Serum Cholesterol from 15 Normal Subjects

Subject	1	2	3	4	5	6	7	8	9	10	11	12	13	14	15
Cholesterol	165	188	194	197	200	202	205	210	214	215	227	231	239	249	297

a statistical test can be applied to determine if the extreme values should be rejected.

Dixon has proposed a test for outlying values which can easily be calculated [1]. The set of observations are first ordered according to magnitude. A calculation is then performed of the *ratio* of the difference of the extreme value from one of its nearest neighboring values to the range of observations as defined below.

The formula for the *ratio*, r, depends on the sample size, as shown in Table IV.8. The calculated ratio is compared to appropriate tabulated values in Table IV.8. If the ratio is equal to or greater than the tabulated value, the observation is considered to be an outlier at the 5% level of significance.

The ordered observations are denoted as X_1, X_2, X_3, . . . , X_N, for N observations, where X_1 is an extreme value and X_N is the opposite extreme. When N = 3 to 7, for example, the ratio r = $(X_2 - X_1)/(X_N - X_1)$ is calculated. For the five (5) values 1.5, 2.1, 2.2, 2.3, and 3.1, where 3.1 is the suspected outlier,

$$r = \frac{3.1 - 2.3}{3.1 - 1.5} = 0.5$$

The ratio must be equal to or exceed 0.642 to be significant at the 5% level for N = 5 (Table IV.8). Therefore, 3.1 is not considered to be an outlier (0.5 < 0.642).

The cholesterol values in Table 10.8 contain two possible outliers, 165 and 297. According to Table IV.8, for a sample size of 15 (N = 15), the test ratio is

$$r = \frac{X_3 - X_1}{X_{N-2} - X_1} \tag{10.3}$$

where X_3 is the third ordered value, X_1 is the smallest value, and X_{N-2} is the third largest value (two removed from the largest value).

$$r = \frac{194 - 165}{239 - 165} = \frac{29}{74} = 0.39$$

The tabulated value for N = 15 (Table IV.8) is 0.525. Therefore, the value 165 cannot be rejected as an outlier.

The test for the largest value is similar, reversing the order (highest to lowest) to conform to Eq. (10.3). X_1 is 297, X_3 is 239, and X_{N-2} is 194.

$$r = \frac{239 - 297}{194 - 297} = \frac{58}{103} = 0.56$$

Since 0.56 is greater than the tabulated value of 0.525, 297 can be considered to be an outlier, and rejected.

Consider an example of the results of an assay performed in triplicate,

94.5, 100.0, 100.3

Is the low value, 94.5, an outlier? As discussed earlier, triplicate assays have an intuitive appeal. If one observation is far from the others, it is often discarded, considered to be the result of some overt, but not obvious error. Applying Dixon's criterion (N = 3),

$$r = \frac{100 - 94.5}{100.3 - 94.5} = 0.93$$

Surprisingly, the test does not find the "outlying" value small enough to reject the value at the 5% level. The ratio must be at least equal to 0.941 in order to reject the possible outlier for a sample of size 3. In the absence of other information, 94.5 is not obviously an outlier. The moral here is that what seems obvious is not always so. When one value of three appears to be "different" from the others, think twice before throwing it away.

After omitting a value as an outlier, the remaining data may be tested again for outliers, using the same procedure as described above with a sample size of N − 1.

10.2.2   The T Procedure

Another highly recommended test for outliers, the *T method*, is also calculated as a ratio, designated T_n, as follows:

$$T_n = \frac{X_n - \overline{X}}{S} \tag{10.4}$$

where X_n is either the smallest or largest value, $\overline{X}$ is the mean, and S is the standard deviation. If the extreme value is not anticipated to be high or low, prior to seeing the data, a test for the outlying value is based on the tabulation in Table IV.9. If the calculated value of T_n is equal to or exceeds the tabulated value, the outlier is rejected as an extreme value ($P \leqslant 0.05$). A more detailed table is given in Ref. 8.

For the cholesterol data in Table 10.7, T_n is calculated as follows:

$$T_n = \frac{297 - 215.5}{30.9} = 2.64$$

where 297 is the suspected outlier, 215.5 is the average of the 15 cholesterol values, and 30.9 is the standard deviation of the 15 values. According to Table IV.9, T_n is significant at the 5% level, agreeing with the conclusions of the Dixon test. The Dixon text and the T_n test may not exactly agree with regard to acceptance or rejection of the outlier, particularly in cases where the extreme value results in tests that are close to the 5% level. To maintain a degree of integrity in situations where more than one test is available, one should decide which test to use prior to seeing the data. On the other hand, for any statistical test, if alternative acceptable procedures are available, any difference in conclusions resulting from the use of the different procedures is usually of a small degree. If one test results in significance ($P < 0.05$) and the other just misses significance (e.g., $P = 0.06$), one can certainly consider the latter result close to being statistically significant at the very least.

10.2.3 Winsorizing

An interesting approach to the analysis of data to protect against distortion caused by extreme values is the process of Winsorization [1]. In this method, the extreme values, both low and high, are changed to the values of their closest neighbors. This procedure provides some protection against the presence of outlying values and, at the same time, very little information is lost. For the cholesterol data (Table 10.7), the extreme values are 165 and 297. These values are changed to that of their nearest neighbors, 188 and 249, respectively. This manipulation results in a data set with a mean of 213.9, compared to a mean of 215.5 for the untransformed data.

Winsorized estimates can be useful when *missing* values are known to be *extreme* values. For example, suppose that the two highest values of the cholesterol data from Table 10.7 were lost. Also, suppose that we know that these two missing values would have been the highest values in the data set, had we had the opportunity to observe them. Perhaps, in this example, the subjects whose values were missing had extremely high measurements in previous analyses; or perhaps, a very rough assay was available from the spilled sample scraped off of the floor showing high levels of cholesterol. A reasonable estimate of the mean would be obtained by substituting 239 (the largest value after omitting 249 and 297) for the two missing values. Similarly, we could replace 165 and 188 by the third lowest value, 194. The new mean is now equal to 213.3, compared to a mean of 215.5 for the original data.

KEY TERMS

Arcsin transformation
Back-transformation
Coefficient of variation
Dixon's test for outliers
Exploratory data analysis
Fisher-Behrens test
Geometric mean
Log transformation
Nonparametric analyses
Ordered observations

Outliers
Parametric analyses
Ratios
Reciprocal transformation
Residuals
Skewed data
Square-root transformation
T procedure
Winsorizing

EXERCISES

1. Convert the data in Table 10.2, data set B, to logs and construct a histogram of the transformed data.
2. Fit the least squares line for the averages of log assay versus
   log drug concentration for the average data in Table 10.4.

Log X	Log Y
1.602	1.578
1.778	1.787
1.903	1.897

   If an unknown sample has a reading of 47, what is the estimate
   of the drug concentration?
3. Perform a t test for the data of Table 10.5 using the ratio B/A
   (H_0: R = 1), and log B − log A (H_0: log B − log A = 0).
   Compare the values of t in these analyses to the similar analyses
   shown in the text for A/B and log A − log B.
4. Ten tablets were assayed with the following results: 51, 54,
   46, 49, 53, 50, 49, 62, 47, 53. Is the value 62 an outlier?
   When averaging the tablets to estimate the batch average,
   would you exclude this value from the calculation? (Use both
   the Dixon method and the T method to test the value of 62 as
   an outlier.)
5. Consider 62 to be an outlier in Problem 4 and calculate the
   Winzorized average. Compare this to the average with 62
   included.
6. A tablet product was manufactured using two different processes,
   and packaged in bottles of 1000 tablets. Five bottles were
   sampled from each batch (process) with the following results:

	Number of defective tablets per bottle									
	Process 1 Bottle					Process 2 Bottle				
	1	2	3	4	5	1	2	3	4	5
No. of defects	0	6	1	3	4	0	1	1	0	1

Perform a t test to compare the average results for each process. Transform the data and repeat the t test. What transformation did you use? Explain why you used the transformation. [Hint: see transformations for Poisson variables.]

REFERENCES

1. Dixon, W. J. and Massey, F. J., Jr., *Introduction to Statistical Analysis*, 3rd ed., McGraw-Hill, New York, 1969.
2. Westlake, W. J., *Statistical Issues in Drug Research and Development* (K. E. Peace, ed.), Marcel Dekker, New York, 1990.
3. Mosteller, F. and Youtz, C., *Biometrika, 48*, 433, 1961.
4. Sokal, R. R. and Rohlf, F. J., *Biometry*, W. H. Freeman, San Francisco, 1969.
5. Weisberg, S., *Applied Linear Regression*, Wiley, New York, 1980.
6. Ostle, B., *Statistics in Research*, 3rd ed., Iowa State University Press, Ames, Iowa, 1981.
7. Youden, W. J., *Statistical Methods for Chemists*, Wiley, New York, 1964.
8. E-178-75, American National Standards Institute, Z1.14, 1975, p. 183.

11
Experimental Design in Clinical Trials

The design and analysis of clinical trials is fertile soil for statistical applications. The use of sound statistical principles in this area is particularly important because of close FDA involvement, in addition to crucial public health issues which are consequences of actions based on the outcomes of clinical experiments. Principles and procedures of experimental design, particularly as applied to clinical studies, are presented. Relatively few different experimental designs are predominantly used in controlled clinical studies. In this chapter we discuss several of these important designs and their applications.

11.1 INTRODUCTION

Both pharmaceutical manufacturers and FDA personnel have had considerable input in constructing guidelines and recommendations for good clinical protocol design and data analysis. In particular, the FDA has published a series of guidelines for the clinical evaluation of a variety of classes of drugs. Those persons involved in clinical studies have been exposed to the constant reminder of the importance of design in these studies. Clinical studies must be carefully devised and documented to meet the clinical objectives. Clinical studies are very expensive indeed, and before embarking, an all-out effort should be made to ensure that the study is on a sound footing. Clinical studies designed to "prove" or demonstrate efficacy and/or safety for FDA approval should be controlled studies, as far as is possible. A controlled study is one in which an adequate control group is present (placebo or active control), and in which measures are taken to avoid bias. The following excerpts from *General Considerations for the Clinical Evaluation of*

Drugs show the FDA's concern for good experimental design and statistical procedures in clinical trials [1]:

1. Statistical expertise is helpful in the planning, design, execution, and analysis of clinical investigations and clinical pharmacology in order to ensure the validity of estimates of safety and efficacy obtained from these studies.
2. It is the objective of clinical studies to draw inferences about drug responses in well defined target populations. Therefore, study protocols should specify the target population, how patients or volunteers are to be selected, their assignment to the treatment regimens, specific conditions under which the trial is to be conducted, and the procedures used to obtain estimates of the important clinical parameters.
3. Good planning usually results in questions being asked which permit direct inferences. Since studies are frequently designed to answer more than one question, it is useful in the planning phase to consider listing of the questions to be answered in order of priority.

The following are general principles that should be considered in the conduct of clinical trials.

1. Clearly state the objective(s).
2. Document the procedure used for randomization.
3. Include a suitable number of patients (subjects) according to statistical principles (see Chap. 6).
4. Include concurrently studied comparison (control) groups.
5. Use appropriate blinding techniques to avoid patient and physician bias.
6. Use objective measurements when possible.
7. Define the response variable.
8. Describe and document the statistical methods used for data analysis.

11.2 SOME PRINCIPLES OF EXPERIMENTAL DESIGN

Although many kinds of ingenious and complex statistical designs have been used in clinical studies, many experts feel that *simplicity* is the key in clinical study design. The implementation of clinical studies is extremely difficult. No matter how well designed or how well intentioned, clinical studies are particularly susceptible to Murphy's law: "If something can go wrong, it will!" Careful attention to protocol procedures and symmetry in design (e.g., equal number of patients per treatment group) often is negated as the study proceeds, due to patient dropouts, missed visits, carelessness, misunderstood directions, and so on. If severe, these deviations can result in extremely difficult analyses and interpretations. Although the experienced researcher anticipates the problems of human research, such problems can be minimized by careful planning.

We will discuss a few examples of designs commonly used in clinical studies. The basic principles of good design should always be kept in mind when considering the experimental pathway to the study objectives. In *Planning of Experiments*, Cox discusses the requirements for a good experiment [2]. When designing clinical studies, the following factors are important:

1. Absence of bias
2. Absence of systematic error (use of controls)
3. Adequate precision
4. Choice of patients
5. Simplicity and symmetry

11.2.1   Absence of Bias

As far as possible, known sources of bias should be eliminated by blinding techniques. If a double-blind procedure is not possible, careful thought should be given to alternatives that will suppress, or at least account for possible bias. For example, if the physician can distinguish two comparative drugs, an in an open study, perhaps the evaluation of the response and the administration of the drug can be done by other members of the investigative team (e.g., a nurse) who are not aware of the nature of the drug being administered.

In a double-blind study, both the observer and patient (or subject) are unaware of the treatment being given during the course of the study. Human beings, the most complex of machines, can respond to drugs (or any stimulus, for that matter) in amazing ways as a result of their psychology. This is characterized in drug trials by the well-known "placebo effect." Also, a well-known fact is that the observer (nurse, doctor, etc.) can influence the outcome of an experiment if the nature of the different treatments is known. The subjects of the experiment can be influenced by words and/or actions, and unconscious bias may be manifested in the recording and interpretation of the experimental observations. For example, in analgesic studies, as many as $30-40\%$ of patients may respond to a placebo treatment.

The double-blind method is accomplished by manufacturing alternative treatment dosage forms to be as alike as possible in terms of shape, size, color, odor, and taste. Even in the case of dosage forms that are quite disparate, ingenuity can always provide for double-blinding. For example, in a study where an injectable dosage form is to be compared to an oral dosage form, the *double-dummy technique* may be used. Each subject is administered both an oral dose and an injection. In one group, the subject receives an active oral dose and a placebo injection, whereas in the other group, each subject receives a placebo oral dose and an active injection. There are occasions where blinding is so difficult to achieve or is so inconvenient to the patient that studies are best left "unblinded." In these cases, every effort should be made to reduce possible biases. For example, in some cases, it may be convenient for one person to administer the study drug, and a second person, unaware of the treatment given, to make and record the observation.

Examples of problems that occur when trials are not blinded are given by Rodda et al. [3]. In a study designed to compare an angiotensin converting enzyme (ACE) inhibitor with a Beta-Blocker, unblinded investigators tended to assign patients who had been previously unresponse to Beta-blockers to the ACE group. This allocation results in a treatment bias. The ACE group may contain the more seriously ill patients.

An important feature of clinical study design is randomization of patients to treatments. This topic has been discussed in Chap. 4, but bears repetition. The randomization procedure as applied to various designs will be presented in the following discussion. Randomization is an integral and essential part of the implementation and design of clinical studies. Randomization will help to reduce potential bias in clinical experiments, and is the basis for valid calculations of probabilities for statistical testing.

11.2.2 Absence of Systematic Errors

Cox gives some excellent examples in which the presence of a systematic error leads to erroneous conclusions [2]. In the case of clinical trials, a systematic error would be present if one drug was studied by one investigator and the second drug was studied by a second investigator. Any observed differences between drugs could include "systematic" differences between the investigators. This ill-designed experiment can be likened to Cox's example of feeding two different rations to a group of animals, where each group of animals is kept together in separate pens. Differences in pens could confuse the ration differences. In the examples above, the experimental units (patients, animals, etc.) are not independent. Although the problems of interpretation resulting from the designs in the examples above may seem obvious, sometimes the shortcomings of experimental procedures are not obvious. We have discussed the deficiencies of a design in which a baseline measurement is compared to a posttreatment measurement in the absence of a control group. Any change in response from baseline to treatment could be due to changes in conditions during the intervening time period. To a great extent, systematic errors in clinical experiments can be avoided by the inclusion of an appropriate control group and random assignment of patients to the treatment groups.

11.2.3 Adequate Precision

Increased precision in a comparative experiment means less variable treatment effects and more efficient estimate of treatment differences. Precision can always be improved by increasing the number of patients in the study. Because of the expense and ethical questions raised by using large numbers of patients in drug trials, the sample size should be based on medical and statistical considerations which will achieve the experimental objectives described in Chap. 6.

Often, an appropriate choice of experimental design can increase the precision. Use of baseline measurements or use of a crossover design rather than a parallel design, for example, will usually increase the precision of treatment comparisons. However, in statistics as in life, we do not get something for nothing. Experimental designs have their shortcomings as well as advantages. Properties of a particular design should be carefully considered before the final choice is made. For example, the presence of carryover effects will negate the advantage of a crossover design as presented in Sec. 11.4.

Blocking is another way of increasing precision. This is the basis of the increased precision accomplished by use of the two-way design discussed in Sec. 8.4. In these designs, the patients in a block have similar (and relevant) characteristics. For example, if age and sex are variables that affect the therapeutic response of two comparative drugs, patients may be "blocked" on these variables. Thus if a male of age 55 years is assigned to drug A, another male of age approximately 55 years will be assigned treatment B. In practice, patients of similar characteristics are grouped together in a block and randomly assigned to treatments.

11.2.4 Choice of Patients

In most clinical studies, the choice of patients covers a wide range of possibilities (e.g., age, sex, severity of disease, concomitant diseases, etc.). In general, inferences made regarding drug effectiveness are directly related to the restrictions (or lack of restrictions) placed on patient eligibility. This is an important consideration in experimental design, and great care should be taken to describe which patients may be qualified or disqualified from entering the study.

11.2.5 Simplicity and Symmetry

Again we emphasize the importance of *simplicity*. More complex designs have more restrictions, and a concurrent lack of flexibility. The gain resulting from a more complex design should be weighed against the expense and problems of implementation often associated with more sophisticated, complex designs.

Symmetry is an important design consideration. Often, the symmetry is obvious. In most (but not all) cases, experimental designs should be designed to have equal number of patients per treatment group, equal number of visits per patient, balanced order of administration, and an equal number of replicates per patient. Some designs, such as balanced incomplete block and partially balanced incomplete block designs, have a less obvious symmetry; these are not treated in this book.

11.3 PARALLEL DESIGN

In a parallel design, two or more drugs are studied, drugs being randomly assigned to different patients. Each patient is assigned a single drug. In the example presented here, a study was proposed to compare the response of patients to a new formulation of an anti-anginal agent and a placebo with regard to exercise time on a stationary bicycle at fixed impedance. An alternative approach would be to use an existing product rather than placebo as the comparative product. However, the decision to use placebo was based on the experimental objective: to demonstrate that the new formulation produces a measurable and significant increase in exercise time. A difference in exercise time between the drug and placebo is such a measure. A comparison of the new formulation with a positive control (an active drug) would not achieve the objective directly.

In this study, a difference in exercise time between drug and placebo of 60 seconds was considered to be of clinical significance. The standard deviation was estimated to be 65 based on change from baseline data observed in previous studies. The sample size for this study, for an alpha level of 0.05 and power of 0.90 (beta = 0.10), was estimated as 20 patients per group (see Exercise Problem 7). Therefore forty patients were entered into the study, 20 each randomly assigned to placebo and active treatment. A randomization that obviates a long consecutive run of patients assigned to one of the treatments was used as described in Chap. 4. Patients were randomly assigned to each treatment in groups of 10, with 5 patients to be randomly assigned to each treatment. This randomization was applied to each of the 4 subsets of 10 patients (40 patients total). From Table IV.1, starting in the fourth row, third column, patients are randomized into the two groups as follows, placebo if an odd number appears and New Formulation if an even number appears:

	Placebo	New formulation
Subset 1	2, 6, 8, 9, 10	1, 3, 4, 5, 7
Subset 2	13, 14, 17, 19, 20	11, 12, 15, 16, 18
Subset 3	21, 23, 25, 26, 27	22, 24, 28, 29, 30
Subset 4	32, 35, 36, 37, 38	31, 33, 34, 39, 40

The first subset is assigned as follows. The first number is 2; patient 1 is assigned to the New Formulation (NF). The second number is (reading down) 9; patient 2 is assigned to placebo. The next 3 numbers (0, 0, 8) are all even; patients 3, 4, 5 are assigned to NF. The next number is odd (9); patient 6 is assigned to placebo. The next number is even and patient 7 is assigned to NF. Patients 8, 9, and 10 are assigned to placebo to balance the first group of 10 patients. Patient 11 is assigned to NF, etc.

An alternative randomization is to number patients consecutively from 1 to 40 as they enter the study. Using a table of random numbers, patients are assigned to placebo if an odd number appears, and assigned to the test product (new formulation) if an even number appears. Starting in the eleventh column of Table IV.1, the randomization scheme is as follows:

Placebo	New formulation
1, 6, 7, 8,	2, 3, 4, 5
12, 13, 14	9, 10, 11
15, 18, 20	16, 17, 19
21, 22, 26	23, 24, 25
27, 28	29, 30, 31
32, 34, 35	33, 38, 39
36, 37	40

For example, the first number in column 11 is 7; patient number 1 is assigned to placebo. The next number in column 11 is 8; the second patient is assigned to the new formulation; and so on.

Patients were first given a predrug exercise test to determine baseline values. The test statistic is the time of exercise to fatigue or an anginal episode. Tablets were prepared so that the placebo and active drug products were identical in appearance. Double-blind conditions prevailed. One hour after administration of the drug, the exercise test was repeated. The results of the experiment are shown in Table 11.1.

The key points in this design are:

1. There are two independent groups (placebo and active, in this example). An equal number of patients are randomly assigned to each group.
2. A baseline measurement and a single posttreatment measurement are available.

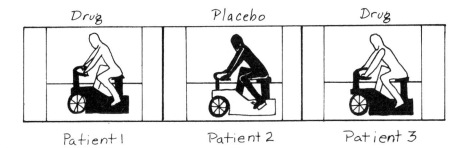

This design corresponds to a one-way analysis of variance, or in the case of two treatments, a two-independent-groups t test. Since, in general, more than two treatments may be included in the experiment, the analysis will be illustrated using ANOVA.

When possible, pretreatment (baseline) measurements should be made in clinical studies. The baseline values can be used to help increase the precision of the measurements. For example, if the treatment groups are compared using differences from baseline, rather than the posttreatment exercise time, the variability of the measurements will usually be reduced. Using differences, we will probably have a better chance of detecting treatment differences, if they exist (increased power). "Subtracting out" the baseline helps to reduce the between-patient variability which is responsible for the variance (the "within mean square") in the statistical test. A more complex, but more efficient analysis is *analysis of covariance*. Analysis of covariance takes baseline readings into account and assumes that the slope of the response vs. baseline is the same for all treatment groups. Also, the interpretation is more difficult than the simple "difference from baseline" approach. Analysis of

Table 11.1 Results of the Exercise Test Comparing Placebo to Active Drug: Time (Sec) to Fatigue or Angina

Placebo				Active drug (new formulation)			
	Exercise time				Exercise time		
Patient	Pre	Post	Post - Pre	Patient	Pre	Post	Post - Pre
1	377	345	-32	2	232	372	140
6	272	310	38	3	133	120	-13
7	348	347	-1	4	206	294	88
8	348	300	-48	5	140	258	118
12	133	150	17	9	240	340	100
13	102	129	27	10	246	393	147
14	156	110	-46	11	226	315	89
15	205	251	46	16	123	180	57
18	296	262	-34	17	166	334	168
20	328	297	-31	19	264	381	117
21	315	278	-37	23	241	376	135

22	133	124	-9
26	223	289	66
27	256	303	47
28	493	487	-6
32	336	309	-27
34	299	281	-18
35	140	186	46
36	161	125	-36
37	259	236	-23
Mean	259	256	-3.05
s.d.	102	95	36.3

24	74	264	190
25	400	541	141
29	320	410	90
30	216	301	85
31	153	143	-10
33	193	348	155
38	330	440	110
39	258	365	107
40	353	483	130
Mean	226	333	107.2
s.d.	83	106	51.5

covariance is described in many statistical textbooks, but is beyond the scope of the present discussion [4].

To illustrate the results of the analysis with and without baseline readings, the data in Table 11.1 will be analyzed in two ways: (a) using only the posttreatment response, posttreatment exercise time, and (b) comparing the difference from baseline for the two treatments. The reader is reminded of the assumptions underlying the t test and analysis of variance: the variables should be independent, normally distributed with homogeneous variance. These assumptions are necessary for both posttreatment and difference analyses. Possible problems with lack of normality will be less severe in the difference analysis. The difference of independent nonnormal variables will tend to be closer to normal than are the original individual data.

Before proceeding with the formal analysis, it is important to test the equivalence of the baseline averages for the two treatment groups. This test, if not significant, gives some assurance that the two groups are "comparable." We will use a two-independent groups t test to compare baseline values (see Sec. 5.2.2).

$$t = \frac{\overline{X}_1 - \overline{X}_2}{S_p \sqrt{1/N_1 + 1/N_2}}$$

$$= \frac{259 - 226}{S_p \sqrt{1/20 + 1/20}} = \frac{33}{93\sqrt{1/10}} = 1.12$$

Note that the pooled standard deviation (93) is the pooled value from the baseline readings, $\sqrt{(102^2 + 83^2)/2}$. From Table IV.4, a t value of approximately 2.03 is needed for significance (38 d.f.) at the 5% level. Therefore, the baseline averages are not significantly different for the two treatment groups. If the baseline values are significantly different, one would want to investigate further the effects of baseline on response in order to decide on the best procedure for analysis of the data (e.g., covariance analysis, ratio of response to baseline, etc.).

11.3.1 Analysis of Variance Using Only Posttreatment Results

The average results for exercise time after treatment are 256 sec for placebo and 333 sec for the new formulation of active drug, a difference of 77 sec (Table 11.1). Although the averages can be compared using a t test as in the case of baseline readings (above),

Table 11.2 ANOVA Table for Posttreatment Readings for the
Data of Table 11.1

Source	d.f.	SS	MS	F
Between groups	1	59,213	59,213	$F_{1,38} = 5.86*$
Within groups	38	383,787	10,099.7	
Total	39	443,000		

*P < 0.05.

the equivalent ANOVA is given in Table 11.2. The reader is directed to Exercise Problem 1 for the detailed calculations. According to Table IV.6, between groups (active and placebo) is significant
at the 5% level.

11.3.2 Analysis of Variance of Differences from the Baseline

When the baseline values are taken into consideration, the active
drug shows an increase in exercise time over placebo of 110.25 sec
[107.2 − (−3.05)]. The ANOVA is shown in Table 11.3. The data
analyzed here are the (post − pre) values in Table 11.1. The F
test for treatment differences is 61.3! There is no doubt about the
difference between the active drug and placebo. The larger F value
is due to the considerable reduction in variance as a result of including the baseline values in the analysis. The within-groups error
term represents *within*-patient variation in this analysis. In the
previous analysis for posttreatment results only, the within-groups

Table 11.3 Analysis of Variance for Differences from
Baseline (Table 11.1)

Source	d.f.	SS	MS	F
Between groups	1	121,551	120,551	$F_{1,38} = 61.3*$
Within groups	38	75,396	1,984	
Total	39	196,947		

*P < 0.01.

error term represents the *between*-patient variation, which is considerably larger than the within-patient error. Although both tests are significant (P < 0.05) in this example, one can easily see that situations may arise in which treatments may not be *statistically* different based on a significance test if between-patient variance is used as the error term, but would be significant based on the smaller within-patient variance. Thus designs that use the smaller within-patient variance as the error term for treatments are to be preferred, other things being equal.

11.4 CROSSOVER DESIGNS AND BIOAVAILABILITY/ BIOEQUIVALENCE STUDIES

In a typical crossover design, each subject takes each of the treatments under investigation on different occasions. Comparative bioavailability* or bioequivalence studies, in which two or more formulations of the same drug are compared, are usually designed as crossover studies. Perhaps the greatest appeal of the crossover design is that each patient acts as his or her own control. This feature allows for the direct comparison of treatments, and is particularly efficient in the presence of large interindividual variation. However, caution should be used when considering this design in studies where carryover effects or other interactions are anticipated. Under these circumstances, a parallel design may be more appropriate.

11.4.1 Description of Crossover Designs: Advantages and Disadvantages

The crossover (or changeover) design is a very popular, and often desirable, design in clinical experiments. In these designs, typically, two treatments are compared, with each patient or subject taking each treatment in turn. The treatments are taken on two occasions, often called *visits*, *periods*, or *legs*. The order of treatment is randomized; that is, either A is followed by B or B is followed by A, where A and B are the two treatments.

| A ⟶ B | or | B ⟶ A |
| First week   Second week | | First week   Second week |

---

*A bioavailability study, in our context, is defined as a comparative study of a drug formulation compared to an optimally absorbed (intravenous or oral solution) formulation.

This design may also be used for the comparison of more than two treatments. The present discussion will be limited to the comparison of two treatments, the most common situation in clinical studies. Crossover designs have great appeal when the experimental objective is the comparison of the performance, or effects, of two drugs or product formulations. Since each patient takes each product, the comparison of the products is based on *within*-patient variation. The *within*- or intrasubject variability will be smaller than the *between*- or intersubject variability used for the comparison of treatments in the one-way or parallel-groups design. Thus crossover experiments usually result in greater precision than the parallel-groups design, where different patients comprise the two groups. Given an equal number of observations, the crossover design is more powerful than a parallel design in detecting product differences.

The crossover design is a type of Latin square. In a Latin square the number of treatments equals the number of patients. In addition, another factor, such as order of treatment, is included in the experiment in a balanced way. The net result is an N × N array (where N is the number of treatments or patients) of N letters such that a given letter appears only once in a given row or column. This is most easily shown pictorially. A Latin square for four subjects taking four drugs is shown in Table 11.4. For randomizations of treatments in Latin squares, see Ref. 4.

For the comparison of two formulations, a 2 × 2 Latin square (N = 2) consists of two patients each taking two formulations (A and B) on two different occasions in two "orders" as follows:

Table 11.4   4 × 4 Latin Square: Four Subjects Take Four Drugs

| Subject | Order in which drugs[a] are taken | | | |
	First	Second	Third	Fourth
1	A	B	C	D
2	B	C	D	A
3	C	D	A	B
4	D	A	B	C

[a]Drugs are designated as A, B, C, D.

Patient	Occasion (period)	
	First	Second
1	A	B
2	B	A

The balancing of order (A–B or B–A) takes care of time trends or other "period" effects, if present. (A period effect is a difference in response due to the occasion on which the treatment is given, independent of the effect due to the treatment.)

The 2 × 2 Latin square shown above is familiar to all who have been involved in bioavailability/bioequivalence studies. In these studies, the 2 × 2 Latin square is repeated several times to include a sufficient number of patients (see also Table 11.5). Thus the crossover design can be thought of as a repetition of the 2 × 2 Latin square.

The crossover design has an advantage, previously noted, of increased precision relative to a parallel-groups design. Also, the crossover is usually more economical: one-half the number of patients or subjects have to be recruited to obtain the same number of observations as in a parallel design. (Note that each patient takes *two* drugs in the crossover.) Often, a significant part of the expense in terms of both time and money is spent recruiting and processing patients or volunteers. The advantage of the crossover design in terms of cost depends on the economics of patient recruiting, cost of experimental observations, as well as the relative within-patient/between-patient variation. The smaller the within-patient variation relative to the between-patient variation, the more efficient will be the crossover design. Hence, if a repeat observation on the same patient is very variable (nonreproducible), the crossover may not be very much better than a parallel design, cost factors being equal. This problem is presented and quantitatively analyzed in detail by Brown [6].

There are also some problems associated with crossover designs. A crossover study may take longer to complete than a parallel study because of the extra testing period. It should be noted, however, that if recruitment of patients is difficult, the crossover design may actually save time, because fewer patients are needed to obtain equal power compared to the parallel design. Another disadvantage of the crossover design is that missing data pose a more serious problem than in the parallel design. If an observation is lost in one of the legs of the two-period crossover, the data for that person carries very little information. Since each subject must supply data on *two occasions* (compared to a single occasion in the parallel design), the chances of observations being lost to the analysis are greater in the crossover study. When data are missing in the crossover design, the statistical analysis is more difficult and the design loses some efficiency. Finally, the administration of crossover designs in terms of management and patient compliance is somewhat more difficult than that of parallel studies.

Perhaps the most serious problem with the use of crossover designs is one common to all Latin square designs, the *possibility of interactions*. The most common interaction that may be present in crossover design is a *differential carryover* or residual effect. This effect occurs when the response on the second period (leg) is dependent on the response in the first period, and this dependency differs depending on which of the two treatments is given during the first period. Differential carryover is illustrated in Fig. 11.1A, where the short interval between administration of dosage forms X and Y is not sufficient to rid the body of drug when formulation X is given first. This results in an apparent larger blood level for formulation Y when it is given subsequent to formulation X. In the presence of such interactions, the data cannot be properly analyzed except by the use of more complex designs. These special designs are not easily accommodated to clinical studies [5].

Figure 11.1B illustrates an example where a sufficiently long washout period ensures that carryover of blood concentration of drug is absent. The results depicted in Fig. 11.1A show a carryover effect which could easily have been avoided if the study had been carefully planned. This example only illustrates the problem; often, carryover effects are not as obvious. These effects can be caused by such uncontrolled factors as psychological or physiological states of the patients, or by external factors such as the weather, clinical setting, assay techniques, and so on.

Grizzle has published an analysis to detect carryover (residual) effects [7]. When differential carryover effects are present, the usual interpretation and statistical analysis of crossover studies are invalid. Only the first period results can be used, resulting in a smaller, less sensitive experiment. An example of Grizzle's analysis is shown in this chapter in the discussion of bioavailability studies (Sec. 11.4.2). Brown concludes that most of the time, in these cases, the parallel design is probably more efficient [6]. Therefore, if carryover effects are suspected prior to implementation of the study, an alternative to the crossover design should be considered.

Because of the "built-in" individual-by-individual comparisons of products provided by the crossover design, the use of such designs in comparative clinical studies often seems very attractive. However, in many situations, where patients are being treated for a disease state, the design is either inappropriate or difficult to implement. In acute diseases, patients may be cured or so much improved after the

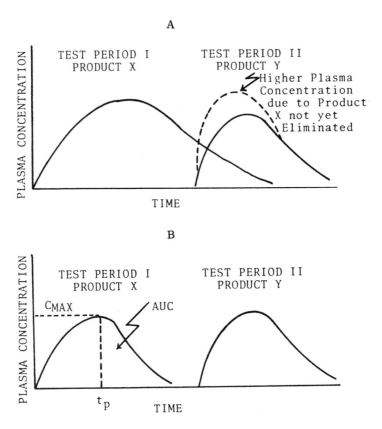

Figure 11.1   Carryover in a bioequivalence study.

first treatment that a "different" condition or state of illness is being treated during the second leg of the crossover. Also, psychological carryover has been observed, particularly in cases of testing
psychotropic drugs.

The longer study time necessary to test two drugs in the crossover design can be critical if the testing period of each leg is of
long duration. Including a possible *washout period* to avoid possible
carryover effects, the crossover study will take at least twice as
long as a parallel study to complete. In a study of long duration,
there will be more difficulty in recruiting and maintaining patients
in the study. One of the most frustrating (albeit challenging)
facets of data analysis is data with "holes," missing data. Long-
term crossover studies will inevitably have such problems.

11.4.2   Bioavailability Studies

Bioavailability/bioequivalence studies are particularly amenable to crossover designs.   Virtually all such studies make use of this design.   Most bioavailability studies involve single doses of drugs given to normal volunteers, and are of short duration.   Thus the disadvantages of the crossover design in long term, chronic dosing studies are not apparent in bioavailability studies.   With an appropriate washout period between doses, the crossover is ideally suited for comparative bioavailability studies.   A washout period of seven half-lives is recommended, ensuring that less than 1% of drug from the first leg remains in the plasma at the time the second dose is administered.   Westlake [8] has noted that significant carry-over effects occur about 5% of the time, just what would be expected when such effects are absent.

An important part of the planning and design of bioavailability studies is determination of a suitable sample size.   The FDA has recommended that the study have 80% power to detect a difference of 20% or more between the comparative products at the 5% level of significance.   Together with the specifications above, the sample size depends on the variability (error) of the comparison.   The variability can be estimated from preliminary experiments or from published data on similar products.   The question of sample-size determination is discussed in Chap. 6.

Crossover designs are planned so that each treatment is given an equal number of times in each period.   This is most efficient and yields unbiased estimates of treatment differences if a period effect is present.   A period effect is an effect on the treatment response

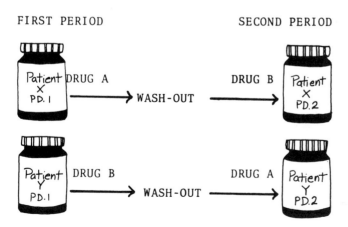

FIRST PERIOD   SECOND PERIOD

Table 11.5 Data for the Bioequivalence Study Comparing Drugs A and B

Subject	Order	AUC		Peak concentration		Time to peak	
		A	B	A	B	A	B
1	AB	290	210	30	18	8	8
2	BA	201	163	22	19	10	4
3	AB	187	116	18	11	6	6
4	AB	168	77	20	14	10	3
5	BA	200	220	18	21	3	3
6	BA	151	133	25	16	4	6
7	AB	294	140	27	14	4	10
8	BA	97	190	16	23	6	6
9	BA	228	168	20	14	6	6
10	AB	250	161	28	19	6	4
11	AB	293	240	28	18	6	12
12	BA	154	188	16	20	8	8
	Mean	209.4	167.2	22.3	17.3	6.4	6.3
	Sum	2513	2006	268	207	77	76

resulting from the period in which the treatment is tested. Such period effects should affect both treatments equally in a balanced crossover design.

A Worked Example

The results of a typical single-dose bioequivalence study is shown in Table 11.5. These data were obtained from drug plasma level versus time determinations similar to that illustrated in Fig. 11.1B. Area under the plasma level versus time curve (AUC, a measure of absorption), time to peak plasma concentration (t_p), and peak of maximum concentration (C_{max}) are the parameters which are usually of most interest in the comparison of the bioavailability of different formulations of the same drug moiety.

The typical ANOVA for crossover studies will be applied to the AUC data to illustrate the procedure used to analyze the experimental results. A critical assumption for the correct interpretation of the analysis is the *absence* of differential carryover effects, as discussed previously. Otherwise, the usual assumptions for ANOVA should hold. FDA statisticians encourage a careful statistical analysis of crossover designs. In particular, they condemn the use of a simple t test which ignores the possible presence of period and/or carryover effects.* If period effects are present, and not accounted for in the statistical analysis, the analysis will be less sensitive. The error mean square in the ANOVA will be inflated due to inclusion of the period variance, and the formulation differences will be more difficult to detect. If differential carryover effects are present, the estimate of treatment differences will be biased (see Sec. 11.4.1).

The usual analysis of variance separates the total sum of squares into four components: subjects, periods, treatments, and error (residual). In the absence of differential carryover effects, the statistical test of interest is for treatment differences. The subject and period sum of squares are separated from the error term which then represents "intrasubject" variation.

The sum of squares for treatments and subjects are computed exactly the same way as for a two-way analysis of variance (see Sec. 8.4). The only new calculation is the computation of the "period" sum of squares, which has 1 degree of freedom. Two new columns are prepared for this calculation. One column contains the data from the first period, and the second column contains data from the second period. For example, for the AUC data in Table 11.5, the data for the first period are obtained by noting the order of administration. Subject 1 took product A during the first period (290); subject 2 took B during the first period (163); and so on. Therefore, the first period observations are

---

*In bioavailability studies, carryover effects are usually due to an inadequate washout period.

Table 11.6 Analysis of Variance Table for the Crossover Bioequivalence Study (AUC)

Source	d.f.	SS	MS	P
Subjects	11	43,560.5	3,960.0	
Period	1	13,490.5	13,490.0	$F_{1,10} = 12.6$*
Treatment	1	10,710.4	10,710.4	$F_{1,10} = 10.0$*
Error	10	10,670.1	1,067.0	
Total	23	78,430.96		

*$P < 0.05$.

290, 163, 187, 168, 220, 133, 294, 190, 168, 250, 293, and 188
(sum = 2544)

The second period observations are

210, 201, 116, 77, 200, 151, 140, 97, 228, 161, 240, 154
(sum = 1975)

The "period" sum of squares may be calculated as follows:

$$\frac{(\Sigma \; X_1)^2 + (\Sigma \; X_2)^2}{N} - C.T. \tag{11.1}$$

where $\Sigma \; X_1$ and $\Sigma \; X_2$ are the sums of observations in the first and second periods, respectively, N is the number of subjects, and C.T. is the correction term. The following analysis of variance and Table 11.6 will help clarify the calculations.

Calculations for ANOVA:

$\Sigma \; X_t$ is the sum of all observations $\quad = \quad$ 4,519

$\Sigma \; X_A$ is the sum of observations for product A = 2,513

$\Sigma \; X_B$ is the sum of observations for product B = 2,006

$\Sigma \; P_1$ is the sum of observations for period 1 $\quad = \quad$ 2,544

$\Sigma \; P_2$ is the sum of observations for period 2 $\quad = \quad$ 1,975

$\Sigma \; X_T^2$ is the sum of the squared observations $\quad = $ 929,321

C.T. is the correction term $\dfrac{(\Sigma \, X_t)^2}{N_t} = \dfrac{(4519)^2}{24} = 850{,}890.04$

$\Sigma \, S_i$ is the sum of the observations for subject i (e.g., 500 for first subject)

Total sum of squares $= \Sigma \, X_t^2 - C.T. = 78{,}430.96$

Subject sum of squares

$$= \dfrac{\Sigma(\Sigma \, S_i)^2}{2} - C.T. = \dfrac{500^2 + 364^2 + \cdots + 342^2}{2} - C.T.$$

$$= 43{,}560.46$$

Period sum of squares $= \dfrac{2544^2 + 1975^2}{12} - C.T. = 13{,}490.0$

Treatment sum of squares $= \dfrac{2513^2 + 2006^2}{12} - C.T.$

$$= 10{,}710.4$$

Error sum of squares

$= $ total SS $-$ subject SS $-$ period SS $-$ treatment SS

$= 78{,}430.96 - 43{,}560.46 - 13{,}490 - 10{,}710.38$

$= 10{,}670.1$

Note that the degrees of freedom for error is equal to 10. The usual two-way ANOVA would have 11 degrees of freedom for error (subjects $-$ 1) $\times$ (treatments $-$ 1). In this design, the error sum of squares is diminished by the *period sum of squares*, which has 1 degree of freedom.

Test for Carryover Effects

Dr. James Grizzle detailed the analysis of crossover designs and presented a method for testing carryover effects (sequence effects in his notation) [7]. Some controversy exists regarding the usual analysis of crossover designs, particularly with regard to the assumptions underlying this analysis. Before using the Grizzle analysis, the reader should examine the original paper by Grizzle as well as the discussion by Brown, in which some of the problems of crossover designs are summarized [6].

One of the key assumptions necessary for a valid analysis and interpretation of crossover designs is the absence of differential carryover effects as has been previously noted. The analysis will be illustrated using the data for AUC from Table 11.5. These data were previously analyzed using the typical crossover analysis, assuming that differential carryover was absent. Table 11.5 is reproduced as Table 11.7 to illustrate the computations needed for the Grizzle analysis.

The test for carryover, or sequence, effects is performed as follows:

1. Compute the sum of squares due to carryover effects by comparing the results for group I to group II. (Note that these two groups, groups I and II, which differ in the order of treatment are designated as treatment "sequence" by Grizzle.) It can be demonstrated that in the absence of sequence effects, the average result for group I (A first, B second) is expected to be equal to the average result for group II (B first, A second). The sum of squares is calculated as

$$\frac{(\Sigma \ \text{group I})^2}{N_1} + \frac{(\Sigma \ \text{group II})^2}{N_2} - \text{C.T.}$$

Table 11.7   Data for the Bioequivalence Study Comparing Drugs A and B

Group I (Treatment A first, B second)				Group II (Treatment B first, A second)			
Subject	A	B	Total	Subject	A	B	Total
1	290	210	500	2	201	163	364
3	187	116	303	5	200	220	420
4	168	77	245	6	151	133	284
7	294	140	434	8	97	190	287
10	250	161	411	9	228	168	396
11	293	240	533	12	154	188	342
Total	1482	944	2426	Total	1031	1062	2093

In our example the sequence sum of squares is (1 d.f.)

$$\frac{(2426)^2}{12} + \frac{(2093)^2}{12} - \frac{(2426 + 2093)^2}{24} = 4620.375$$

2. The proper error term to test the sequence effect is the within-group (sequence) mean square, represented by the sum of squares between subjects within groups (sequence). This sum of squares is calculated as follows:

$$\frac{1}{2} \Sigma \text{ (subject total)}^2 - (C.T.)_I - (C.T.)_{II}$$

where $C.T._I$ and $C.T._{II}$ are the correction terms for groups I and II, respectively. In our example, the within-group sum of squares is

$$\frac{1}{2}(500^2 + 303^2 + 245^2 + \cdots + 364^2 + 420^2 + \cdots 342^2)$$

$$- \frac{(2426)^2}{12} - \frac{(2093)^2}{12} = 38,940.08$$

This within-group (or within-sequence) SS has 10 d.f., 5 from each group. The mean square is $38,940/10 = 3894$.

3. Test the sequence effect by comparing the sequence mean square square to the within-group mean square (F test).

$$F_{1,10} = \frac{4620.375}{3894} = 1.19$$

Referring to Table IV.6, the effect is not significant at the 5% level. If the sequence (carryover) effect is not significant, one would proceed with the usual analysis and interpretation as shown in Table 11.6.

If the carryover effect is significant, the usual analysis is not valid. The recommended analysis uses only the first period results, deleting the data contaminated by the carryover, the second period results. Grizzle recommends that the preliminary test for carryover be done at the 10% level (see also the discussion by Brown [6]). For the sake of this discussion, we will compute the analysis as if the data revealed a significant sequence effect in order to show the calculations. Using only the first-period data, the analysis is appropriate for a one-way analysis of variance design (Sec. 8.1). We have two "parallel" groups, one on product A and the other on product B. The data for the first period are as follows:

Subject	A	Subject	B
1	290	2	163
3	187	5	220
4	168	6	133
7	294	8	190
10	250	9	168
11	293	12	188
Mean	247		177
S^2	3204.8		870.4

The analysis of variance table is as follows:*

	d.f.	SS	MS	F
Between treatments	1	14,700	14,700	7.21
Within treatments	10	20,376	2,037.6	

Referring to Table IV.6, an F value of 4.96 is needed for significance at the 5% level (1 and 10 d.f.). Therefore, in this example, the analysis leads to the conclusion of significant treatment differences.

The discussion and analysis above should make it clear that sequence or carryover effects are undesirable in crossover experiments. Although an alternative analysis is available, one-half of the data are lost (second period) and the error term for the comparison of treatments is usually larger than that which would have been available in the absence of carryover (within-subject versus between-subject variation). One should thoroughly understand the nature of treatments in a crossover experiment in order to avoid differential carryover effects if at all possible.

Since the test for carryover was set at 5% in a priori, we will proceed with the interpretation, assuming that carryover effects are absent. Both period and treatment effects are significant ($F_{1,10}$ = 12.6 and 10.0, respectively). The AUC values tend to be

---

*This analysis is identical to a two-sample independent-groups t test.

higher during the first period (on the average). This period (or order) effect does not interfere with the conclusion that product A has a higher average AUC than that of product B. The balanced order of administration of the two products in this design compensates equally for both products for systematic differences due to the period or order. Also, the ANOVA subtracts out the sum of squares due to the period effect from the error term, which is used to test treatment differences.

If the design is not symmetrical, because of missing data, dropouts, or poor planning, a statistician should be consulted for the data analysis and interpretation. In an asymmetrical design, the number of observations in the two periods is different for the two treatment groups. This will always occur if there is an odd number of subjects. For example, the following scheme shows an asymmetrical design for seven subjects taking two drug products, A and B. In such situations, computer software programs can be used, which adjusts the analysis and mean results for the lack of symmetry [9].

Subject	Period 1	Period 2
1	A	B
2	B	A
3	A	B
4	B	A
5	A	B
6	B	A
7	A	B

The statistical analysis in the example above was performed on AUC, which is a measure of relative absorption. The FDA recommends that plasma or urine concentrations be determined out to at least three half-lives, so that practically all the area under the curve will be included when calculating this parameter (by the trapezoidal rule, for example). Other measures of the rate and extent of absorption are time to peak and peak concentration.

Much has been written and discussed about the expression and interpretation of bioequivalancy/bioavailability data as a measure of rate and extent of absorption. When are the parameters AUC, t_p, and C_{max} important, and what part do they play in bioequivalency? The FDA has stated that products may be considered equivalent in the presence of different rates of absorption, particularly if these differences are designed into the product [10]. For example, for a drug that is used in chronic dosing, the extent of absorption is probably a much more important parameter than the rate of absorption.

It is not the purpose of this presentation to discuss the merits of these parameters in evaluating equivalence, but only to alert the reader to the fact that bioequivalence interpretation need not be fixed and rigid.

Confidence Intervals

The analysis illustrated above was a test of the hypothesis of the equality of the AUCs for the two formulations (H_0: $AUC_A = AUC_B$). Arguments have been presented that hypothesis testing may not be an appropriate statistical approach to bioavailability/bioequivalence studies. Two *different* formulations are apt to be different with regard to bioavailability parameters such as AUC. Proposals have been made that a more informative statement about equivalence would be to present a "range" of equivalence, a lower and upper limit of the "equivalence" of two products. Then the user or prescriber of the drug can make an educated decision regarding the equivalence of the alternative products. In the example given here the confidence interval for the *difference* of the AUCs is calculated as follows (see Chap. 5 for a discussion of confidence intervals).

95% confidence interval for AUC difference

$$= \overline{\Delta} \pm t \ \sqrt{EMS \left(\frac{1}{N_1} + \frac{1}{N_2} \right)}$$

$$42.25 \pm 2.23 \ \sqrt{\frac{1067}{6}} \ = \ 42.25 \pm 29.74 \ = \ 12.51 \text{ to } 71.99$$

where 42.25 is the average difference of the AUCs, 2.23 the t value with 10 d.f., 1067 the variance estimate (Table 11.6), and $1/6 = 1/N_1 + 1/N_2$. The confidence interval can be expressed as an approximate percentage relative bioavailability by dividing the lower and upper limits for the AUC difference by the average AUC for product B, the reference product as follows:

Average AUC for drug product B   =   167.2

Approximate 95% confidence interval for A/B

$$= \ (167.2 + 12.51)/167.2 \text{ to } (167.2 + 71.99)/167.2$$

$$= \ 1.075 \text{ to } 1.431$$

Product A is between 7.5 and 43.1% more bioavailable than product B.

11.4.3   Miscellaneous Comments

More recently, the FDA has advocated the use of two one-sided t tests to evaluate bioequivalency [11,12]. The tests are performed each at the 5% level with the null hypotheses:

$$H_0: \frac{A}{B} < 0.8 \qquad \text{and} \qquad H_0: \frac{A}{B} > 1.20$$

If both tests are rejected, the products are considered to have a ratio of AUC and/or C_{max} between 0.8 and 1.2 and are taken to be equivalent. The outcome of the test is equivalent to forming a 90% symmetric confidence interval about the mean difference, and accepting equivalence if the limits of the interval lie between 0.8 and 1.2. If either test (or both) is not rejected, the products are not considered to be equivalent. In the example from Table 11.5, a 90% confidence interval for the difference of the AUCs for the two products is

$$42.25 \pm 1.81 \sqrt{1067/6} \ = \ 18.11 \text{ to } 66.39$$

The 90% confidence limits for the ratio of the AUC of test product/ standard product is calculated as:

$$\frac{167.2 + 18.11}{167.2} \ = \ 1.108$$

$$\frac{167.2 + 66.39}{167.2} \ = \ 1.397$$

The test product would not pass the FDA equivalency test because the upper limit exceeds 1.2. For the two one-sided t tests, we test the observed difference vs. the hypothetical difference needed to reach 80% and 120% of the standard product. In this example, a difference from the standard product of ±33.4 would result in limits of 1.2 and 0.8, respectively. The observed difference of 42.25 clearly results in a ratio of test to standard product exceeding 1.2 and the test vs. the upper limit is clearly not rejected.

$$H_0: \frac{A}{B} > 1.2$$

This is sufficient to call the products inequivalent.

If the test product had an average AUC of 175 and the error were 1067, the product would pass the FDA criterion. The 90% confidence limits would be

$$175 - 167.2 \pm 1.81 \sqrt{1067/6} = -16.34 \text{ to } 31.94$$

The 90% confidence limits for the ratio of the AUC of test product/ standard product is calculated as:

$$\frac{(167.2 - 16.34)}{167.2} = 0.902$$

$$\frac{(167.2 + 31.94)}{167.2} = 1.191$$

The limits are within 0.8 and 1.20.
The two one-sided t tests are:

$$H_0: \frac{A}{B} < 0.8 \qquad t = \frac{175 - 167.2 - [-33.4]}{\sqrt{1067/6}} = 3.09$$

$$H_0: \frac{A}{B} > 1.2 \qquad t = \frac{175 - 167.2 - [33.4]}{\sqrt{1067/6}} = -1.92$$

Since both t values exceed 1.81, the table t for a one-sided test at the 5% level, the products are deemed to be equivalent.

Westlake has discussed the application of a confidence interval that is symmetric about the ratio 1.0, the value that defines equivalent products. The construction of such an interval is described in Sec. 5.1.

Because of the FDA's recommendation of 80% bioavailability for a claim of bioequivalence, the ratio of AUCs is often statistically analyzed rather than the differences of AUCs. An alternative to this analysis often preferred by statisticians for theoretical reasons is to analyze the logarithms of the AUC (see Sec. 10.1.1 and Ref. 8). Note that the *difference* of the logarithms is equivalent to the logarithm of the *ratio* [i.e., log A − log B = log (A/B)]. The antilog of the average difference of the logarithms is an estimate of the ratio of AUCs.

The ANOVA for the ln transformed data is shown below:

Source	d.f.	SS	MS	F
Subjects	11	1.39	0.127	
Periods	1	0.45	0.45	10.02[a]

Source	d.f.	SS	MS	F
Treatments	1	0.29	0.29	6.44^b
Error	10	0.45	0.045	
Total	23	2.58		

[a] $P < 0.01.$

[b] $P < 0.05.$

The averages ln values for the test and standard products are

$$\overline{A} = 5.29751$$
$$\overline{B} = 5.07778$$
$$\overline{A} - \overline{B} = 5.29751 - 5.0778 = 0.21973$$

The anti-ln of this difference, corresponding to the geometric mean of the individual ratios, is 1.246. This compares to the ratio of $\overline{A}/\overline{B}$ for the untransformed values of 1.252.

The 90% confidence limits for $A - B$ are

$$0.21973 \pm 1.81 \ \sqrt{0.045/6} = 0.06298 \text{ to } 0.37648$$

The anti-ln of these limits are 1.065 to 1.457. The 90% confidence limits for the untransformed data are 1.075 to 1.431.

It is not surprising that both analyses give similar results and conclusions. However, in situations where the upper and lower limits are close to 1.2 and 0.8, respectively, the data should be considered carefully so that the correct analysis can be applied.

Recently, the FDA suggested an alternative criterion for proof of bioequivalence: that 75% of the subjects should show at least 75% of the availability for a test product compared to the reference or standard formulation. This is called the *75/75 rule*. If 75% of the population *truly* shows at least 75% relative absorption of the test formulation compared to the standard, a sample of subjects in a clinical study will have a 50% chance of failing the test based on the FDA criterion. This criterion has little statistical basis and has fallen into disrepute.

11.5 **REPEATED MEASURES (SPLIT-PLOT) DESIGNS

Many clinical studies take the form of a baseline measurement followed by observations at more than one point in time. For example,
a new antihypertensive drug is to be compared to a standard, marketed drug with respect to diastolic blood pressure reduction. In
this case, after a baseline blood pressure is established, the patients
are examined every other week for 8 weeks, a total of four observations (visits) after treatment is initiated.

11.5.1 Experimental Design

Although this antihypertensive drug study was designed as a multiclinic study, the data presented here represent a single clinic.
Twenty patients were randomly assigned to the two treatment groups,
10 to each group (see Sec. 11.3 for the randomization procedure).
Prior to drug treatment, each patient was treated with placebo, and
blood pressure determined on three occasions. The average of these
three measurements was the baseline reading.

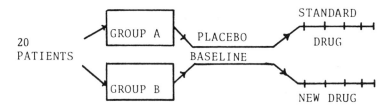

The baseline data were examined to ensure that the three baseline
readings did not show a time trend. For example, a placebo effect
could have resulted in decreased blood pressure with time during
this preliminary phase.

Treatment was initiated after the baseline blood pressure was
established. Diastolic blood pressure was measured every 2 weeks
for 8 weeks following initiation of treatment. (The dose was one
tablet each day for the standard and new drug.) Two patients
dropped out in the "standard drug" group, and one patient was lost
to the "new drug" group, resulting in eight and nine patients in
each treatment group. The results of the study are shown in
Table 11.8 and Fig. 11.2.

The design described above is commonly known in the pharmaceutical industry as a *repeated measures* or *split-plot* design. (This
design is also denoted as an incomplete three-way or a partially
hierarchical design.) This design is common in clinical or preclinical
studies, where two or more products are to be compared with multiple

Table 11.8 Results of a Comparison of Two Antihypertensive Drugs

| | Standard drug | | | | | | New drug | | | | | |
| | | | Week | | | | | | | Week | | | |
Patient	Baseline	2	4	6	8	Patient	Baseline	2	4	6	8
1	102	106	97	86	93	3	98	96	97	82	91
2	105	103	102	99	101	4	106	100	98	96	93
5	99	95	96	88	88	6	102	99	95	93	93
9	105	102	102	98	98	8	102	94	97	98	85
13	108	108	101	91	102	10	98	93	84	87	83
15	104	101	97	99	97	11	108	110	95	92	88
17	106	103	100	97	101	12	103	96	99	88	86
18	100	97	96	99	93	14	101	96	96	93	89
						16	107	107	96	93	97
Mean	103.6	101.9	98.9	94.6	96.6	Mean	102.8	99.0	95.2	91.3	89.4

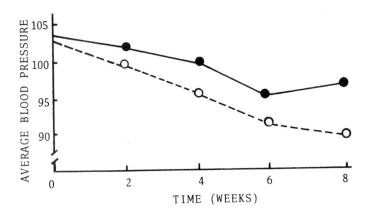

Figure 11.2   Plot of mean results from antihypertensive drug study.
● —— standard drug; ○ ----- new drug.

observations over time. The design can be considered as an extension of the one-way or parallel-groups design. In the present design (repeated measures), data are obtained at more than one time
point. The result is two or more two-way designs, as can be seen
in Table 11.8, where we have two two-way designs. The two-way
designs are related in that observations are made at the same time
periods. *The chief features of the repeated measures design* as
presented here are:

1. Different patients are randomly assigned to the different treat-
    ment groups, i.e., a patient is assigned to only one treatment
    group.
2. The number of patients in each group need not be equal. Equal
    numbers of patients per group, however, result in optimum
    precision when comparing treatment means. Usually, these
    studies are designed to have the same number of patients in
    each group, but dropouts usually occur during the course of
    the study.
3. Two or more treatment groups may be included in the study.
4. Each patient provides more than one measurement over time.
5. The observation times (visits) are the same for all patients.
6. Baseline measurements are usually available.
7. The usual precautions regarding blinding and randomization
    are followed.

Although the analysis tolerates lack of symmetry with regard to the
number of patients per group (see feature 2), the statistical analysis

can be difficult if patients included in the study have missing data for one or more visits. In these cases, a statistician should be consulted regarding data analysis [13].

The usual assumptions of normality, independence, and homogeneity of variance for each observation hold for the split-plot analysis. In addition, there is another important assumption with regard to the analysis and interpretation of the data in these designs. The assumption is that the data at the various time periods (visits) are not correlated, or that the correlation is of a special form [14]. Although this is an important assumption, often ignored in practice, moderate departures from the assumption can be tolerated. Correlation of data during successive time periods often occurs such that data from periods close together are highly correlated compared to the correlation of data far apart in time. For example, if a person has a high blood pressure reading at the first visit of a clinical study, we might expect a similar reading at the subsequent visit if the visits are close in time. The reading at the end of the study is apt to be less related to the initial reading. The present analysis assumes that the correlation of the data is the same for all pairs of time periods, and that the pattern of the correlation is the same in the different groups (e.g., drug groups) [14]. If these assumptions are substantially violated, the conclusions based on the usual statistical analysis will not be valid. The following discussion assumes that this problem has been considered and is negligible [13].

11.5.2 Analysis of Variance

The data of Table 11.8 will be subjected to the typical repeated measures (split-plot) ANOVA. As in the previous examples in this chapter, the data will be analyzed, corrected for baseline, by subtracting the baseline measurement from each observation. The measurements will then represent *changes from baseline*. The more complicated analysis of covariance is an alternative method of treating such data [13,14]. More expert statistical help will usually be needed when applying this technique, and the use of a computer is almost mandatory. Subtracting out the baseline reading is easy to interpret and, generally, results in conclusions very similar to that obtained by covariance analysis. Table 11.9 shows the "changes from baseline" data derived from Table 11.8. For example, the first entry in this table, 2 weeks for the standard drug, is $106 - 102 = 4$.

When computing the ANOVA by hand (use a calculator), the simplest approach is to first compute the two-way ANOVA for each treatment group, "standard drug" and "new drug." The calculations are described in Sec. 8.4. The results of the analysis of variance are shown in Table 11.10. Only the sums of squares need be calculated for this preliminary computation.

Table 11.9 Changes from Baseline of Diastolic Pressure for the Comparison of Two Antihypertensive Drugs

	Standard drug					New drug			
	Week					Week			
Patient	2	4	6	8	Patient	2	4	6	8
1	4	-5	-16	-9	3	-2	-1	-16	-7
2	-2	-3	-6	-4	4	-6	-8	-10	-13
5	-4	-3	-11	-11	6	-3	-7	-9	-9
9	-3	-3	-7	-7	8	-8	-5	-4	-17
13	0	-7	-17	-6	10	-5	-14	-11	-15
15	-3	-7	-5	-7	11	2	-13	-16	-20
17	-3	-6	-9	-5	12	-7	-4	-15	-17
18	-3	-4	-1	-7	14	-5	-5	-8	-12
					16	0	-11	-14	-10
Mean	-1.75	-4.75	-9	-7	Mean	-3.8	-7.6	-11.4	-13.3
Sum	-14	-38	-72	-56	Sum	-34	-68	-103	-120

Table 11.10 ANOVA for Changes from Baseline for Standard Drug and New Drug

Source	Standard drug		New drug	
	d.f.	Sum of squares	d.f.	Sum of squares
Patients	7	57.5	8	114.22
Weeks	3	232.5	3	486.97
Error	21	255.5	24	407.78
Total	31	545.5	35	1008.97

The final analysis combines the separate two-way ANOVAs and has two new terms, "weeks × drugs" interaction and "drugs," the variance represented by the difference between the drugs. The calculations are described below, and the final ANOVA table is shown in Table 11.11.

Patients' sum of squares: Pool the sum of squares from the separate ANOVAs (57.5 + 114.22 = 171.72 with 7 + 8 = 15 d.f.).

Table 11.11 Repeated Measures (Split-Plot) ANOVA for the Antihypertensive Drug Study

Source	d.f.[a]	SS	MS	
Patients	15	171.7	11.45	
Weeks	3	669.7	223.23	
Drugs	1	196.2	196.2	$F_{1,15} = \dfrac{196.2}{11.45}$
Weeks × drugs	3	49.8	16.6	$= 17.1*$
Error (within treatments)	45	663.3	14.74	$F_{3,45} = \dfrac{16.6}{14.74}$
	67	1750.6		$= 1.1$

[a]Degrees of freedom for "patients" and "error" are the d.f. pooled from the two-way ANOVAs. For "weeks" and "drugs," the d.f. are (weeks - 1) and (drugs - 1), respectively. For "weeks × drugs," d.f. are (weeks - 1) × (drugs - 1).
*P < 0.01.

Weeks' sum of squares: This term is calculated by combining all of the data, resulting in four columns (weeks), with 17 observations per column, 8 from the standard drug and 9 from the new drug. The calculation is

$$\frac{\Sigma \, C^2}{R_1 + R_2} - C.T.$$ where C = column sums of combined data
$R_1 + R_2$ = sum of the number of rows

$$= \frac{(-48)^2 + (-106)^2 + (-175)^2 + (-176)^2}{17} - \frac{(-505)^2}{68}$$

$$= \; 4420.1 - 3750.4 \; = \; 669.7$$

Drug sum of squares: Drug sum of squares = $(C.T._{SP})$ + $(C.T._{NP}) - (C.T._T)$, where $C.T._{SP}$ is the correction term for the standard drug, $C.T._{NP}$ is the correction term for the new product, and $C.T._T$ is the correction term for the combined data.

$$\text{Drug sum of squares} \; = \; \frac{(-180)^2}{32} + \frac{(-325)^2}{36} - \frac{(-505)^2}{68}$$

$$= \; 196.2$$

Weeks × drugs sum of squares: This interaction term (see below for interpretation) is calculated as the pooled sum of squares from the "week" terms in the separate two-way ANOVAs above, minus the week term for the final combined analysis, 669.7.

Weeks × drug sum of squares   = $232.5 + 486.97 - 669.7 = 49.8$

Error sum of squares: The error sum of squares is the pooled error from the two-way ANOVAs, $255.5 + 407.8 = 663.3$.

Interpretation and Discussion

The terms of most interest are the "drugs" and "weeks × drugs" components of the ANOVA. "Drugs" measures the difference between the overall averages of the two treatment groups. The average change of blood pressure was $(-180/32) - 5.625$ mmHg for standard drug, and $(-325/36) - 9.027$ mmHg for the new drug. The F test for "drug" differences is (drug MS)/(patients MS) equal to 17.1 (1 and 15 d.f.; see Table 11.11). This difference is highly significant ($P < 0.01$). The significant result indicates that on the average, the new drug is superior to the standard drug with regard to lowering diastolic blood pressure.

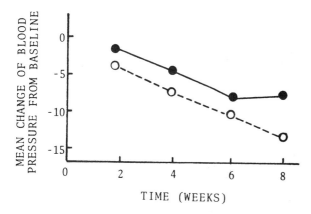

Figure 11.3 Plot from the data of Table 11.9 showing lack of significant interaction of weeks and drugs in experiment comparing standard and new antihypertensive drugs. ●——— standard drug; ○----- new drug.

The significant difference between the standard and new drugs is particularly meaningful if the difference is constant over time. Otherwise, the difference is more difficult to interpret. "Weeks × drugs" is a measure of interaction (see also Chap. 9). This test compares the parallelism of the two "change from baseline" curves as shown in Fig. 11.3. The F test for "weeks × drugs" uses a different error term than the test for "drugs." The F test with 3 and 45 d.f. is 16.6/14.74 = 1.1, as shown in Table 11.11. This nonsignificant result suggests that the pattern of response is not very different for the two drugs. A reasonable conclusion based on this analysis is that the new drug is effective (superior to the standard drug), and that its advantage beyond the standard drug is approximately maintained during the course of the experiment.

A significant nonparallelism of the two "curves" in Fig. 11.3 would be evidence for a "weeks × drugs" interaction. For example, if the new drug showed a lower blood pressure than the standard drug at 2 weeks, and a higher blood pressure at 8 weeks (the curves cross one another), interaction of weeks and drugs would more likely be significant. Interaction, in this example, would suggest that drug differences are dependent on the time of observation.

If interaction is present or the assumptions underlying the analysis are violated (particularly concerning the form of the covariance matrix) [13], a follow-up or an alternative is to perform p

one-way ANOVAs at each of the p points in time. In the previous
example, analyses would be performed at each of the 4 posttreatment weeks. A conclusion is then made based on the results
of these individual analyses (see Exercise Problem 8).

11.6 MULTICLINIC STUDIES

Most clinical studies carried out during late phase 2 or phase 3
periods of drug testing involve multiclinic studies. In these investigations, a common protocol is implemented at more than one study
site. This procedure, recommended by the FDA, serves several purposes. It may not be possible to recruit sufficient patients in a
study carried out by a single investigator. Thus multiclinic studies
are used to "beef up" the sample size. Another very important
consideration is that multiclinic studies, if performed at various
geographic locations with patients representing a wide variety of
attributes, such as age, race, socioeconomic status, and so on,
yield data that can be considered representative under a wide
variety of conditions. Multiclinic studies, in this way, guard
against the possibility of a result peculiar to a particular single clinical site. For example, a study carried out at a single Veterans'
Administration hospital would probably involve older males of a particular economic class. Also, a single investigator may implement
the study in a unique way which may not be typical, and the results would be peculiar to his or her methods. Thus, if a drug is
tested at many locations and the results show a similar measure of
efficacy at all locations, one has some assurance of the general ap-
plicability of the drug therapy.

However, there are instances where a drug has been found to
be efficaceous in the hands of some investigators and not for others.
When this occurs, the drug effect is in some doubt unless one can
discover the cause of such results. This problem is statistically apparent in the form of a treatment × site interaction. The comparative treatments (drug and placebo, for example) are not differentiated equally at different sites. A treatment × site interaction may
be considered very serious when one treatment is favored at some
clinical sites and the other favored at different sites. Less serious
is the case of interaction where all clinics favor the same treatment,
but some favor it more than others. These two examples of interaction are illustrated in Fig. 11.4.

When interaction occurs, the design, patient population, clinical
methods, protocol, and other possible problems should be carefully
investigated and dissected, to help find the cause. The cause will
not always be readily apparent, if at all. See Sec. 8.4.3 for a
further example and discussion of interactions in clinical studies.

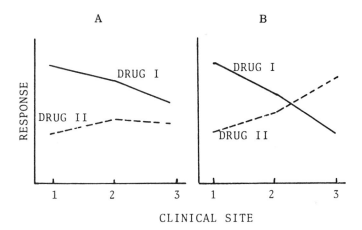

Figure 11.4 Two kinds of interaction: (A) one drug always better than another, but the difference changes for different clinical sites; (B) one drug better than another at sites 1 and 2 and worse at site 3.

An important feature of multiclinic studies, as noted above, is that the same protocol and design should be followed at all sites.

Since one can anticipate missing values due to dropouts, missed visits recording errors, and so on, an important consideration is that the design should not be so complicated that missing data will cause problems with the statistical interpretation or that the clinicians will have difficulty following the protocol. A simple design that will achieve the objectives is to be preferred. Since parallel-groups designs are the most simple in concept, these should be preferred to some more esoteric design. Nevertheless, there are occasions where a more complex design would be appropriate providing that the study is closely monitored and the clinical investigators thoroughly educated.

KEY TERMS

Analysis of covariance
AUC (area under curve)
Balance
Baseline measurements
Between-patient variation
   (error)

Bias
Bioavailability
Bioequivalence
Blinding
Carryover
Changeover design

C_{max} Objective measurements
Controlled study   Parallel design
Crossover design   Period (visit)
Differential carryover   Placebo effect
Double-blind   Positive control
Double dummy   Randomization
75 – 75 rule   Repeated measures
Experimental design   Split plot
Grizzle analysis   Symmetry
Incomplete three-way ANOVA   Systematic error
Interaction T_p
Latin square   Washout period
Log transformation   Within-patient variation (error)
Multiclinic   80% power to detect 20% difference

EXERCISES

1. (a) Perform the calculations for the ANOVA table (Table 11.2) from the data in Table 11.1.

   (b) Perform a t test comparing the differences from baseline for the two groups in Table 11.1. Compare the t value to the F value in Table 11.3.

2. Using the data in Table 11.5, test to see if the values of t_p are different for formulations A and B (5% level).

3. (a) Using the data in Table 11.5, compare the values of C_{max} for the two formulations (5% level). Calculate a confidence interval for the difference in C_{max}.

   **(b) Analyze the data for C_{max} using the Grizzle method. Is a differential carryover effect present?

4. Analyze the AUC data in Table 11.5 using ratios of AUC (A/B). Find the average ratio and test the average for significance. (Note that H_0 is $AUC_A/AUC_B = 1.0$.) Assume no period effect.

5. Analyze the AUC data in Table 11.5 using logarithms of AUC. Compare the antilog of the average difference of the logs to the average ratio determined in Problem 4. Put a 95% confidence interval on the average difference of the logs. Take the antilogs of the lower and upper limit and express the interval as a ratio of the AUCs for the two formulations.

**6. In a pilot study, two acne preparations were compared by measuring subjective improvement from baseline (10-point scale). Six patients were given a placebo cream and six different patients were given a cream with an active ingredient. Observations were made once a week for 4 weeks. Following are the results of this experiment:

Placebo					Active				
	Week					Week			
Patient	1	2	3	4	Patient	1	2	3	4
1	2	2	4	3	1	2	2	3	3
2	3	2	3	3	2	4	4	5	4
3	1	4	3	2	3	1	3	4	5
4	3	2	1	0	4	3	4	4	7
5	2	1	3	2	5	2	2	3	6
6	4	4	5	3	6	3	4	6	5

A score of 10 is complete improvement. A score of 0 is no improvement (negative scores mean a worsening of the condition). Perform an analysis of variance (split plot). Plot the data as in Fig. 11.3. Are the two treatments different? If so, how are they different?

7. For the exercise study described in Sec. 11.3, the difference considered to be significant is 60 minutes with an estimated standard deviation of 55 minutes. Compute the sample size if the Type I (alpha) and Type II (beta) error rates are set at 0.05 and 0.10, respectively.

8. From the data in Table 11.9, test for a difference ($\alpha = 0.05$) between the two drugs at week 4.

9. Perform the ANOVA on the ln transformed bioavailability data (Sec. 11.4.3).

REFERENCES

1. Dept. of Health, Education and Welfare, Pub. HEW(FDA)77-3040, *General Considerations for the Clinical Evaluation of Drugs* (GPO 017-012-00245-5), FDA Bureau of Drugs, Clinical Guidelines, U.S. Government Printing Office, Washington, D.C.
2. Cox, D. R., *Planning Experiments*, Wiley, New York, 1958.
3. Rodda, B. E. et al., *Statistical Issues in Drug Research and Development* (K. E. Peace, ed.), Marcel Dekker, New York, 1990.
4. Snedecor, G. W. and Cochran, W. G., *Statistical Methods*, 7th ed., Iowa University Press, Ames, Iowa, 1980.
5. Cochran, W. G. and Cox, G. M., *Experimental Designs*, 2nd ed., Wiley, New York, 1957.
6. Brown, B. W., Jr., *Biometrics, 36*, 69, 1980.

7. Grizzle, J. E., *Biometrics, 21*, 467, 1965; *30*, 727, 1974.
8. Westlake, W. J., *Statistical Issues in Drug Research and Development* (K. E. Peace, ed.), Marcel Dekker, New York, 1990.
9. SAS Institute, Inc., Cary, North Carolina.
10. FDA Bioavailability/Bioequivalence Regulations, *Fed. Reg. 42*, 1624, 1977.
11. Schuirman, D. L., *Biometrics, 37*, 617 (abstract).
12. Schuirman, D. L., *J. Pharmacokinet. Biopharm., 15*, 657–680, 1987.
13. Chinchill, V. M., *Statistical Issues in Drug Research and Development* (K. E. Peace, ed.), Marcel Dekker, New York, 1990.
14. Winer, B. J., *Statistical Principles in Experimental Design*, 2nd ed., McGraw-Hill, New York, 1971.

12
Quality Control

The science of quality control is largely statistical in nature, and entire books have been devoted to the application of statistical techniques to quality control. Statistical quality control is a key factor in process validation and the manufacture of pharmaceutical products. In this chapter we discuss some common applications of statistics to quality control. These applications include Shewhart control charts, sampling plans for attributes, operating characteristic curves, and some applications to assay development, including components of variance analysis. The applications to quality control make use of standard statistical techniques, many of which have been discussed in previous portions of this book.

12.1 INTRODUCTION

Starting from raw materials to the final packaged container, quality control departments have the responsibility of assuring the integrity of a drug product with regard to safety, potency, and biological availability. If each and every item produced could be tested (100% testing), there would be little need for statistical input in quality control. Those individual dosage units that are found to be unsatisfactory could be discarded, and only the good items would be released for distribution. Unfortunately, conditions exist which make 100% sampling difficult, if not impossible. For example, if every dosage unit could be tested, the expense would probably be prohibitive both to manufacturer and consumer. Also, it is well known that attempts to test individually every item from a large batch (several million tablets, for example), result in tester fatigue, which can cause misclassifications of items and other errors. If testing is destructive, such as would be the case for assay of individual tablets, 100% testing is, obviously, not a practical procedure. However, 100% testing is not necessary to determine product quality precisely. Quality can be accurately and precisely estimated by testing only part of the total material (a sample). In general, quality control procedures require relatively small samples for inspection or analysis. Data obtained from this sampling can then be treated statistically to estimate population parameters such as potency, tablet hardness, dissolution, weight, impurities, content uniformity (variability), as well as to ensure the quality of attributes such as color, appearance, and so on.

Statistical techniques are also used to monitor processes. In particular, control charts are commonly used to ensure that the average and variability of a pharmaceutical operation are stable. Control charts can be applied during *in-process* manufacturing operations, for *finished* product characteristics, and in *research and development* for repetitive procedures. Control charts are one of the most important statistical applications to quality control.

12.2   CONTROL CHARTS

Probably the best known application of statistics to quality control which has withstood the test of time is the Shewhart control chart. Important attributes of the control chart are its simplicity and the visual impression which it imparts. The control chart allows for judgments based on an easily comprehended graph. The basic principles underlying the use of the control chart are described below.

12.2.1   Statistical Control

A process under statistical control is one in which the process is susceptible to variability due only to inherent, but unknown and uncontrolled *chance* causes. According to Grant [1]: "Measured quality of manufactured product is always subject to a certain amount of variation as a result of chance. Some stable system of chance causes is inherent in any particular scheme of production and inspection. Variation within this stable pattern is inevitable. The reasons for variation outside this stable pattern may be discovered and corrected."

Using tablet manufacture as an example, where tablet weights are being monitored, it is not reasonable to expect that each tablet should have an identical weight, precisely equal to some target value. A tablet machine is simply not capable of producing identical tablets. The variability is due, in part, to (a) the variation of compression force, (b) variation in filling the die, and (c) variation in granulation characteristics. In addition, the balance used to weigh the tablets cannot be expected to give exactly reproducible weighings, even if the tablets could be identically manufactured. Thus the weight of any single tablet will be subject to the vagaries of chance from the foregoing uncontrollable sources of error, in addition to other identifiable sources which we have not mentioned.

12.2.2 Constructing Control Charts

The process of constructing a control chart depends, to a great extent, on the process characteristics and the objectives that one wishes to achieve. A control chart for tablet weights can serve as a typical example. In this example, we are interested in ensuring that tablet weights remain close to a target value, under "statistical control." To achieve this objective, we will periodically sample a group of tablets, measuring the mean weight and variability. The mean weight and variability of each sample (*subgroup*) are plotted sequentially as a function of time. The control chart is a graph that has time or order of submission of sequential lots on the X axis and the average test result on the Y axis. The process average together with upper and lower limits are specified as shown in Fig. 12.1. The preservation of order with respect to the observations is an important feature of the control chart. Among other things, we are interested in attaining a state of statistical control and detecting *trends* or changes in the process average and variability. One can visualize such trends (mean and range) easily with the use of the control chart. The "consistency" of the data as reflected by the deviations from the average value is not only easily seen, but the chart provides a record of batch performance. This record is useful for regulatory purposes as well as for an in-house source of data.

As will be described subsequently, variability can be calculated on the basis of the standard deviation or the range. The range is easier to calculate than the standard deviation. Remember: The range is the difference between the lowest and highest value. If the sample size is not large (<10), the range is an efficient estimator of the standard deviation. Figure 12.1 shows an example of an "$\overline{X}$" (X bar or average) and "range" chart for tablet weights determined from consecutive tablet production batches.

Rational Subgroups

The question of how many tablets to choose at each sampling time (*rational subgroups*) and how often to sample is largely dependent on the nature of the process and the level of precision required. The larger the sample and the more frequent the sampling, the greater the precision, but also the greater will be the cost. If tablet samples are taken and weights averaged over relatively long

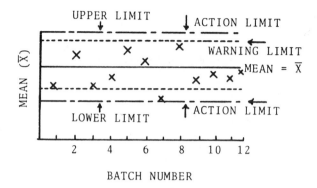

BATCH NUMBER

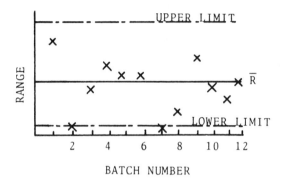

BATCH NUMBER

Figure 12.1   Quality control $\overline{X}$ and range charts.

periods of time, significant fluctuations which may have been observed with samples taken at shorter time intervals could be obscured.   The subgroups should be as homogeneous as possible relative to the overall process.   Subgroups are usually (but not always)
taken as units manufactured close in time.   For example, in the case
of tablet production, consecutively manufactured tablets may be
chosen for a subgroup.   If possible, the subgroup sample size
should be constant.   Otherwise, the construction and interpretation
of the control chart is more difficult.   Four to five items per subgroup is usually an adequate sample size.   Procedures for selecting
samples should be specified under SOPs (standard operating procedures) in the quality control manual.   In our example, 10 consecutive tablets are individually weighed at approximately 1 hour intervals.   Here the subgroup sample size is larger than the "usual"
four or five, principally because of the simple and inexpensive
measurement (weighing tablets).   The average weight and range

are calculated for each of the subgroup samples. One should understand that under ordinary circumstances the variation between individual items (tablets in this example) within a subgroup is due only to chance causes, as noted above. In this example, the 10 consecutive tablets are made almost at the same time. The granulation characteristics and tablet press effects are similar for these 10 tablets. Therefore, the variability observed can be attributed to causes that are not under our control (i.e., the inherent variability of the process).

Establishing Control Chart Limits

The principal use of the control chart is as a means of monitoring the manufacturing process. As long as the mean and range of the 10 tablet samples do not vary "too much" from subgroup to subgroup, the product is considered to be in control. To be "in control" means that the observed variation is due only to the random, uncontrolled variation inherent in the process, as discussed previously. We will define *upper and lower limits* for the mean and range of the subgroups. Values falling outside these limits are cause for alarm. The construction of these limits is based on normal distribution theory. We know, from Chap. 3 that individual values from a normal distribution will be within 1.96 standard deviations of the mean 95% of the time, and within 3.0 (or 3.09) standard deviations of the mean 99.73% (or 99.8%) of the time (see Table IV.2). Therefore, the probability of observing a value outside these limits is small; only 1 in 20 in the former case and 2.7 in 1000 in the latter case. Two limits are often used in the construction of $\overline{X}$ (mean) charts as "warning" and "action" limits, respectively (see Fig. 12.1). The warning limits are narrower than the action limits and do not require immediate action. If a process is subject only to random, chance variation, a value far from the mean is unlikely. In particular, a value more than 3.0 standard deviations from the mean is highly unlikely (2.7/1000), and can be considered to be probably due to some *systematic, assignable* cause. Such a "divergent" observation should signal the quality control unit to modify the process and/or initiate an investigation into its cause. Of course, the "abberant" value may be due only to chance. If so, subsequent means should fall close to the process average as expected. In some circumstances, one may wisely make an observation on a new subgroup before the scheduled time, in order to verify the initial result. If two successive averages are outside the acceptable limits, chances are extremely high that a problem exists. An investigation to detect the cause and make a correction may then be initiated.

The procedure for constructing control charts will be illustrated using data on tablet weights as shown in Table 12.1 and Fig. 12.2.

Table 12.1   Tablet Weights and Ranges
from a Tablet Manufacturing Process[a]

Date	Time	Mean, $\overline{X}$	Range
3/1	11 a.m.	302.4	16
	12 p.m.	298.4	13
	1 p.m.	300.2	10
	2 p.m.	299.0	9
3/5	11 a.m.	300.4	13
	12 p.m.	302.4	5
	1 p.m.	300.3	12
	2 p.m.	299.0	17
3/9	11 a.m.	300.8	18
	12 p.m.	301.5	6
	1 p.m.	301.6	7
	2 p.m.	301.3	8
3/11	11 a.m.	301.7	12
	12 p.m.	303.0	9
	1 p.m.	300.5	9
	2 p.m.	299.3	11
3/16	11 a.m.	300.0	13
	12 p.m.	299.1	8
	1 p.m.	300.1	8
	2 p.m.	303.5	10
3/22	11 a.m.	297.2	14
	12 p.m.	296.2	9
	1 p.m.	297.4	11
	2 p.m.	296.0	12

[a]Data are the average and range of 10
tablets.

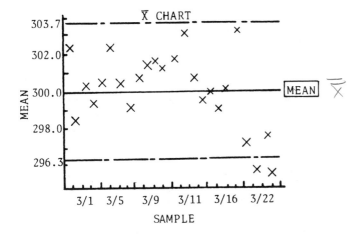

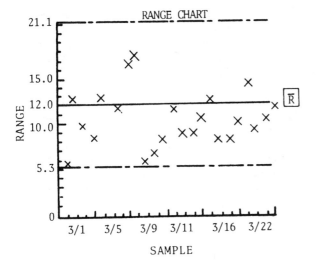

Figure 12.2 Control chart for tablet averages and range data from Table 12.1.

Note that the $\overline{X}$ chart consists of an "average" or "standard" line along with upper and lower lines which represent the *action* lines. The *average* line may be determined from the history of the product, with regular updating, or may be determined from the product specifications. In this example, the average line is defined by the quality control specifications (standards) for this product, a target value of 300 mg. The *action* lines are constructed to represent ±3 standard deviations from the target value. This is also known as "3σ limits." Observations that lie outside these limits are a cause for action. (Note the 12 p.m. observation on 3/22.) Adjustments or other corrective action should *not* be implemented if the averages are within the action limits. Tampering with equipment and/or changing other established procedures while the process remains within limits should be avoided. Such interference will often result in increased variation.

In order to establish the *upper* and *lower* limits for the mean ($\overline{X}$), we need an estimate of the standard deviation, if it is not previously known. The standard deviation can be obtained from the replicates (10 tablets) of the subgroup samples which generate the means for the control chart. By pooling the variability from many subgroups (N = 10), a very good estimate of the true standard deviation, σ, can be obtained (see App. I). Note that an estimate of the standard deviation or range is needed before limits for the $\overline{X}$ chart can be established. If a "range" chart is used in conjunction with the $\overline{X}$ chart, the upper and lower limits for the $\overline{X}$ chart can be obtained from the range according to Table IV.10 (column A). These factors are derived from theoretical calculations relating the range and standard deviation. For example, in the long run, the range can be shown to be equal to *3.078* times the standard deviation for samples of size 10. If we wish to establish 3σ limits about the *mean* of samples of size 10 ($3σ/\sqrt{10}$) using the range, the following relationship leads to the value 0.31 in Table IV.10 (see column A):

$$\overline{X} \pm \frac{3σ}{\sqrt{10}} = \overline{X} \pm \frac{3(\overline{R})}{(3.078)\sqrt{10}} = \overline{X} \pm 0.31\overline{R}$$

$\overline{R}/3.078$ is the average range divided by 3.078 which on the average is equal to σ. Thus, if the average range is 12 for samples of size 10, the upper and lower control chart limits for $\overline{X}$ are

$$\overline{X} \pm 0.31\overline{R} = \overline{X} \pm 0.31(12) = \overline{X} \pm 3.72 \tag{12.1}$$

Note that the average range is simply the usual average of the range values, obtained in a manner similar to that for calculating the process average. Ranges obtained during the control charting process are averaged and updated as appropriate.

Table IV.10 also has factors for upper and lower limits for a *range chart*. The values in columns D_L and D_U are multiplied times the average range to obtain the lower and upper limits for the range. Usually, a range that exceeds the upper limit is a cause for action. A small value of the range shows good precision and may be disregarded in many situations. In the present example, the average range is set equal to 12 based on previous experience. For samples of size 10, D_L and D_U are 0.441 and 1.76, respectively. Therefore, the lower and upper limits for the range are

Lower limit: $0.441 \times 12 = 5.3$ (12.2)

Upper limit: $1.76 \times 12 = 21.1$

These limits are shown in the control chart for the range in Fig. 12.2. Note that unlike the limits for the mean, the upper and lower limits for the range are not symmetrical about the mean range. See Fig. 12.1 for another example of a Range chart. Ordinarily, the sample size should be kept constant. If sample size varies from time to time, the limits for the control chart will change according to the sample size. If the sample sizes do not vary greatly, one solution to this problem is use an average sample size [9].

Having established the *mean* and the average *range*, the process is considered to be under control as long as the average and range of the subgroup samples fall within the lower and upper limits. If either the mean or range of a sample falls outside the limits, a possible "assignable" cause is suspected. The reason for the deviation should be investigated and identified, if possible. One should appreciate that a process can change in such a way that (a) only the average is affected, (b) only the variability is affected, or (c) both the average and variability are affected. These possibilities are illustrated in Fig. 12.3.

In the example of tablet weights, one might consider the following as possible causes for the results shown in Fig. 12.3. A change in average weight may be caused by a misadjustment of the tablet press. Increased variability may be due to some malfunction of one or more punches. Since 10 consecutive tablets are taken for measurement, if one punch gives very low weight tablets, for example, a large variability would result. A combination of lower weight and increased variability probably would be quickly detected if half of the punches were *sticking* in a random manner. Under these circumstances, the average ($\overline{X}$) would be substantially reduced and the range would be substantially increased relative to the values expected under *statistical control*.

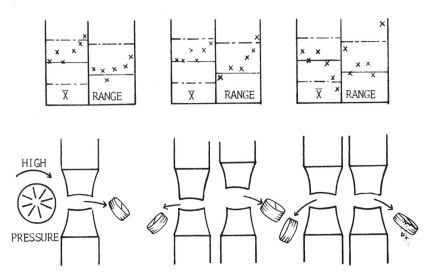

Figure 12.3   Representation of possible process changes as may be detected in a control chart procedure.

The control charts shown in Fig. 12.2 are typical. For the $\overline{X}$ chart, the mean was taken as 300 mg based on the target value as set out in the quality control standards. The upper and lower action limits were calculated on the basis of an average range of 12 and factor A in Table IV.10. The lower and upper action limits are 300 ± 3.72 mg or approximately 296.3 to 303.7 mg, respectively. The process is out of control during the production of the batch produced on 3/22. This will be discussed further below. The range control chart shows that the process is in control with respect to this variable. One value of the range falls below the lower limit revealing increased precision. One would be concerned about this value, for example, if an investigation into effects that might *improve* the precision were to be pursued.

When the *standard deviation* rather than the range is computed for purposes of constructing control charts, the factors for calculating the limits for the $\overline{X}$ chart are different. The vaiability is monitored via a chart of the standard deviation of the subgroup rather than the range. Factors for setting limits for both $\overline{X}$ charts and "sigma" (standard deviation) charts may be found in Ref. 1.

If an outlying observation ($\overline{X}$, R) is eliminated because an assignable cause has been found, that observation should be eliminated from future updating of the $\overline{X}$ and R charts.

12.2.3 Between-Batch Variation as a Measure of Variability (Moving Averages)

The discussion of control charts above dealt with a system that is represented by a regular schedule of production batches. The action limits for $\overline{X}$ were computed using the "within"-batch variation as measured by the variability between items in a "rational subgroup." The subgroup consists of a group of tablets manufactured under very similar conditions. For the manufacture of unit dosage forms with inherent heterogeneity, such as tablets, attempts to construct control charts which include different batches, based on within subgroup variation, may lead to apparently excessive product failure and frustration. Sometimes, this unfortunate situation may result in the discontinuation of the use of control charts as an impractical statistical device. However, the nature of the manufacture of a heterogeneous mixture, such as the bulk granulations used for manufacturing tablets, lends itself to new sources of uncontrolled error. This error resides in the variability due to the different (uncontrolled) conditions under which different tablet batches are manufactured. One would be hard put to describe exactly why batch-to-batch differences should exist, or to identify the sources of these differences. Perhaps the dies and punches of the tablet press are subject to wear and erosion. Perhaps a new employee involved in the manufacturing process performs the job in a slightly different manner from his or her predecessor. Whatever the reason, such interbatch variation may exist.* In these cases, the within-subgroup variation underestimates the variation, and many readings will appear out of control. This is exemplified by the last batch in Table 12.1 and Fig. 12.2.

Thus, when significant interbatch variation exists, the usual control chart will lead to many batches being out of control. If the cause of this variation cannot be identified or controlled, and the product consistently passes the official quality control specifications, other methods than the usual control chart may be used to monitor the process.

Use of the "Control Chart for Individuals" [1,9] seems to be one reasonable approach to monitoring such processes. The limits for the $\overline{X}$ chart are based on a moving range using two consecutive samples (see Table 12.2). For example, the first value for the two-batch moving range is the range of batches 1 and 2 = 1.1 (399.5 − 398.4). The second moving range is 399.5 − 398.8 = 0.7, etc. The average moving range is 1.507. The average tablet weight of the 30 batches is 400.01. The average range is based on samples

---

*Process validation investigates and identifies such variation.

Table 12.2 Average Weight of 50 Tablets from 30 Batches of a Tablet Product: Example of the Moving Average

Batch	Batch average (mg)	Two-batch moving range	Three-batch moving average	Three-batch moving range
1	398.4	—	—	—
2	399.5	1.1	—	—
3	398.8	0.7	398.9	1.1
4	397.4	1.4	398.6	2.1
5	402.7	5.3	399.6	5.3
6	400.5	2.2	400.2	5.3
7	401.0	0.5	401.4	2.2
8	398.5	2.5	400.0	2.5
9	399.5	1.0	399.7	2.5
10	400.1	0.6	399.4	1.6
11	399.0	1.1	399.5	1.1
12	401.7	2.7	400.3	2.7
13	395.4	6.3	398.7	6.3
14	400.7	5.3	399.3	6.3
15	401.6	0.9	399.2	6.2
16	401.4	0.2	401.2	0.9
17	401.5	0.1	401.5	0.2
18	400.4	1.1	401.1	1.1
19	401.0	0.6	401.0	1.1
20	402.1	1.1	401.2	1.7
21	400.9	1.2	401.3	1.2
22	400.8	0.1	401.3	1.3
23	401.5	0.7	401.1	0.7
24	398.6	2.9	400.3	2.9
25	398.4	0.2	399.5	3.1
26	398.8	0.4	398.6	0.4
27	399.9	1.1	399.0	1.5
28	400.9	1.0	399.9	2.1
29	399.9	1.0	400.2	1.0
30	399.5	0.4	400.1	1.4

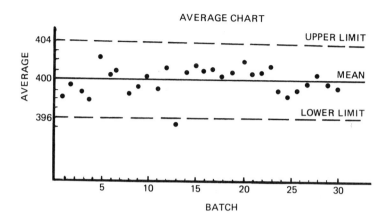

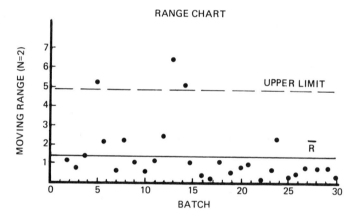

Figure 12.4   Control charts for individuals from Table 12.2.

of 2.   To estimate the standard deviation from the average range of samples of size 2, it can be shown that we should divide the average range by 1.128 (Table IV.10).   The 3 sigma limits are $\overline{X} \pm 3 \ (\overline{R}/1.128) = 400.01 \pm 3(1.507/1.128) = 400.01 \pm 4.01$.   The range chart has an upper limit of $3.27(1.507) = 4.93$.   These charts are shown in Fig. 12.4.   Batch 13 is out of limits based on both the average and range charts.

The moving average method is another approach to construct control charts that can be useful in the presence of inter-batch variation.   In this method, we use only a single mean value for each

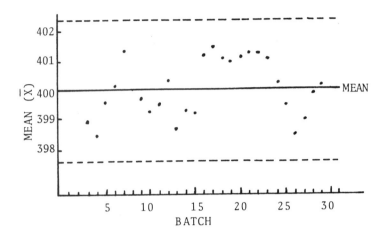

Figure 12.5   Moving average plot for tablet weight means from
Table 12.2.

batch, ignoring the individual values within the subgroup, if they
are available. Thus the data consist of a series of means over
many batches as shown in Table 12.2. A three-batch moving average consists of averaging the present batch with the two immediately
preceding batches. For example, starting with batch 3, the first
value for the moving average chart is

$$\frac{398.4 + 399.5 + 398.8}{3} = 398.9$$

The second value is (399.5 + 398.8 + 397.4)/3 = 398.6. The calculation is similar to that used for the two-batch moving range in the
example of the Control Chart for Individuals. The moving average
values are plotted as in the ordinary control chart. Limits for the
control chart are established from the moving range, which is calculated in a similar manner. The range of the present and the two
immediately preceding batches is calculated for each batch. The
average of these ranges is $\overline{R}$, the limits for the control chart are
computed from Table IV.10. The computations of the moving
average and range for samples of size 3 are shown in Table 12.2,
and the data charted in Fig. 12.5. The average weight was set at
the targeted weight of 400 mg. The average moving range (from
Table 12.2) is 2.35. The limits for the moving average chart are
determined using the average range and the factor from Table IV.10
for samples of size 3.

$$400 \pm 1.02(2.35) \;=\; 400 \pm 2.4$$

All of the moving average values fall within the limits based on the average moving range. In this analysis, the suspect batch number 13 is "smoothed" out when averaged with its neighboring batches. The upper limit for the range chart is $2.57(3.35) = 6.04$, which would be cause to investigate the conditions under which batch number 13 was produced (see Table 12.2). For further details of the construction and interpretation of moving average charts, see Refs. 1 and 3.

Another approach to the problem of between batch variation is the difference chart. A good standard lot is set aside as the control. Each production lot is compared to the standard lot by taking samples of each. Both the control and production lots are measured and the difference of the means is plotted. The limits are computed as

$$0 \pm \frac{3}{\sqrt{n}} \; \sqrt{S_c^2 + S_p^2}$$

where S_c^2 and S_p^2 are the estimates of the variances of the control and production lots, respectively.

12.2.4 Quality Control Charts in Research and Development

Control charts may be advantageously conceived and used during assay development and validation, in preliminary research of formulation studies, and in routine pharmacological screening procedures. During the development of assay methodology and validation, for example, by keeping records of assay results, an initial estimate of the assay standard deviation is available. The initial estimate can then be updated as data accumulate.

The following example shows the usefulness of control charts for control measurements in a drug screening procedure. This test for screening potential anti-inflammatory drugs measures improvement of inflammation (guinea pig paw volume) by test compounds compared to a control treatment. A control chart was established to monitor the performance of the control drug (a) to establish the mean and variability of the control, and (b) to ensure that the results of the control for a given experiment are within reasonable limits (a validation of the assay procedure). The average paw volume difference (paw volume before treatment − paw volume after treatment) and the average range for a series of experiments are shown in Table 12.3. The control chart is shown in Fig. 12.6.

Table 12.3   Average Paw Volume Difference and Range for a Screening Procedure (Four Guinea Pigs per Test Group)

Test number	Mean	Range	Test number	Mean	Range
1	38	4	11	28	12
2	43	3	12	41	10
3	34	3	13	40	22
4	48	6	14	34	5
5	38	24	15	37	4
6	45	4	16	43	14
7	49	5	17	37	6
8	32	9	18	45	8
9	48	5	19	32	7
10	34	8	20	42	13

As in the control charts for quality control, the mean and average range of the "process" were calculated from previous experiments. In this example, the screen had been run 20 times previous to the data of Table 12.3. These initial data showed a mean paw volume difference of 40 and a mean range ($\overline{R}$) of 9, which were used to construct the control charts shown in Fig. 12.6. The subgroups consist of 4 animals each. Using Table IV.10, the action limits for the $\overline{X}$ and range charts were calculated as follows:

$$\overline{X} \pm 0.73\overline{R} = 40 \pm 0.73(9) = 33.4 \text{ to } 46.6 \ (\overline{X} \text{ chart})$$

$$\overline{R}(2.28) = 9(2.28) = 20.5 \text{ the upper limit for the range}$$

Note that the lower limit for the range of subgroups consisting of four units is zero. Six of the twenty means are out of limits. Efforts to find a cause for the larger inter-test variation failed. The procedures were standardized and followed carefully, and the animals appeared to be homogeneous. Because different shipments of animals were needed to proceed with these tests over time, the researchers felt that there was no way to "tighten up" the procedure. Therefore, as in the tablet weight example discussed in the preceding section, a new control chart was prepared based on the variability between test means. A moving average was recommended using *four*

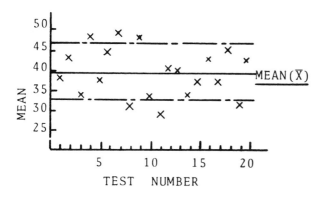

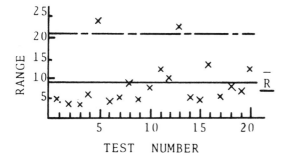

Figure 12.6 Control chart for means and range for control group in a pharmacological screening procedure.

successive averages. Based on historical data, $\overline{X}$ was calculated as 39.7 with an average moving range of 12.5. The limits for the moving average graph are

$$39.7 \pm 0.73(12.5) = 30.6 \text{ to } 48.8$$

The factor 0.73 is obtained from Table IV.10 for subgroup samples of size 4.

12.2.5 Quality Control Charts for Proportions

Table 12.4 shows quality control data for the inspection of tablets where the measurement is an attribute, a binomial variable. Three hundred tablets are inspected each hour to detect various problems,

Table 12.4 Proportion of Chipped Tablets of 300 Inspected
During Tablet Manufacture

	Time			
Batch	10 a.m.	11 a.m.	12 p.m.	1 p.m.
1	0.060	0.053	0.087	0.055
2	0.073	0.047	0.060	0.047
3	0.040	0.067	0.033	0.053
4	0.033	0.040	0.030	0.027
5	0.040	0.013	0.023	0.040
6	0.025	0.000	0.027	0.013

such as specks, chips, color uniformity, logo, and so on. For this
example, the defect under consideration is a chipped tablet. According to quality control specifications, this type of defect is considered of minor importance and an average of 5% chipped tablets is
tolerable. This problem of chipped tablets was of recent origin, and
the control chart was implemented as an aid to the manufacturing
and research and development departments, who were looking into
the cause of this defect. In fact, the 5% average had been written
into the specifications as a result of the persistent appearance of
the chipped tablets in recent batches. The data in Table 12.4 represent the first six batches where this attribute was monitored.

For the control chart, 5% defects was set as the average value.
The action limits can be calculated from the standard deviation of a
binomial. In this example, where 300 tablets were inspected, N =
300, p = 0.05, and q = 0.95 [$\sigma = \sqrt{pq/N}$, Eq. (3.11)].

$$\sigma = \sqrt{\frac{(0.05)(0.95)}{300}} = 0.0126$$

The limits are $0.05 \pm 3\sigma = 0.05 \pm 3(0.0126) = 0.012$ to 0.088. Proportions below the lower limit indicate an improvement in the process
in this example. Note that we can use the normal approximation to
the binomial when calculating the 3σ limits, because both Np and Nq
are greater than 5 (see Sec. 3.4.3). The control chart is shown in
Fig. 12.7. The chart clearly shows a trend with time toward less
chipping. The problem seems to be lessening. Although no specific
cause was found for this problem, increased awareness of the problem among manufacturing personnel may have resulted in more care
during the tableting process.

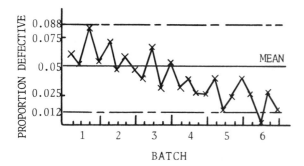

PROPORTION DEFECTIVE

0.088
0.075
0.05
0.025
0.012

MEAN

1 2 3 4 5 6

BATCH

Figure 12.7 Control chart for proportion of tablets chipped.

12.2.6 Runs in Control Charts

The most important feature of the control chart is the monitoring of
a process based on the average and control limits. In addition,
control charts are useful as an aid in detecting trends that could
be indicative of a lack of control. This is most easily seen as a
long consecutive series of values that are within the control limits
but (a) stay above (or below) the average or (b) show a steady increase (or decline). Statistically, such occurrences are described
as "runs." For example, a run of 7 successive values that lie above
the average constitutes a run of size 7. Such an event is probably
not random because if the observed values are from a symmetric
distribution and represent random variation about a common mean,
the probability of 7 successive values being above the mean is
$(1/2)7 = 1/128$. In fact, the occurrence of such an event is considered to be suggestive of a trend and the process should be carefully watched or investigated.

In general, when looking for runs in a long series of data, the
problem is that significant runs will be observed by chance when
the process is under control. Nevertheless, with this understanding, it is useful to examine data to be forewarned of the possibility
of trends and potential problems. The test for the number of runs
above and below the median of a consecutive series of data is described in Chap. 15, Sec. 15.7. For the consecutive values 9.54,
9.63, 9.42, 9.86, 9.40, 9.31, 9.79, 9.56, 9.2, 9.8, and 10.1, the
median is 9.56. The number of runs above and below the median is
8. According to Table IV.14, this is not an improbable event at the
5% level. If the consecutive values observed were 9.63, 9.86, 9.79,
9.8, 10.1, 9.56, 9.54, 9.42, 9.40, 9.31, and 9.2, the median is still
9.56, but the number of runs is 2. This shows a significant lack
of randomness ($p < 0.05$). Also see Exercise Problem 12.

Duncan [9] describes a runs test that looks at the longest run occurring above or below the median. The longest run is compared to the values in Table IV.15. If the longest run is equal to or greater than the table value, the data is considered to be non-random. For the data of Table 12.1, starting with the data on the date 3/5 (ignore the data on 3/1 for this example), the median is 300.35. The longest run is 7. There are 7 consecutive values above the median starting at 11 a.m. on 3/9. For N = 20, the table value in Table IV.15 is 7, and the data is considered to be significantly non-random (p < 0.05). Note that this test allows a decision of lack of control at the 5% level if a run of 7 is observed in a sequence of 20 observations.

For other examples of the application of the runs test, see Reference 9. Also see Sec. 15.7 and Exercise Problem 11 in Chap. 15.

In addition to the aforementioned criteria, i.e., a point outside the control limits, a significant number of runs, or a single run of sufficient length, other rules of thumb have been suggested to detect lack of control. For example, a run of 2 or 3 outside the 2σ limits but within the 3σ limits, and runs of 4 or 5 between 1σ and 2σ limits can be considered cause for concern.

Cumulative sum control charts (cusum charts) are more sensitive to process changes. However, the implementation, construction, and theory of cusum charts are more complex than the usual Shewhart control chart. Reference 10 gives a detailed explanation of the use of these control charts.

For more examples of the use of control charts, see Chap. 13, Validation.

12.3   ACCEPTANCE SAMPLING AND OPERATING CHARACTERISTIC CURVES

Finished products or raw materials (including packaging components) which appear as separate units are inspected or analyzed before release for manufacturing purposes or commercial sale. The sampling and analytical procedures are specified in official standards or compendia (e.g., the USP), or in in-house quality control standards. The quality control procedure known as *acceptance sampling* specifies that a number of items be selected according to a scheduled sampling plan, and be inspected for attributes or quantitatively analyzed. The chief purpose of acceptance sampling is to make a decision regarding the acceptability of the material. Therefore, based on the inspection, a decision is made, such as "the material or lot is either accepted or rejected." Sampling plans for variables (quantitative measurements such as chemical analyses for potency) and attributes (qualitative inspection) are presented in detail in the

U.S. government documents MIL-STD-414 and MIL-STD-105D, respectively [2,3].

A single *sampling plan* for *attributes* is one in which N items are selected at random from the population of such items. Each item is classified as defective or not defective with respect to the presence or absence of the attribute(s). If the sample size is small relative to the population size, this is a binomial process, and the properties of sampling plans for attributes can be derived using the binomial distribution. For example, consider the inspection of finished bottles of tablets for the presence of an intact seal. This is a binomial event; the seal is either intact or it is not intact. The sampling plan states the number of units to be inspected and the number of defects which, if found in the sample, leads to rejection of the lot. A typical plan may call for inspection of 100 items; if two or more are defective, reject the lot (batch). If one or less are defective, accept the lot. (The acceptance number is equal to one.) Theoretically, "100% inspection" will separate the good and defective items (seals in our example). In the absence of 100% inspection, there is no guarantee that the lot will have 0% (or any specified percentage) defects. Thus underlying any sampling plan are two kinds of risks:

1. The *producer's or manufacturer's risk*. This is the risk or probability of rejecting (not releasing) the product, although it is really good. By "good" we mean that had we inspected every item, the batch would meet the criteria for release or acceptance. This risk reflects an unusually high number of defects appearing in the sample taken for inspection, by chance. The producer's risk can be likened to the α error, that is, rejecting the batch, even though it is good.
2. The *consumer's risk*, This is the probability that the product is considered acceptable (released), although, in truth, it would not be acceptable were it 100% inspected. The consumer's risk can be likened to the β error, that is, the batch is accepted even though it has a more than acceptable number of defects.

There are any number of possible sampling plans which, in addition to economic considerations, depend on:

1. The number of items sampled
2. The producer's risk
3. The consumer's risk

MIL-STD-105D is an excellent compilation of such plans [3]. Each plan gives the number of items to be inspected, and the number of defects in the sample needed to cause rejection of the lot. Each

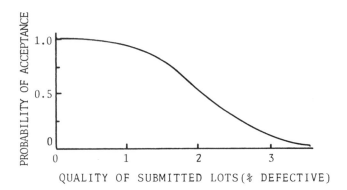

Figure 12.8   Operating characteristic curve for sampling plan:
sample 500 items — accept if 10 or less defective.

plan is accompanied by an *operating characteristic* (OC) *curve*.   The
OC curve shows the probability of accepting a lot based on the
sampling plan specifications, given the true proportion of defects in
the lot.   A typical OC curve is shown in Fig. 12.8.

The OC curve is a form of power curve (see Sec. 6.5).   The
OC curve in Fig. 12.8 is derived from a sampling plan (plan N from
MIL-STD-105D) in which 500 items (bottles) are inspected from a
lot that contains 30,000 items.   If 11 or more items inspected are
found to be defective, the lot is rejected.   Inspection of Fig. 12.8
shows that if the batch truly has 1% defects, the probability of accepting the lot is close to 99% when plan N is implemented.   This
plan is said to have an *acceptable quality level* (AQL) of 1%.   An
AQL of 1% means that the consumer will accept most of the product
manufactured by the supplier if the level of defects is not greater
than 1%, the specified AQL (i.e., 1%).   In this example, with the
AQL equal to approximately 1%, about 99% of the batches will pass
this plan if the percent defects is 1% or less.

The plan actually chosen for a particular product and a particular attribute depends on the lot size and the nature of the attribute.   If the presence (or absence) of an attribute (such as the
integrity of a seal) is critical, then a stringent plan (a low AQL)
should be adopted.   If a defect is considered of minor importance,
inspection for the presence of a defect can make use of a less stringent plan.   MIL-STD-105D describes various plans for different lot
(population) sizes, which range from less stringent for minor defects to more stringent for critical defects.   These are known as
levels of inspection, level I, II, or III.   This document also includes criteria for contingencies for switching to more or less tight

plans depending on results of prior inspection. A history of poor quality will result in a more stringent sampling plan and vice versa. If 2 of 5 consecutive lots are rejected, the normal plan is switched to the tightened plan. If 5 consecutive lots are accepted under the tightened plan, the normal plan is reinstated. If quality remains very good, reduced plans may be administered as described in MIL-STD-105D. The characteristics of the plan are defined by the AQL and the OC curve. For example, for lot sizes of 10,001 to 35,000, the following are two of the possible plans recommended by MIL-STD-105D:

Plan	Sample size	Reject number[a] if AQL =	
		0.4%	1%
K	125	2	4
N	500	6	11

[a]Reject the lot if the reject number de- fects (or more) are observed.

Plan N is a more "discriminating" plan than plan K. The larger sample size results in a greater probability of rejecting lots with more than AQL percentage of defects. For plan N, if there are 2% defects in the lot, the lot will be accepted approximately 57% of the time. For plan K, with 2% defects in the lot, the lot will be accepted 75% of the time. (See MIL-STD 105D [3] for OC curves. The OC curve for an AQL of 1% for plan N is shown in Fig. 12.8.)

In the present example, a defective seal is considered a critical defect and plan N will be implemented with an AQL of 0.025%. This means that lots with 0.025% (25 defects per 100,000 bottles) are considered acceptable. According to MIL-STD-105D, if one or more defects are found in a sample of 500 bottles, the lot is rejected.* This means that the lot is passed only if all 500 bottles are good. The OC curve for this plan is shown in Fig. 12.9.

The calculations of the probabilities needed to construct the OC curve are not very difficult. These calculations have been presented in the discussion of the binomial distribution in Chap. 3. As an illustration we will calculate the probability of rejecting a lot using

---

*If the result of inspection calls for rejection, 100% inspection is a feasible alternative to rejection.

Table 12.5 Sample Size Code Letter: K (Chart shows operating characteristic curves for single sampling plans)[a]

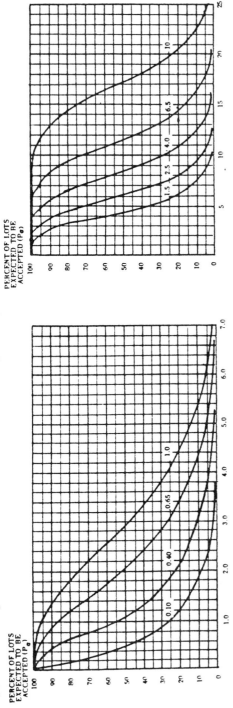

Tabulated values for operating characteristic curves for single sampling plans

P_a	Acceptable quality levels (normal inspection)											
	0.10	0.40	0.65	1.0	1.5	2.5	X	4.0	X	6.5	X	10
99.0	0.0081	0.119	0.349	0.658	1.43	2.33	2.81	3.82	4.88	5.98	8.28	10.1
95.0	0.0410	0.284	0.654	1.09	2.09	3.19	3.76	4.94	6.15	7.40	9.95	11.9
90.0	0.0840	0.426	0.882	1.40	2.52	3.73	4.35	5.62	6.92	8.24	10.9	13.0
75.0	0.230	0.769	0.382	2.03	3.38	4.77	5.47	6.90	8.34	9.79	12.7	14.9
50.0	0.554	1.34	2.14	2.94	4.54	6.14	6.94	8.53	10.1	11.7	14.9	17.3
25.0	1.11	2.15	3.14	4.09	5.94	7.75	8.64	10.4	12.2	13.9	17.4	20.0
10.0	1.84	3.11	4.26	5.35	7.42	9.42	10.4	12.3	14.2	16.1	19.8	22.5
5.0	2.40	3.80	5.04	6.20	8.41	10.5	11.5	13.6	15.6	17.5	21.4	24.2
1.0	3.68	5.31	6.73	8.04	10.5	12.8	18.3	16.1	18.3	20.4	24.5	27.5
	0.15	0.65	1.0	1.5	2.5	4.0	—	—	6.5	—	10	—
	Acceptable quality levels (tightened inspection)											

Sampling plans for sample size code letter K

		Acceptable quality levels (normal inspection)																																		
Type of sampling plan	Cumulative sample size	Less than 0.10		0.10		0.15		—		0.25		—		0.40		0.65		1.0		1.5		2.5		—		4.0		—		6.5		—		10		Higher than 10	
		Ac	Re	Ac	Re	Ac	Re	Ac	Re	Ac	Re	Ac	Re	Ac	Re	Ac	Re	Ac	Re	Ac	Re	Ac	Re	Ac	Re	Ac	Re	Ac	Re	Ac	Re	Ac	Re	Ac	Re	Ac	Re
Single	125	▽		0	1	Use letter J		Use letter M		Use letter L				1	2	2	3	3	4	5	6	7	8	8	9	10	11	12	13	14	15	18	19	21	22	△	
Double	80	▽		*										0	2	0	3	1	4	2	5	3	7	3	8	5	9	6	10	7	11	9	14	11	16	△	
	160													1	2	3	4	4	5	6	7	8	9	11	12	12	13	15	16	18	19	23	24	26	27		
Multiple	32	▽		*										#	2	#	2	#	3	#	4	0	4	0	4	0	5	0	6	1	7	1	8	2	9	△	
	64													#	2	0	3	0	3	1	5	1	6	2	7	3	8	3	9	4	10	6	12	7	14		
	96													0	2	0	3	1	4	2	6	3	8	4	9	6	10	7	12	8	13	11	17	13	19		
	128													0	3	1	4	2	5	3	7	5	10	6	11	8	13	10	15	12	17	16	22	19	25		
	160													1	3	2	4	3	6	5	8	7	11	9	13	11	15	14	17	17	20	22	25	25	29		
	192													1	4	3	5	4	6	7	9	10	12	12	15	14	17	18	20	21	23	27	29	31	33		
	224													2	3	4	5	6	7	9	10	13	14	16	17	18	19	21	22	25	26	32	33	37	38		
		Less than 0.15		0.15		—		—		0.25		—		0.40		0.65		1.0		1.5		2.5		—		4.0		—		6.5		—		10		Higher than 10	
		Acceptable quality levels (tightened inspection)																																			

[a] Quality of submitted lots (p, in percent defective for AQLs ⩽ 10; in defects per hundred units for AQLs > 10).

Note: Figures on curves are acceptable quality levels (AQLs) for normal inspection. Curves for double and multiple sampling are matched as closely as practicable.

△ = Use next preceding sample size code letter for which acceptance and rejection numbers are available.

▽ = Use next subsequent sample size code letter for which acceptance and rejection numbers are available.

Ac = Acceptance number.

Re = Rejection number.

* = Use single sampling plan above (or alternatively use letter N).

= Acceptance not permitted at this sample size.

Table 12.6 Sample Size Code Letter N (Chart N shows operating characteristic curves for single sampling plans)[a]

(Curves for double and multiple sampling are matched as closely as practicable)

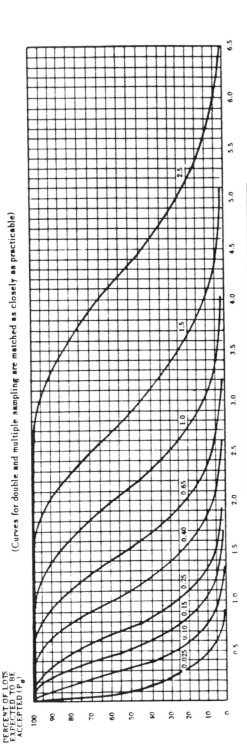

Tabulated Values for Operating characteristic curves for single sampling plans

P_a	Acceptable quality levels (normal inspection)											
	0.025	0.10	0.15	0.25	0.40	0.65	X	1.0	X	1.5	X	2.5
99.0	0.0020	0.030	0.087	0.165	0.357	0.581	0.701	0.954	1.22	1.50	2.07	2.51
95.0	0.0103	0.071	0.164	0.273	0.523	0.796	0.939	1.23	1.54	1.85	2.49	2.98
90.0	0.0210	0.106	0.220	0.349	0.630	0.931	1.09	1.40	1.73	2.06	2.73	3.25
75.0	0.0576	0.192	0.345	0.507	0.844	1.19	1.37	1.72	2.08	2.45	3.18	3.74
50.0	0.139	0.336	0.535	0.734	1.13	1.53	1.73	2.13	2.53	2.93	3.73	4.33
25.0	0.277	0.539	0.784	1.02	1.48	1.94	2.16	2.60	3.04	3.48	4.35	4.99
10.0	0.461	0.778	1.06	1.34	1.86	2.35	2.60	3.08	3.56	4.03	4.95	5.64
5.0	0.599	0.949	1.26	1.55	2.10	2.63	2.89	3.39	3.89	4.38	5.34	6.05
1.0	0.921	1.328	1.68	2.01	2.62	3.20	3.48	4.03	4.56	5.09	6.12	6.87
	0.040	0.15	0.25	0.40	0.65	—	1.0	—	1.5	—	2.5	—
	Acceptable quality levels (tightened inspection)											

Sampling plans for sample size code letter N

Acceptable quality levels (normal inspection)

In the table below each acceptable quality level (AQL) column gives the acceptance number (Ac) and rejection number (Re). The "Use letter M / Q / P" entries span the Single, Double and Multiple rows.

Type of sampling plan	Cum. sample size	<0.025	0.025	0.040	—	0.065	0.10	0.15	0.25	0.40	0.65	—	1.0	—	1.5	—	2.5	Higher than 2.5	Cum. sample size
Single	500	△	0 1	Use letter M	Use letter Q	Use letter P	1 2	2 3	3 4	5 6	7 8	8 9	10 11	12 13	14 15	18 19	21 22	△	500
Double	315	▽	*				0 2	0 3	1 4	2 5	3 7	4 8	5 9	6 10	7 11	9 14	11 16	△	315
	630						1 2	3 4	4 5	6 7	8 9	10 11	12 13	15 16	18 19	23 24	26 27		630
Multiple	125	▽	*				# 2	# 2	# 3	# 4	0 4	0 4	0 5	0 6	1 7	1 8	2 9	△	125
	250						# 2	0 3	0 3	1 5	1 6	2 7	3 8	3 9	4 10	6 12	7 14		250
	375						0 3	0 3	1 4	2 6	3 8	4 9	6 10	7 12	8 13	11 17	13 19		375
	500						0 3	1 4	2 5	3 7	5 10	6 11	8 13	10 15	12 17	16 22	19 25		500
	625						1 3	2 4	3 6	5 8	7 11	9 12	11 15	14 17	17 20	22 25	25 29		625
	750						1 3	3 5	4 6	7 9	10 12	12 14	14 17	18 20	21 23	27 29	31 33		750
	875						2 3	4 5	6 7	9 10	13 14	14 15	18 19	21 22	25 26	32 33	37 38		875

Acceptable quality levels (tightened inspection) — the same body, read against the AQL header:
Less than 0.040 | 0.040 | — | 0.065 | 0.10 | 0.15 | 0.25 | 0.40 | 0.65 | — | 1.0 | — | 1.5 | — | 2.5 | Higher than 2.5

[a] Quality of submitted lots (p, in percent defective for AQLs ≤ 10; in defects per hundred units for AQLs > 10).

Note: Figures on curves are acceptable quality levels (AQLs) for normal inspection. Curves for double and multiple sampling are matched as closely as practicable.

△ = Use next preceding sample size code letter for which acceptance and rejection numbers are available.

▽ = Use next subsequent sample size code letter for which acceptance and rejection numbers are available.

Ac = Acceptance number.

Re = Rejection number.

* = Use single sampling plan above (or alternatively use letter R).

= Acceptance not permitted at this sample size.

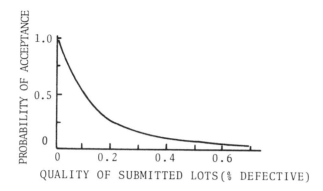

Figure 12.9 Operating characteristic curve for plan N: AQL = 0.025%.

plan N with an AQL of 0.025%. As noted above, the lot will be rejected if one or more defects are observed in a sample of 500 items. Thus the probability of accepting a lot with 0.025% defects is the probability of observing zero defects in a sample of 500. This probability can be calculated from Eq. (3.9).

$$\binom{N}{X} p^X q^{N-X} = \binom{500}{0} p^0 q^{500} = (0.00025)^0 (0.99975)^{500} = 0.88$$

where 500 is the sample size, p the probability of a defect (0.00025), and q the probability of observing a bottle with an intact seal (0.99975). Thus, using this plan, lots with *0.025% defects will be passed 88% of the time.* A lot with 0.4% (4 defects per 1000 items) will be accepted with a probability of

$$\binom{500}{0} (0.004)^0 (0.996)^{500} = 0.13 \text{ (i.e., 13%)}$$

Copies of Sampling Plans K and N from MIL-STD-105D are shown in Tables 12.5 and 12.6.

In addition to the single sampling plans discussed above, MIL-STD-105D also presents *multiple sampling plans.* These plans use less inspection than single sampling plans, on the average. After the first sampling, one of three decisions may be made:

1. Reject the lot
2. Accept the lot
3. Take another sample

In a double-sampling plan, if a second sample is necessary, the final decision of acceptance or rejection is based on the outcome of the second sample inspection.

The theory underlying acceptance sampling for *variables* is considerably more complex than that for sampling for attributes. In these schemes, actual measurements are taken, such as assay results, dimensions of tablets, weights of tablets, measurement of containers, and so on. Measurements are usually more time consuming and more expensive than the observation of a binomial attribute. However, quantitative measurements are usually considerably less variable. Thus there is a trade-off between expense and inconvenience, and precision. Many times, there is no choice. Official procedures may specify the type of measurement. Readers interested in plans for variable measurements are referred to MIL-STD-414 [2] and the book, "Quality Control and Industrial Statistics" [9] for details.

12.4 STATISTICAL PROCEDURES IN ASSAY DEVELOPMENT

Statistics can play an important role in assisting the analytical chemist in the development of assay procedures. A subcommittee of PMA (Pharmaceutical Manufacturers Association) statisticians developed a comprehensive scheme for documenting and verifying the equivalence of alternative assay procedures to a standard [4]. The procedure is called the *Greenbriar procedure* (named after the location where the scheme was developed). This approach includes a statistical design which identifies sources of variation such as that due to different days and different analysts. The design also includes a range of concentration of drug. The Greenbriar document emphasizes the importance of a thoughtful experimental design in assay development, a design that will yield data to answer questions raised in the study objectives. The procedure is too detailed to present here. However, for those who are interested, it would be a good exercise to review this document, a good learning experience in statistical application.

For those readers interested in pursuing statistical applications in assay and analytical development, two books, *Statistical Methods for Chemists* by Youden [5] and *The Statistical Analysis of Experimental Data* , by Mandel [6], are recommended. Both of these statisticians had long tenures with the National Bureau of Standards.

In this book we have presented some applications of regression analysis in analytical methodology (see Chaps. 7 and 13). Here we will discuss the application of simple designs to identify and quantify factors that contribute to assay variability (components of variance).

**12.4.1   Components of Variance

During the discussion of the one-way ANOVA design (Sec. 8.1), we noted that the "between-treatment mean square" is a variance estimate which is composed of two different (and *independent*) variances: (a) that due to variability among units *within* a treatment group, and (b) that due to variability due to differences *between* treatment groups. If treatments are, indeed, identical, the ANOVA calculations are such that observed differences between treatment means will probably be accounted for by the within-treatment variation. In the ANOVA table, the ratio of the between-treatment mean square to the within-treatment mean square (F = BMS/WMS) will be approximately equal to 1 on the average when treatments are identical.

WITHIN TREATMENT VARIABILITY   BETWEEN TREATMENT VARIABILITY
Repeat Assays Using the
Same Method   METHOD A   METHOD B

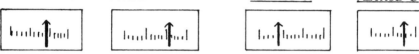

In certain situations (particularly when treatments are a random effect), one may be less interested in a statistical test of treatment differences, but more interested in separately estimating the variability due to different treatment groups *and* the variability within treatment groups. We will consider an example of a quality control procedure for the assay of finished tablets. Here we wish to characterize the assay procedure by estimating the sources of variation that make up the variability of the analytical results performed on different, distinct tablets. This variability is composed of two parts: (a) that due to analytical error, and (b) that due to tablet heterogeneity. A one-way ANOVA design such as that shown in Table 12.7

Table 12.7   Design to Analyze Components of Variance for the Tablet Assay

	Tablets (treatment groups)									
	1	2	3	4	5	6	7	8	9	10
Assay	48	49	49	55	48	54	45	47	53	50
Results	51	50	52	55	47	52	49	49	50	51
Mean	49.5	49.5	50.5	55	47.5	53	47	48	51.5	50.5
				Grand average = 50.2						

Table 12.8   Analysis of Variance for the Tablet Assay Data
from Table 12.7

Source	d.f.	SS	MS
Between tablets	9	112.2	12.47
Within tablets	10	27.0	2.70
Total	19	139.2	

will yield data to answer this objective. In the example shown in
the table, 10 tablets are each analyzed in duplicate. Duplicate
determinations were obtained by grinding each tablet separately,
and then weighing two portions of the ground mixture for assay.
The manner in which replicates (duplicates, in this example) are obtained is important, not only in the present situation, but in most
examples of statistical designs. Here we can readily appreciate that
analytical error, the variability due to the analytical procedure only,
is represented by differences in the analytical results of the two
"identical" portions of a homogeneously ground tablet. This variability is represented by the "within" error in the ANOVA table
shown in Table 12.8. The "within" mean square is the pooled variance *within* treatment groups, where a group, in this example, is
a single tablet.

The *between-tablet* mean square is an estimate of both *assay*
(analytical *error*) and the *variability of drug content in different
tablets* (tablet heterogeneity) as noted above. If tablets were
identical, individual tablet assays would still not be the same because of analytical error. In reality, in addition to analytical error,
the drug assay is variable due to the inherent heterogeneity of such
dosage forms. Variability between tablet assays is larger than that
which can be accounted for by analytical error alone. This is the
basis for the F test in the ANOVA [(between mean square)/(within
mean square)]. Large differences in the drug content of different
tablets result in a large value of the between-tablet mean square.
This concept is illustrated in Fig. 12.10, which shows an example
of the distribution of *actual* drug content in a theoretical batch of
tablets. The distribution of tablet assays is more spread out than
the drug content distribution, because the variation based on the
assay results of the different tablets includes components due to
actual drug content variation plus assay error.

Based on the theoretical model for the one-way ANOVA, Sec. 8.1
(random model), it can be shown that the between mean square is a
combination of the assay error and tablet variability as follows:

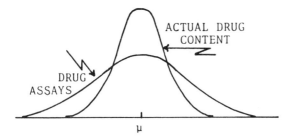

Figure 12.10   Distribution of actual drug content compared to distribution of analytical results of tablets (these are theoretical, hypothetical distributions).

$$\text{BMS} \sim n\sigma_T^2 + \sigma_W^2 \tag{12.3}$$

where n is the number of replicates in the design (based on equal replication in each group, two assays per tablet in our example), σ_T^2 the variance due to tablet drug content heterogeneity, and σ_W^2 is the within-treatment (assay) variance. In our example, n = 2, and the between mean square is an estimate of $2\sigma_T^2 + \sigma_W^2$. The *within-tablet* mean square is an estimate of σ_W^2, equal to 2.70 (Table 12.8). The estimate of σ_T^2 from Eq. (12.3) is $(\text{BMS} - \sigma_W^2)/n$:

$$\text{Estimate of } \sigma_T^2 = \frac{\text{between MS} - 2.70}{2} = \frac{12.47 - 2.70}{2} = 4.9$$

In this manner we have estimated the *two components* of the between-treatment mean square term: $S_W^2 = 2.7$ and $S_T^2 = 4.9$.

The purpose of the experiment above, in addition to estimating the components of variance, would often include an estimation of the overall average of drug content based on the 20 assays (Table 12.7). The average assay result is 50.2 mg. The estimates of the variance components can be used to estimate the variance of an average assay result, consisting of *m* tablets with *n* assay replicates per tablet. We use the fact that the variance of an average is equal to the variance divided by N, where N is equal to *mn*, the total number of observations. According to Eq. (12.3), the variance of the average result can be shown to be equal to

$$\frac{n\sigma_T^2 + \sigma_W^2}{mn} \tag{12.4}$$

The variance estimate of the average assay result (50.2) for the data in Table 12.7, where m = 10 and n = 2, is

$$\frac{2(4.9) + 2.7}{10(2)} = 0.62$$

Note that this result is exactly equal to the between mean square divided by 20.

According to Eq. (12.4), the variance of *single* assays performed on *two* separate tablets, for example, is equal to (m = 2, n = 1)

$$\frac{4.9 + 2.7}{2} = 3.8$$

Note that the variance of a *single assay* of a *single tablet* is $\sigma_T^2 + \sigma_W^2$. Similarly, the variance of the average of two assays performed on a single tablet (m = 1, n = 2) is $(2\sigma_T^2 + \sigma_W^2)/2$ (see Exercise Problem 11). The former method, where *two tablets* were each *assayed once*, has greater precision than duplicate assays on a single tablet. Given the same number of assays, the procedure that uses more tablets will always have better precision. The "best" combination of the number of tablets and replicate assays will depend on the particular circumstances, and includes time and cost factors. In some situations, it may be expensive or difficult to obtain the experimental material (e.g., obtaining patients in a clinical trial). Sometimes, the actual observation may be easily obtained, but the procedure to prepare the material for observation may be costly or time consuming. In the case of tablet assays, it is conceivable that the grinding of the tablets, dissolving, filtration, and other preliminary treatment of the sample for assay might be more expensive than the assay itself (perhaps automated). In such a case, replicate assays on ground material may be less costly than assaying separate tablets, where each tablet must be crushed and ground, dissolved, and filtered prior to assay. However, such situations are exceptions. Usually, in terms of precision, it is cost effective to average results obtained from different tablets.

The final choice of how many tablets to use and the total number of assays will probably be a compromise depending on the precision desired and cost constraints. The same precision can be

obtained by assaying different combinations of numbers of tablets
(m) with different numbers of replicate determinations (n) on each
tablet. Time-cost considerations can help make the choice. Suppose that we have decided that a sufficient number of assays should
be performed so that the variance of the average result is equal to
approximately 1.5. In our example, where the variance estimates
are $S_T^2 = 4.9$ and $S_W^2 = 2.7$, the average of five single-tablet assays
would satisfy this requirement:

$$S_{\overline{X}}^2 = \frac{4.9 + 2.7}{5} = 1.52$$

As noted above, the variance of a single-tablet assay is $S_T^2 + S_W^2$.
An alternative scheme resulting in a similar variance of the mean
result is to assay four tablets, each in duplicate (m = 4, n = 2).

$$S_{\overline{X}}^2 = \frac{2(4.9) + 2.7}{8} = 1.56$$

The latter alternative requires eight assays compared to five assays
in the former scheme. However, the latter method uses only four
tablets compared to the five tablets in the former procedure. The
cost of a tablet would probably not be a major factor with regard to
the choice of the alternative procedures. In some cases, the cost of
the item being analyzed could be of major importance. In general,
for tablet assays, in the presence of a *large assay variation*, if the
analytical procedure is automated and the preparation of the tablet
for assay is complex and costly, the procedure that uses less tablets
with more replicate assays per tablet could be the best choice.

Nested Designs

Designs for the estimation of variance components often fall into a
class called *nested* or completely hierarchical designs. The example
presented above can be extended if we were also interested in ascertaining the variance due to differences in average drug content between *different batches* of tablets. We are now concerned with estimating (a) between-batch variability, (b) between-tablet (within
batches) variability, and (c) assay variability. Between-batch variability exists because, despite the fact that the target potency is
the same for all batches, the actual mean potency varies due to
changing conditions during the manufacture of different batches.
This concept has been discussed under the topic of control charts.
     A design used to estimate the variance components, including
batch variation, is shown in Table 12.9 and Fig. 12.11. In this

Table 12.9 Nested Design for Determination of Variance Components

Batch:	A			B			C			D		
Tablet:	1	2	3	1	2	3	1	2	3	1	2	3
	50.6	49.1	51.1	50.1	51.0	50.2	51.4	52.1	51.1	49.0	47.2	48.9
	50.5	48.9	51.1	49.0	50.9	50.0	51.7	52.0	51.9	49.0	47.6	48.5
	50.8	48.5	51.4	49.4	51.6	49.8	51.8	51.4	51.6	48.5	47.6	49.2

ANOVA

Source	d.f.	SS	MS	Expected MS[a]
Between batches	3	48.6875	16.229	$\sigma_W^2 + 3\sigma_T^2 + 9\sigma_B^2$
Between tablets (within batches)	8	17.52	2.195	$\sigma_W^2 + 3\sigma_T^2$
Between assays (within tablets)	24	2.50	0.104	σ_W^2

[a]Coefficient for σ_T^2 = replicate assays; coefficient for σ_B^2 = replicate assays times the number of tablets per batch.

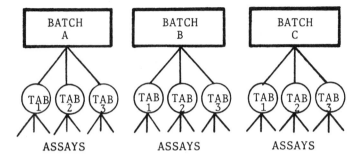

Figure 12.11 A nested or completely hierarchical design to estimate variance components.

example, four batches are included in the experiment, with three tablets selected from each batch (tablets nested in batches), and three replicate assays of each tablet (replicate assays nested in tablets). This design allows the estimate of variability due to batch differences, tablet differences, and analytical error. The calculations for the ANOVA will not be detailed (see Ref. 8) but the arithmetic is straight forward and is analogous to the analysis in the previous example.

The *mean squares* (MS) calculated from the *ANOVA estimate* the *true variances* indicated in the column "expected MS." The coefficients of the variances from the expected mean squares and the estimates of the three "sources" of variation can be used to estimate the components of variance. The variance components, σ_B^2, σ_T^2, and σ_W^2 may be estimated as follows from the mean square and expected mean square columns in Table 12.9:

$$S_W^2 = 0.104$$

$$S_W^2 + 3S_T^2 = 2.195 \qquad\qquad S_T^2 = 0.697$$

$$S_W^2 + 3S_T^2 + 9S_B^2 = 16.229 \qquad\qquad S_B^2 = 1.559$$

An estimate of the variance of single-tablet assays randomly performed within a single batch is $S_W^2 + S_T^2 = 0.801$. If tablets are randomly selected from different batches, the variance estimate of single-tablet assays is $S_W^2 + S_T^2 + S_B^2 = 2.36$.

Nested designs should be symmetrical to be easily analyzed and interpreted. The symmetry is reflected by the equal number of tablets from each batch, and the equal number of replicates per tablet. Missing or lost data results in difficulties in estimating the variance components.

KEY TERMS

Acceptance sampling	Operating characteristic (OC)
Action limits	Power curve
AQL	Producer's (manufacturer's) risk
Batch variation	Proportion (P) charts
Between- and within-batch	Range chart
variation	Rational subgroups
Chance variation	Runs
Components of variance	Sampling for attributes
Consumer's risk	Sampling for variables
Control chart for differences	Sampling plan
Control chart for individuals	Statistical control
Control chart	Upper and lower limits
Expected mean square	Warning limits
Moving average chart	$\overline{X}$ charts
Nested designs	100% inspection

EXERCISES

1. Duplicate assays are performed on a finished product as part of the quality control procedure. The average of assays over many batches is 9.95 and the average range of the duplicates is 0.10 mg. Calculate upper and lower limits for the $\overline{X}$ chart and and the range chart.

2. Past experience has shown the percentage of defective tablets to be 2%. What are the lower and upper 3σ limits for samples of size 1000?

3. A raw material assay shows an average percentage of 47.6% active with an average range of 1.2 based on triplicate assays. Construct a control chart for the mean and range.

4. What is the probability of rejecting a batch of product that truly has 1.0% rejects (defects) if the sampling plan calls for sampling 100 items and rejecting the batch if two or more defects are found?

5. The initial data for the assay of tablets in production runs are as follows (10 tablets per batch):

Batch	Mean	Range
1	10.0	0.3
2	9.8	0.4
3	10.2	0.4
4	10.0	0.2
5	10.1	0.5
6	9.8	0.4
7	9.9	0.2
8	9.9	0.5
9	10.3	0.3
10	10.2	0.6

Construct an $\overline{X}$ and range chart based on this "initial" data. Comment on observations out of limits.

6. A sampling plan for testing sterility of a batch of 100,000 ampuls is as follows. Test 100 ampuls selected at random. If there are no rejects, pass the batch. If there are one or more rejects, reject the batch. If 50 of the 100,000 ampuls are not sterile, what is the probability that the batch will pass?

**7. A new method was tried by four analysts in triplicate.

1	2	3	4
115	105	131	129
120	130	152	121
112	106	141	130

Perform an analysis of variance (one-way). Estimate the components of variance (between-analyst and within-analyst variance). What is the variance of the mean assay result if three analysts each perform four assays (a total of 12 assays)? What is the variance if four analysts each perform duplicate assays (a total of eight assays)? If the first analysis by an analyst costs $5 and each subsequent assay by that analyst costs $1, which of the two alternatives is more economical?

8. Construct an $\overline{X}$ chart for the data of Table 12.2, using the moving average procedure. Use the moving average to obtain $\overline{X}$ and $\overline{R}$ for the graph, from the first 15 batches. Plot results for first 15 batches only.

9. Duplicate assays were run for quality control purposes for production batches. The first 10 days of production resulted in the following data: (a) 10.1, 9.8; (2) 9.6, 10.0; (3) 10.0, 10.1; (4) 10.3, 10.3; (5) 10.2, 10.8; (6) 9.3, 9.9; (7) 10.1, 10.1; (8) 10.4, 10.6; (9) 10.9, 11.0; (10) 10.3, 10.4.

   (a) Calculate the mean, average range, and average standard deviation.

   (b) Construct a control chart for the mean and range and plot the data on the chart.

10. What are the lower and upper limits for the range for the example of the moving average discussed at the end of Section 12.2.3?

11. What is the variance of the average of duplicate assays performed on the same tablet where the between tablet variance is 4.9 and the within tablet variance is 2.7? Compare this to the variance of the average of singles assays performed on two different tablets.

12. How did 8 runs arise from the data in the example discussed in Sec. 12.2.5?

REFERENCES

1. Grant, E. L., *Statistical Quality Control*, 4th ed., McGraw-Hill, New York, 1974.
2. MIL-STD-414, Sampling Plans, Superintendent of Documents, U.S. Government Printing Office, Washington, D.C.
3. MIL-STD-105D, Military Sampling Procedures and Tables for Inspections by Attributes, Superintendent of Documents, U.S. Government Printing Office, Washington, D.C.
4. Haynes, J. D., Pauls, J., and Platt, R., Statistical Aspects of a Laboratory Study for Substantiation of the Validity of an Alternate Assay Procedure, "The Greenbriar Procedure," Final Report of the Standing Committee on Statistics to the PMA/QC Section, March 14, 1977.
5. Youden, W. J., *Statistical Methods for Chemists*, Wiley, New York, 1964.
6. Mandel, J., *The Statistical Analysis of Experimental Data*, Interscience, New York, 1964.
7. Box, G. E., Hunter, W. G., and Hunter, J. S., *Statistics for Experimenters*, Wiley, New York, 1978.
8. Bennet, C. A. and Franklin, N. L., *Statistical Analysis in Chemistry and the Chemical Industry*, Wiley, New York, 1963.
9. Duncan, A. J., *Quality Control and Industrial Statistics*, 5th Ed., Irwin, Homewood, Illinois, 1986.

13
Validation

Although validation of analytical and manufacturing processes has always been important in pharmaceutical quality control, recent emphasis on their documentation by the FDA has resulted in a more careful look at the implementation of validation procedures. The FDA defines process validation as ". . . a documented program which provides a high degree of assurance that a specific process will consistently produce a product meeting its predetermined specification and quality attributes" [1]. Pharmaceutical process validation consists of well documented, written procedures that define processes which ensure that a specific pharmaceutical technology is capable of and is attaining that which is specified in official or in-house specifications, e.g., a specified precision and accuracy of an assay procedure or the characteristics of a finished pharmaceutical product. Validation can be categorized as either *prospective* or *retrospective*. Prospective validation should be applied to new drug entities or formulations in anticipation of the product's requirements and expected performance. Berry [2] and Nash [3] have reviewed the physical—chemical and pharmaceutical aspects of process validation.

Retrospective validation is often the most convenient and effective way of validating processes for an existing product. Data concerning the key in-process and finished characteristics of an existing product are always available from previously manufactured batches. Usually, there is sufficient information available to demonstrate whether or not the product is being manufactured in a manner that meets the specifications expected of it.

13.1 PROCESS VALIDATION

In order to achieve a proper validation, an in-depth knowledge of the pharmaceutical process is essential. Since the end result of the process is variable (e.g., sterility, potency assay, tablet hardness, dissolution characteristics), statistical input is essential to validation procedures. For example, experimental design and data analysis are integral parts of assay and process validation. Because of the diverse nature of pharmaceutical products and processes, one cannot give a template method of validation procedures and analyses. Usually, however, relatively simple and straightforward statistical methods can be used. Several examples will be given with solutions to illustrate the "validation" train of thought. There is no unique statistical approach to any single problem in most practical situations. In validation procedures, in particular, there will be more than one way of attacking a problem. What is most needed is a clear idea of the problem and some common sense. In all of the following examples, statistical methods will be used that have been discussed elsewhere in this book.

Example 1. Retrospective validation. Quality control data are available for an ointment that has been manufactured during a period of approximately one year. The in-process (bulk) product is assayed in triplicate for each batch (top, middle, and bottom of the mixing tank). The finished product consists of either a 2-ounce container or a 4-ounce container, or both. A single assay is performed on each size of the finished product. The assay results for the eight batches manufactured are shown in Table 13.1.

The following questions must be answered to pursue the process validation of this product:

1. Are the assays within limits as stated in the in-house specifications?
2. Do the average results differ for the top, middle, and bottom of the bulk? This can be considered as a measure of drug homogeneity. If the results are (statistically or practically) different in different parts of the bulk container, mixing heterogeneity is indicated.
3. Are the average drug concentration and homogeneity in the bulk mix different from the average concentration and homogeneity of the product in the final container?
4. Are batches in control based on the charting of averages using control charts?

Answers:

Question 1. The in-house specifications call for an average assay between 100 and 120%. All batches pass based on the average results of both the bulk and finished products. Batch 8 has a relatively high assay, but still falls within the specifications.

Question 2. A two-way analysis of variance (Chap. 8) is used to test for equality of means from the top, middle, and bottom of

Table 13.1   Results of Bulk and Finished Tablet Assays of 8
Batches

Batch	In-process bulk material (%)				Finished Product (%)		
	Top	Middle	Bottom	Average	2 oz	4 oz	Average
1	105	106	106	105.7	104	101	102.5
2	105	107	103	105.0	108	107	107.5
3	102	109	105	105.3	−	107	107.0
4	105	104	104	104.3	105	107	106.0
5	106	104	107	105.7	107	102	104.5
6	110	108	107	108.3	108	107	107.5
7	103	105	105	104.3	102	104	103
8	108	112	114	111.3	113	−	113
Avg.	105.5	106.9	106.4	106.24	106.7	105	106.38
s.d.	2.56	2.75	3.38	2.40	−	−	3.31

the bulk container. The average results are shown in Table 13.1,
and the ANOVA table is shown in Table 13.2. The F test shows
lack of significance at the 5% level, and the product can be considered to be homogeneous. The assay of top, middle, and bottom are
treated as *replicate assays* for purposes of determining within batch
variability. (Some statisticians may not recommend a two-step procedure where a preliminary statistical test is used to set the conditions for a subsequent test. However, in this case for purposes of
validation in the absence of true replicates, there is little choice.)
Note that if the average results of top, middle, and bottom showed
significant differences, a mixing problem would be indicated. This
would trigger a study to optimize the mixing procedure and/or equipment to produce a relatively homogeneous product. We understand
that a heterogeneous system, as exemplified by an ointment, can
never be perfectly homogeneous. The aim is to produce a product
that has close to the same concentration of material in each part.
From Table 13.2, the within-batch variation is obtained by pooling
the between position (top, middle, bottom) sum of squares and the
error sum of squares. The within-batch error (variance) estimate
is 64.67/16 = 4.04 with 16 d.f. The standard deviation is the square

Table 13.2   ANOVA for Top, Middle, and Bottom of
Bulk

Source	d.f.	SS	MS	F
Batches	7	121.8	17.4	—
Top −middle −bottom	2	7.75	3.88	0.95
Error	14	56.92	4.07	—
Total	23	186.5		

root of the variance, 2.01. This would be the same error that
would have been obtained had we considered this a one-way ANOVA
with 8 batches and disregarded the "top −middle −bottom" factor.

   Question 3. The comparison of the variability in the bulk and
finished product would be a test of change in homogeneity due to
handling from the bulk to the finished product. Although this may
not be expected in a viscous, semisolid product such as an ointment,
a test to confirm the homogeneity of the finished product should be
carried out if possible. In powdered mixes such as may occur in
the bulk material for tablets, a disruption of homogeneity during the
transformation of bulk material into the final tablet is not an unlikely
occurrence. For example, movement of the material in the containers
during transport, or vibrations resulting in the settling and sifting
of particles in the storage containers prior to tableting, may result
in preferential settling of the materials comprising the tablet mix.

   In order to compare the within-batch variability of the bulk and
finished product, a within-batch error estimate for the finished
product is needed. We can use a similar approach to that used for
the bulk. Compare the average results for the two different
containers (when both sizes are manufactured) and if there is no
significant difference, consider the results for the two finished containers as duplicates. The analysis comparing the average results
for the 2- and 4-ounce containers for the 6 batches where both
were manufactured is shown in Table 13.3. The paired t test shows
no significant difference ($P > 0.05$). The within batch variation is
obtained by pooling the error from each of the 6 pairs, considering
each pair a duplicate determination.

Within mean square =

$$\frac{(104 - 101)^2 + (108 - 107)^2 + \ldots + (102 - 104)^2}{2 \times 6} = 3.67$$

Table 13.3   Paired t Test for Comparison of
2- and 4-Ounce Containers (Omit Batches 3
and 8)

Average of 2 oz =   105.67
Average of 4 oz =   104.67
$\quad$ t = $1/(2.76 \sqrt{1/6})$ = 0.89

This estimate of the within batch variation is very close to that
observed for the bulk material (3.67 vs. 4.04). A formal statistical
test may be performed to compare the within batch variance of the
bulk and finished products for the 6 batches (F test; see Chap. 5,
Sec. 5.3) where estimates of the variability of both the bulk and finished product are available. (We can assume that all variance estimates are independent for purposes of this example.) The results
show no evidence of a discrepancy in homogeneity between the bulk
and finished product. Although this approach may seem complex
and circuitous, in retrospective, undesigned experiments, one
often must make do with what is available, making reasonable and
rational use of the available data.

The average results of the bulk and finished product can be
compared using a paired t test. For this test we first compute the
average result of the bulk and finished material for each batch.
The average results are shown in Table 13.1. The t test (Table
13.4) shows no significant difference between the average results of
the bulk and finished material.

If either or both of the tests comparing bulk and finished product (average result or variance) shows a significant difference, the
data should be carefully examined for outliers or obviously erroneous
data, or research should be initiated to find the cause. In the
present example, where data for only 8 batches are available, if the
cause is not apparent, further data may be collected as subsequent

Table 13.4   Paired t Test Comparing the Average
of the Bulk and Finished Product

$\quad$ Average of bulk = 106.24
Average of finished = 106.38
$\quad$ t = $0.14/(2.03 \sqrt{1/8})$ = 0.20

batches are manufactured to ensure that conclusions based on the 8 batches remain valid.

Question 4. A control chart can be constructed to monitor the process based on the data available. This chart is preliminary (only 8 batches) and should be updated as new data become available. In fact, after a few more batches are produced, the estimates and comparisons described above should also be repeated to ensure that bulk and finished product assays are behaving normally. The usual Shewhart control chart for averages uses the within batch variation as the estimate of the variance (see Chap. 12). Sometimes in the case of naturally heterogeneous products, such as ointments, tablets, etc., a source of variation between batches is part of the process that is difficult to eliminate. In these cases, we may wish to use between-batch variation as an estimate of error for construction of the control chart. As long as this approach results in limits that are reasonable in view of official and/or in-house specifications, we may feel secure. However, to be prudent, one would want to find reasons why batches cannot be more closely reproduced. The within-batch variation for the bulk material was estimated as (s.d.) 2.01. A control chart with 3 sigma limits could be set up as $\overline{X} \pm 3 \times 2.01/\sqrt{3}$ = 106.2 ± 3.5 based on the average of the top, middle, and bottom assays. Because of the presence of between-lot variability, a moving-average control chart may be appropriate for this data. This chart is constructed from the averages of the 3 bulk assays for the 8 batches (Table 13.1) using a control chart with a moving average of size 3. Table 13.5 shows the calculations for this chart.

For samples of size 3, from Table IV.10, the control chart limits are 105.91 ± 1.02(3.02) = 105.44 ± 3.08. Figures 13.1 and 13.2 show the control charts based on within batch variation and that based on the moving average. Note that the moving-average chart shows no out-of-control values and would include batch number 8 within the average control chart limits. The control chart based on within-batch variation finds batch number 8 out of limits. Within-batch variation appears to underestimate the inherent variation that includes between-batch variability. Until other sources of variability can be discovered, the moving-average chart, which includes between-batch variation, appears to accomplish the objective, i.e., to set up a control chart that allows monitoring of the average result of the manufacturing process.

A control chart for the moving range can be constructed using the factor for samples of size 3 in Table IV.10. The upper limit is 2.57 × 3.02 = 7.76.

Another control chart of interest is a "range chart" that monitors within-batch variability. If top, middle, and bottom assays are considered to be replicates, we can chart the range of assays within each batch, a monitoring of product homogeneity. The

Table 13.5 Computations for the
Moving-Average Control Chart
Shown in Figure 13.2

Moving average (N = 3)	Moving range
105.33	0.7
104.87	1
105.1	1.4
106.1	4
106.1	4
107.97	7
Av. 105.91	3.02

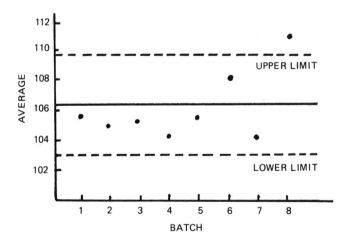

Figure 13.1 Control chart for Table 13.1 data using within-batch
variation to construct limits.

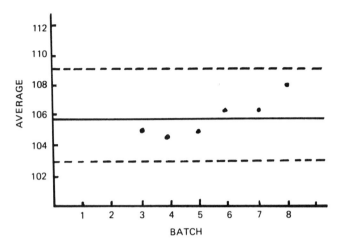

Figure 13.2   Moving average control chart for data of Table 13.1.

construction of range charts is discussed in Chap. 12.   Figure 13.3
shows the range chart for the bulk data from Table 13.1.   (See also
Exercise Problem 1.)

A control chart for the finished product is less easily conceived.
Different batches may have a different number of assays depending
on whether one container or two different size containers are manufactured.   There are several alternatives here including the possibility of using (1) separate control charts for the two different
sizes, (2) a control chart based on an average result, or (3) a
chart with varying limits that depend on the sample size.   Note that
only a single assay was performed for each finished container.   If
separate control charts are used for each product, one may wish to
consider assays from duplicate containers for each size container so
that a range chart to monitor within-batch variability can be constructed.   In the present case, limits for the average control chart
for the finished product would be wider than that for the bulk
average chart since each value is derived from a single (or duplicate)
reading rather than the 3 readings from the bulk.   (Note that if
within variation is appropriate for construction of the control chart,
as may occur with other products, one might use the pooled within
variation from both the finished and bulk assays as an estimate of
the variance to construct limits.)   Exercise Problem 2 asks for the
construction of a control chart for finished containers.

A preliminary control chart using a moving average of size 2 is
shown for the 4-oz container in Fig. 13.4.

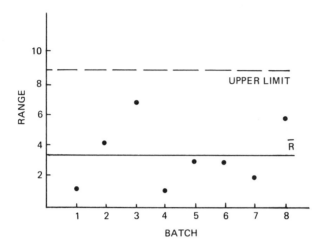

Figure 13.3   Range chart for Table 13.1 data.

Should any values fall outside the control chart limits, appropriate action should be taken.   Refer to the discussion on control
charts in Chap. 12.

Example 2:   *An example of a prospective validation study*.   In
this example, a new manufacturing process is just underway for a

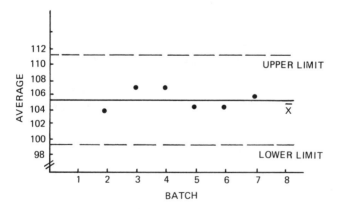

Figure 13.4   Moving average chart for a 4-ounce container from
Table 13.1 data.

tablet formulation of either (1) a new drug entity or (2) reformulation of an existing product. Since it would be difficult to generate data from many batches in a reasonable period of time, a recommended procedure is to carefully collect and analyze data from at least 3 consecutive batches. Of course, this procedure does not negate the necessity of keeping careful in-process and finished-product quality control records to ensure that the quality of the product is maintained.

Prior to the design of the validation procedure, a review of the critical steps in the manufacturing process is necessary. The critical steps will vary from product to product. For the manufacture of tablets, critical steps would include (1) homogeneity and potency after mixing and/or other processes in the preparation of bulk powder prior to tableting, (2) maintenance of homogeneity after storage of the bulk material prior to tableting, (3) the effect of the tableting process on potency as well as other important tablet characteristics such as content uniformity, hardness, friability, disintegration, and dissolution.

In this example, we consider a product in which potency and homogeneity are to be examined as indicators of the validation of the manufacturing process. To this end, both the bulk material and final product are to be tested. We will assume that the critical steps have been identified as (1) the mixing or blending step prior to compression and (2) the manufacture of the finished tablet. Therefore, the product will be sampled both prior to compression in the mixing equipment and after compression, the final manufactured tablet. Three mixing times will be investigated to determine the effect of mixing time on the homogeneity of the mix.

If many variables are considered to be critical, the number of experiments needed to test the effects of these variables may not be feasible from an economic point of view. In these cases, one can restrict the range of many of the variables based on a "knowledge" of their effects from experience. Other options include the use of fractional factorial designs or other experimental screening designs [4].

The question of how many samples to take, as well as where and how to sample is not answered easily. The answer will depend on the nature of the product, the manufacturing procedure, as well as a certain amount of good judgment and common sense. We are interested in taking sufficient samples to answer the questions posed by the validation process:

1. Does the process produce tablets that are uniform?
2. Does the process produce tablets that have the correct potency?

Table 13.6   Analysis of Bulk Mix in Blender and Final Tablets

			5 minutes mixing time			
Location	1	2	3	4	5	6
	101	104	101	104	101	109
	93	110	104	100	105	103
	102	106	96	94	99	105
Average	98.7	106.7	100.3	99.3	101.7	105.7
s.d.	4.93	3.06	4.04	5.03	3.06	3.06

			10 minutes mixing time			
Location	1	2	3	4	5	6
	101	105	100	104	99	103
	103	102	99	100	103	104
	103	104	103	101	102	103
Average	102.3	103.7	100.7	101.7	101.3	103.3
s.d.	1.15	1.53	2.08	2.08	2.08	0.58

			20 minutes mixing time			
Location	1	2	3	4	5	6
	102	100	101	99	101	103
	101	102	104	100	101	98
	104	103	100	102	105	102
Average	102.3	101.7	101.7	100.3	102.3	101.0
s.d.	1.53	1.53	2.08	1.53	2.31	2.65

	Final tablets		
	Beginning	Middle	End
	102	99	102
	98	100	103
	103	105	100
	100	101	100
	103	97	104
	103	102	102
	101	98	100
	100	103	97
	99	102	105
	104	100	101
Average	101.3	100.7	101.4
s.d.	2.00	2.41	2.32

Table 13.7 ANOVA for Table 13.6

Description	Source	d.f.	MS	F
5-minute mix	Between	5	33.79	2.16
	Within	12	15.67	−
10-minute mix	Between	5	4.1	1.45
	Within	12	2.83	−
20-minute mix	Between	5	1.82	0.46
	Within	12	3.94	−
Tablets	Between	2	1.43	0.28
	Within	27	5.06	−

3. Does the variability of the final tablet correspond to the variation in the pre-compression powdered mix?

Usually, samples are taken directly from the mixing equipment to test for uniformity. Samples may be taken from different parts of the mixer depending on its geometry and potential trouble spots. For example, some mixers, such as the ribbon mixer, are known to have "dead" spots where mixing may not be optimal. Such "dead" spots should be included in the samples to be analyzed. The finished tablets can be sampled at random from the final production batch, or sampled as production proceeds. In the present example, 10 samples (tablets) will be taken at each of the beginning, middle, and end of the tableting process.

Data for the validation of this manufacturing process are shown in Table 13.6. Triplicate assay determinations were made at 6 different locations in the mixer after 5, 10, and 20 minutes of mixing. In this example, 6 locations were chosen to represent different parts of the mixture. In other examples, samples may be chosen by a suitable random process. For example, the mixer may be divided into 3-dimensional sectors, and samples taken from a suitable number of sectors at random. In the present case, each sample assayed from the bulk mix was approximately the same weight as the finished tablet. During tablet compression, 10 tablets were chosen at 3 different times in the tablet production run and drug content measured on individual tablets. This procedure was repeated for 3 successive batches to ensure that the process continued to show good reproducibility. We will discuss the analysis of the results of a single batch.

Analysis of variance can be used to estimate the variability and to test for homogeneity of sample averages from different parts of the blender or from different parts of the production run.

For the bulk mix, none of the F ratios for between sampling locations mean squares are significant. This suggests that drug is dispersed uniformly to all locations after 5, 10, and 20 minutes of mixing. However, the within MS is significantly larger in the 5 minute mix compared to the 10- and 20-minute mixes. A test of the equality of variances can be performed using Bartlett's test or a simple F test, whichever is appropriate (see Exercise Problem 3). The data suggest a minimum mixing time of 10 minutes. The homogeneity of the finished tablets is not significantly different from the bulk mixes at 10 and 20 minutes as evidenced by the within MS error term. The tablet variance is somewhat greater than that in the mix (5.06 compared to 2.83 and 3.94 in the 10- and 20-minute bulk mixes). This may be expected, a result of moving and handling of the mix subsequent to the mixing and prior to the tableting operation.

The average results and homogeneity of the final tablets appear to be adequate. Nevertheless, it would be prudent to continue to monitor the average results and the within variation of both the bulk mix and finished tablet during production batches using appropriate control charts. Again, a moving-average chart, where between-batch rather than within-batch variance is the measure of variability, may be necessary in order to keep results for the average chart within limits.

13.2 ASSAY VALIDATION

Validation is an important ingredient in the development and application of analytical methodology for assaying potency of dosage forms or drug in body fluids. Assay validation must demonstrate that the analytical procedure is able to accurately and precisely predict the concentration of unknown samples. This consists of a "documented program which provides a high degree of assurance that the analytical method will consistently result in a recovery and precision within predetermined specifications and limits." To accomplish this, several procedures are usually required. A calibration "curve" is characterized by determining the analytical response (optical density, area, etc.) over a suitable range of known concentrations of drug. Unknown samples are then related to the calibration curve to estimate their concentrations. During the validation procedure, calibration curves may be run in duplicate for several days to determine between- and within-day variation. In most cases, the calibration curve is linear with an intercept close to 0.

The proof of the validity of the calibration curve is that known samples, prepared independently of the calibration samples, and in the same form as the unknown samples (tablets, plasma, etc.), show consistently good recovery based on the calibration curve. By "good," we mean that the known samples show both accurate and precise recovery. These known samples are called quality control (QC) samples and are used in both the assay validation and in real studies where truly unknown samples are to be assayed. Typically, the QC samples are prepared in 3 concentrations that cover the range of concentrations expected in the unknown samples, and are run in duplicate. The QC samples are markers and as long as they show good recovery, the assay is considered to be performing well, as intended.

Good experimental design should be carefully followed in the validation procedure. Careful attention should be paid to the use of proper replicates and statistical analyses. In the following example, the calibration curve consists of 5 concentrations and is run on 3 days. Separate solutions are freshly prepared each day for construction of the calibration curve. A large volume of a set of QC samples at 3 concentrations is prepared from the start to be used throughout the validation and subsequent analyses. A complete validation procedure can be rather complicated in order to cover the many contingencies that may occur to invalidate the assay procedure. In this example, only some of the many possible problems that arise will be presented. The chief purpose of this example is to demonstrate some of the statistical thinking needed when developing and implementing assay validation procedures.

The results of the calibration curves run in duplicate on 3 days are shown in Table 13.8 and Fig. 13.5.

As is typical of analytical data, the variance increases with concentration. For the fitting and analysis of regression lines, a weighted analysis is recommended with each value weighted by $1/X^2$, where X is the concentration. For analysis of variance, either a weighted analysis or a transformation of the data can be used to get rid of the variance heterogeneity (heteroscedascity). Analyses will be run to characterize the reproducibility and linearity of these data. The calibration lines are at the heart of the analytical procedure as these are used to estimate the unknown samples during biological (e.g., clinical) studies or for quality control.

ANOVA: Table 13.9 shows the analysis of variance for the data of Table 13.8 after a log (ln) transformation. The analysis is a three-way ANOVA with factors Days (random), Replicates (fixed), and Concentration (fixed). The two replicates from Table 13.8 are obtained by running all concentrations at the beginning of the day's assays and repeating the procedure at the end of the day. Although the ANOVA for 3 factors has not been explained in any

Table 13.8   Calibration Curve Data for Validation (Peak Area)

Day	Concentration	Replicate 1	Replicate 2	Average	c.v.
1	0.05	0.003	0.004	0.0035	0.0141
	0.20	0.016	0.018	0.017	0.0071
	1.00	0.088	0.094	0.092	0.0042
	10.0	0.920	0.901	0.9105	0.0013
	20.0	1.859	1.827	1.843	0.0011
2	0.05	0.006	0.004	0.005	0.0283
	0.20	0.024	0.020	0.022	0.0141
	1.00	0.108	0.116	0.112	0.0057
	10.0	1.009	1.055	1.032	0.0033
	20.0	2.146	2.098	2.122	0.0017
3	0.05	0.005	0.008	0.0065	0.0424
	0.20	0.019	0.023	0.021	0.0141
	1.00	0.099	0.105	0.102	0.0042
	10.0	1.000	0.978	0.989	0.0016
	20.0	1.998	2.038	2.018	0.0014

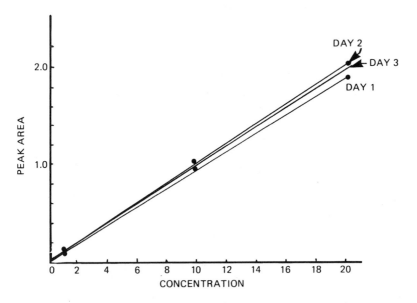

Figure 13.5   Calibration curves from Table 13.8 (weighted least squares fits).

Table 13.9 Analysis of Variance for Calibration Data (Log Transformation)

Source	d.f.	SS	MS	F
Days (A)	2	0.0377	0.019	–
Replicates (B)	1	0.000002	0.0000027	0.02
Concentrations (C)	4	18.137	4.534	630.6*
AB	2	0.00027	0.000135	–
AC	8	0.0575	0.00719	–
BC	4	0.000347	0.0000866	0.20
ABC	8	0.00341	0.000427	–
Total	29	18.236		

detail in this book, the interpretation of the ANOVA table follows the same principles presented in Chaps. 8 and 9, Analysis of Variance and Factorial Designs, respectively.

The terms of interest in Table 13.8 are Replicates and Replicate × Concentration (BC) interaction. If the assay is performing as expected, neither of these terms should be significant. A significant Replicate term indicates that the first replicate is giving consistently higher (or lower) results than the second. This suggests some kind of time trend in the analysis and should be corrected or accounted for in an appropriate manner. A Replicate × Concentration interaction suggests erroneous data or poor procedure. This interaction may be a result of significant differences between replicates in one direction at some concentrations and opposite differences at other concentrations. For example, if the areas were 1.0 and 1.2 for replicates 1 and 2, respectively, at a concentration of 10.0, and 2.3 and 2.1 at a concentration of 20.0, a significant interaction may be detected. Under ordinary conditions, this interaction is unlikely to occur.

A least squares fit should be made to the calibration data to check for linearity and outliers. A weighted regression is recommended as noted above (see also Sec. 7.7). This analysis is performed if the ANOVA (Table 13.9) shows no problems. A single analysis may be performed for all 3 (days) calibration curves, but experience suggests that calibration curves may often vary from day to day. (This is the reason for the use of QC samples, to check the adequacy of each calibration curve.) In the present case,

Table 13.10   ANOVA for Regression Analysis for Calibration Data
from Day 1

Source	d.f.	SS	MS	F
Slope	1	0.056885	0.056889	1653.0
Error	8	0.000275	0.0000344	−
Deviations from regression	3	0.000004	0.0000013	0.02
Within (duplicates)	5	0.000271	0.0000542	−
Total	9	0.057164		

Slope (weighted regression) = 0.09153

Intercept = −0.00109

regression analysis is performed separately for each day's data.
Table 13.10 shows the analysis of variance for the weighted least
squares fit for the calibration data on day 1 (weight = $1/X^2$). Each
concentration is run in duplicate. The computations for the analysis
are lengthy and are not given here. Rather, the interpretation of
the ANOVA table (Table 13.10) is more important.

The important feature of the ANOVA is the test of deviations
from regression (deviations). This is an F test (deviation MS/with-
in MS) with 3 and 5 d.f. The test shows lack of significance
(Table 13.10) indicating that the calibration curve can be taken as
linear. This is the usual, expected conclusion for analytical procedures. If the F test is significant, the regression plot (Fig.
(13.5) should be examined for outliers or other indications that result in nonlinearity (e.g., residual plots, Chap. 7). Sometimes,
even with a significant F test, examination of the plot will reveal
no obvious indication of nonlinearity. This may be due to a very
small within MS error term, for example, and in these cases, the
regression may be taken as linear if the other days' regressions
show linearity. If curvature is apparent as indicated by inspection
of the plot and a significant F test, the data should be fit to a quadratic model, or an appropriate transformation applied to linearize
the concentration−response relationship. The test for linearity is
discussed further in Appendix II.

A control chart may also be constructed for the slope and intercept of each day's calibration curve, starting with the validation
data. This will be useful for detecting trends or outlying data.

Table 13.11   Data for Quality Control Samples (% Recovery)

Day	Concentration	Replicate 1	Replicate 2	Average
1	0.50	106.5	103.9	105.2
	1.50	97.8	102.4	100.1
	15.0	101.6	97.2	99.4
2	0.50	99.4	107.6	103.5
	1.50	104.0	105.4	104.7
	15.0	96.9	100.7	98.8
3	0.50	97.4	100.2	98.8
	1.50	100.6	99.2	99.9
	15.0	104.2	101.8	103.0

A critical step in the assay validation procedure is the analysis of the performance of the quality control (QC) samples. These samples provide a constant standard from day to day to challenge the validity of the calibration curve. In the simplest case, large volumes of QC samples at 3 concentrations are prepared to be used both in the validation and in the real studies. The concentrations cover the greater part of the concentration range expected for the unknown samples. The QC samples are run in duplicate (a total of 6 samples) throughout each day's assays. Usually, the samples will be run at evenly spaced intervals throughout the day with the 3 concentrations (low, medium, and high) run during the first part of the day and then run again during the latter part of the day. Each set of three should be run in random order. For example, the six QC samples may be interspersed with the unknowns in the following random order:

Medium . . . Low . . . High . . . Low . . . High . . . Medium

Table 13.11 shows the results for the QC samples, in terms of percent recovery, during the validation procedure. Percent recovery is used to help equalize the variances for purposes of the statistical analysis. The first step is to perform an ANOVA for the QC results using all of the data. In this example, the factors in the ANOVA are Days (3 days), Concentrations (3 concentrations), and Replicates (2, beginning of run vs. end of run). The ANOVA table is shown in Table 13.12.

Table 13.12   Analysis of Variance for Quality Control Samples

Source	d.f.	SS	MS	F
Days (A)	2	9.418	4.709	–
Replicates (B)	1	5.556	5.556	0.44
Concentrations (C)	2	13.285	6.642	0.31
AB	2	25.498	12.749	–
AC	4	84.675	21.169	–
BC	2	11.231	5.616	0.73
ABC	4	30.956	7.739	–
Total	17	180.618		

Table 13.12 should not indicate problems if the assay is working as expected. No effect should be significant. A significant Replicates effect indicates a trend from the first set of QC samples (beginning of run) to the second set. A significant Replicate × Concentration interaction is also cause for concern, and the data should be examined for errors, outliers, or other causes. Table 13.12 shows no obvious evidence of assay problems.

To test that the assay is giving close to 100% recovery, a t test is performed comparing the overall average of all the QC samples vs. 100%. This is a two-sided test:

$$t = \frac{|\text{Overall average} - 100|}{\sqrt{\text{Days MS}/3}} \tag{13.1}$$

where 3 = number of days. This is a weak test with only 2 d.f. If no significant effects are obvious in the ANOVA, one may perform the t test on all the data disregarding days and replicates (N = 18), and the t test would be:

$$t = \frac{|\text{Overall average} - 100|}{\sqrt{s^2/18}} \tag{13.2}$$

The interpretation of this test should be made with caution because of the assumption of the absence of day, replicate, concentration, and interaction effects.

For the data of Table 13.11, the t tests [Eqs. (13.1) and (13.2)] are:

$$t = \frac{|101.489 - 100|}{\sqrt{4.709/3}} = 1.188 \tag{13.1}$$

$$t = \frac{|101.489 - 100|}{\sqrt{(180.618/17)/18}} = 1.938 \tag{13.2}$$

We can conclude that the assay is showing close to 100% recovery. Should the t test show significance, at least one of the three QC concentrations is showing low or high assay recovery. The data should be examined for errors or outliers, and if necessary, each concentration analyzed separately. The t tests would proceed as above but the data for a single concentration would be used. For the low concentration in Table 13.11, the t test (ignoring the day and replicate effects), would be:

$$t = \frac{|102.5 - 100|}{4.12 \sqrt{1/6}} = 1.486$$

To monitor the assay performance, control charts for QC samples may be constructed starting with the results from the validation data. Control charts may be used for each QC concentration separately or, if warranted, all QC concentrations during a day's run can be considered replicates. In the example to follow, we examine the control chart for each QC concentration separately and use the medium concentration as an example. Probably, the best approach is to use a control chart for individuals or a moving average chart. In this example, a control chart for individuals will be constructed (see Chap. 12). The validation data cover only 3 days. Following the validation, data were available for 6 more days using unknown samples from a clinical study. The data for the medium QC sample from the 3 validation days and the 6 clinical study days are shown in Table 13.13.

The average moving range is 2.62 based on samples of size 2. The overall average (of the "average" column in Table 13.12) is 101.17. The 3 sigma limits are $101.17 \pm 3(2.62/1.128) = 101.17 \pm 6.97$. The control chart is shown in Fig. 13.6. All the results fall within the control chart limits. Another control chart can be constructed for the range for the duplicate assays performed each day. The average range is 2.38. The upper limit for the range chart is 7.78 (see Exercise Problem 4). As for all control charts, the average and limits should be updated as more data become available.

Table 13.13   Data for Medium QC Sample (Concentration = 1.50) for Control Chart

Day	Replicate 1	Replicate 2	Average	Moving range
1	97.8	102.4	100.1	–
2	104.0	105.4	104.7	4.6
3	100.6	99.2	99.9	4.8
4	99.3	97.8	98.55	1.35
5	103.8	101.4	102.6	4.05
6	103.4	103.0	103.2	0.60
7	99.6	102.4	101.0	2.2
8	99.4	103.8	101.6	0.6
9	100.1	97.6	98.85	2.75

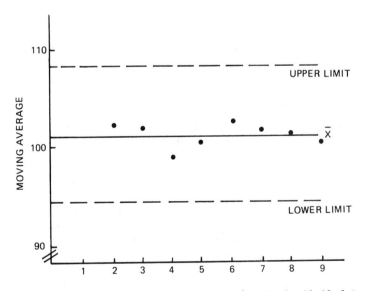

Figure 13.6   Moving average chart for Table 13.13 data.

The control chart for the individual daily averages of the QC samples and the control charts for the slope and intercept, if desired, are used to monitor the process for the analysis of the unknown samples submitted during the clinical studies or for quality control. If QC samples fall out of limits and no obvious errors can be found, the analyses of the samples during that run may be suspect.

13.3   CONCLUDING REMARKS

In this chapter, some examples of statistical analysis and design of validation studies have been presented. As we have noted, statistical input is a necessary part of the design and analysis of validation procedures. The statistical procedures that may be used to analyze such data are not limited to the examples given here, but are dependent on the design of the procedures and the characteristics of the data resulting from these experiments. The design of the experiments needed to validate processes will be dependent on the complexity of the process and the identification of critical steps in the process. This is a most important part of validation and the research scientist should be very familiar with the nature of the process, e.g., a manufacturing process or assay procedure [1,2,3]. The steps in the validation and statistical analysis are best implemented with the cooperation of a scientist familiar with the physical and chemical processes and a statistician. This is one of the many areas where such a joint venture can greatly facilitate project completion.

KEY TERMS

Assay validation	Process validation
Average control chart	Prospective validation
Calibration curve	Quality control samples
Control chart	Range control chart
Critical steps	Refractive validation
Moving average control chart	Weighted analysis
Moving range control chart	

EXERCISES

1. Construct the range chart using within-batch variation for the bulk material in Table 13.1. Assume that the 3 reading within each batch are true replicates.

2. Construct a moving average chart (n = 3) for the 2-oz finished container in Example 2, Table 13.1.
3. Compare the variances during the mixing stage in Example 2 using Bartlett's test. (The variances are estimated from the within m.s. terms in the ANOVAs in Table 13.7.)
4. Construct a range chart for the data of Table 13.12. Use the range of the daily duplicates to construct this chart.
5. Construct a control chart for individuals based on the data for 3 days for the low QC concentration from Table 13.10.

REFERENCES

1. Guideline of General Principles of Process Validation, FDA, Rockville, Maryland, March 1983.
2. Berry, I. R., *Drug Dev. and Ind. Pharmacy, 14,* 377, 1988.
3. Nash, R., *Pharmaceutical Dosage Forms: Tablets,* Vol. 3, edited by N. A. Lieberman and L. Lachman, Marcel Dekker, New York, 2nd Ed., in press.
4. Plackett, R. L. and Burman, J. P., *Biometrika, 33,* 305−325, 1946.

14
Consumer Testing

In this chapter we discuss several approaches to testing consumer acceptance of pharmaceutical products. Here we are more concerned with sensory aspects of a product, such as taste, smell, feel, and appearance, as opposed to efficacy. One should appreciate, however, that sensory and physical attributes of a product may relate to its pharmacological effect from a subliminal, psychological point of view. Also patient compliance may be, at least in part, a function of palatability. Consumer testing is most often applied to "consumer" goods, those products that are widely advertised and promoted, which includes foods and household products as well as drug products. The largest application in the pharmaceutical industry is in the area of over-the-counter (OTC) products, although these testing techniques may be applicable to many prescription drugs as well. The statistical techniques used in consumer testing are not unique to this area. However, the design of consumer studies and the introduction of new terminology specific to this area warrant a separate discussion.

14.1 INTRODUCTION

Before consumer products are marketed, the prudent manufacturer performs one or more tests to assess and confirm consumer acceptance. With regard to pharmaceutical products, oral solid dosage forms for prescription use have less need for formal testing than OTC oral liquid products, such as cough mixtures, or external use preparations, such as lotions and ointments. However, it is not unusual for a manufacturer to test inhalation and injectable dosage forms to ensure patient acceptance. Some large companies have a separate consumer testing group, particularly in those divisions which market OTC consumer products. Often consumer tests can be performed using volunteers from within company ranks. Although convenient, if in-house personnel are used as volunteers, the testing procedure and analysis should be carefully documented. When using only company employees for such tests, certain biases may be introduced if proper precautions are not taken. Principles of sample selection and experimental design are as important in these experiments as in any sophisticated laboratory or clinical experiment.

Consumer testing may be divided into several categories. Here we will consider (a) comparative tests that compare products according to one or more attributes, (b) tests that distinguish products rather than comparing them, and (c) assessing attributes which may subsequently be used for marketing position and promotion.

14.2 PRODUCT COMPARISONS

Different products may be compared one to another for many reasons. The products can be different formulations of the same drug manufactured in the premarketing, testing stage of development. If the product is a cough syrup, for example, various flavors may be under consideration. The formulator may wish to find that particular flavor which is most palatable, or which connotes efficacy. Sometimes, the product may already be successfully marketed, but a formulation change is contemplated, perhaps, because of a raw material shortage (one of its essential components), or to improve the product in some way. An alternative ingredient is used and the two formulations, the original product and its modification, are "put to the test." Perhaps an existing product is not selling according to expectations, and a formulation change is made with the hope of improved consumer acceptability and sales. Perhaps a new product is to be sold to compete with an existing marketed product. A preliminary consumer test to compare the new product with that already on the market would be a prudent step before launching an expensive advertising and retailing introduction of the new product.

In addition to safety and efficacy considerations, a consumer product generally has several attributes that contribute to its acceptance. An antacid tablet may be more or less acceptable, according to its size, shape, color, and taste. Its commercial success can even be dependent on the characteristics of the container and label. A consumer test comparing two brands of antacids, for example, may be directed toward only one of these attributes. However, in most situations, more than one attribute will be under investigation. The expense of recruiting volunteers or subjects to compare products makes it worthwhile to collect as much information as possible without compromising the test. The analysis of multiattribute tests is very complex, often requiring statistical techniques in the realm of multivariate analysis.* These analyses take into account correlations of variables, and use techniques such as factor analysis and multidimensional scaling, topics not included in this book. Our discussion will consider the comparisons of only one variable at a time. However, one should appreciate that in the analysis of data with multivariable observations, analysis of each variable separately does not consider relationships among the variables. For example, when looking at multivariate data, there exist so-called "halo" effects. This means that the answer to a question concerning one attribute, such as color, may very much influence the evaluation of another attribute, such as taste. On the other hand, examining one attribute at a time is simple, and easy to understand and communicate. A written report of results of a consumer test usually addresses each attribute separately as part of the data analysis and discussion of results.

The principal designs used for comparison testing to be presented in the following sections are:

1. *Paired comparisons.* In these tests, the consumer is presented with two or more products simultaneously, and compares all possible pairs in a random or balanced order. Often, the test involves only two products, a test product and standard product, for example. However, testing of three or more products is not uncommon. In the case of three products, A, B, and C, for example, the consumer compares A to B, A to C, and B to C, with respect to one or more attributes. The evaluation can be simply based on preference, or a score can be given to each product according to a rating scale.

2. *Crossover comparisons (sequential monadic tests).* In this design, each subject is given one of the comparative products for use or evaluation, and then rates the product. The second product is then supplied, the order of use of the two products being randomized or balanced. The subject completes a similar evaluation of the second product at the end of the evaluation period. Often, the subject is asked for a preference after the final evaluation.

3. *Monadic tests.* This design is similar to the parallel (one-way ANOVA) design in clinical trials. Each subject evaluates only a single product based on a multivariable questionnaire, usually with a rating scale.

The problems of sample size, blinding, assignment of products to subjects, and other statistical design considerations are similar to those for other comparative studies discussed elsewhere in this

---

*Multivariate analysis may be used when more than one response is observed as a result of an experiment (e.g., color, taste, efficacy) [6].

book. For tests run by the industrial pharmacist, these studies are of limited size. The tests are often conducted in-house, using colleagues as the experimental subjects. One should appreciate that this is not the ideal way to conduct such studies. For example, using the same people repeatedly in different studies results in a bias. The sample is not randomly chosen, and decisions based on the results of the studies will be continually reflected in the attitudes and habits of a select group. Also, the research and development scientist is probably not representative of the typical consumer. On the other hand, if the final test will be performed in a large group of "randomly" selected volunteers, using company personnel for the test panel for a preliminary look at the competing formulations is often convenient and expedient. Contract houses that have access to a large group of volunteers are usually used for the final full-scale tests. Thus, although an in-house test may consist of only a relatively few subjects, the data may give direction to the formulation scientist.

14.2.1   Paired Comparisons

The paired comparison design is very desirable from many points of view. The subject evaluates both products. If the evaluation consists of the choice, "I prefer product A" or "I prefer product B," the study is known as a *preference test*. The paired test is a side-by-side comparison, often easing the problem of making relative decisions about comparative products. The products are given concurrently to the panelist, and sufficient time is allowed for the evaluation. When the subject is presented with two or more products concurrently, position may be important if it affects the preference. As is also true for the order of presentation, position should be balanced with regard to "geometric arrangement of samples" [5]. The product evaluation may consist of a simple preference (as noted above) or the comparison can be derived from a rating scale. Table 14.1 shows an example of a rating scale that can be used for product comparisons.

Some people in the field of consumer research believe that paired tests should involve products that differ according to only one attribute: color, for example. Products whose overall acceptance and characteristics are evaluated based on two or more attributes can cause confusion for the subject (as well as the testor) if one attribute is preferred for one product and another attribute is preferred for the alternate product. In fact, one attribute that might be *unimportant* in terms of the sale of the product could dominate a more important attribute in this regard when tested in the artificial atmosphere of the consumer test. For example, important differences in flavor could be masked by a dramatic color difference

Table 14.1 Example of a Rating Scale for a Paired Test

Evaluation	Score
Product A is much superior to product B	5
Product A is superior to product B	4
Product A is the same as product B	3
Product B is superior to product A	2
Product B is much superior to product A	1

which may have little effect on the eventual commercial potential of the product.

Data from a typical in-house paired comparison test are shown in Table 14.2. In this example, an OTC antacid product that was shown to be very efficacious in vivo was lagging in sales compared to products that were clearly less effective. The color of the tablet was thought to be one of the factors involved in the failure of the product. The marketed tablet was blue–green and the marketing management recommended a change to a yellow tablet. Twelve members of the company research and manufacturing staff who suffered from gastrointestinal distress volunteered to evaluate the two products. They were presented with two identical-appearing packages (labeled as the marketed product), one containing the marketed blue–green tablet and the other containing the new yellow tablet. Otherwise, the products contained the same ingredients. The panelists were told that these two products were both new variations of the established formulation. *Prior* to using the products, the subjects were requested to indicate which of the two formulations they *thought* would be a better antacid. The subjects were then asked to use each of the products during the next 2 weeks and to report which product they thought was most effective for relieving their gastrointestinal distress. The products were to be used alternatively. Thus we have two sets of data: preference regarding color and preference regarding efficacy. Since both products were identical except for color, perceived differences in efficacy would be expected to reflect color preference (correlation of attributes, the *halo* effect).

The analysis of preference data for the comparison of two products is the same as the analysis of paired data using the "sign test" (see Sec. 15.2). The null hypothesis,

$$H_0: \quad P_1 = P_2 = 0.5$$

Table 14.2 Results of a Preference Test for a
New Antacid Preparation Versus a Standard
Product with only a Color Difference

	Preference for:	
Subject	Color	Efficacy
1	New	New
2	New	No preference
3	New	New
4	New	No preference
5	Standard	Standard
6	New	Standard
7	Standard	New
8	New	New
9	New	New
10	New	New
11	New	Standard
12	New	New

states that the preference for product 1 is equal to the preference
for product 2, both equal to 0.5 (i.e., half of the population prefers each product). This is a two-sided test because, a priori, a
preference for either product is possible and relevant. The statistical test is a one-sample test for a proportion. In this example,
the hypothetical value of P is 0.5. According to Table 14.2, the
preference for color is in favor of the new yellow-colored formulation, 10 to 2. The normal approximation to the binomial can be
used, with a continuity correction [see Sec. 5.2.4, Eq. (5.16)]:

$$Z = \frac{|p - 0.5| - 1/(2N)}{\sqrt{(0.5)(0.5)/N}}$$

$$= \frac{|0.833 - 0.5| - 1/24}{\sqrt{(0.5)(0.5)/12}} = 2.02$$

Note that the observed proportion is $10/12 = 0.833$. According to Table IV.2, a value of Z greater than or equal to 1.96 is needed for significance at the 5% level. Therefore, we can conclude that the yellow color is significantly preferred ($P < 0.05$) for this product.

The significance test for preference in terms of efficacy is performed in the same manner. For purposes of this test, we ignore ties (no preference signifies a tie; see Sec. 15.2). In this example, "no preference" means that the person likes (or dislikes) each product equally. Such a decision supplies no information with regard to the evaluation of preference. However, when reporting the results of preference tests, it is a good idea to include the number of no preference judgments in order to put the results in proper perspective. In our example, the statement that 70% of the panelists, among those who expressed a preference, preferred the new product for efficacy (7 of 10 preferences for the new product, Table 14.2) has a different meaning from that which would result from an experiment that included 30 subjects, 20 of whom expressed "no preference" and 7 of whom preferred the new product.

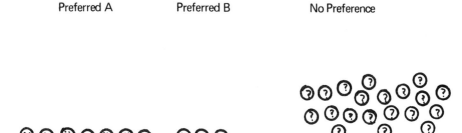

"70% PREFERRED PRODUCT A"

Preferred A   Preferred B   No Preference

Preferred A   Preferred B   No Preference

The test for the preference data regarding efficacy is not significant at the 5% level. Seven preferences for the new color out of 10 total preferences is not enough of a preponderance to reach the 5% level of significance [Eq. (5.16)].

$$Z = \frac{|0.7 - 0.5| - 1/20}{\sqrt{(0.5)(0.5)/10}} = 0.95$$

Table 14.3   Correlation of Preference for Color and Efficacy of an Antacid Tablet[a]

		Color	
		Preferred yellow tablet	Preferred marketed tablet
Efficacy	Preferred yellow tablet	6 (7)	1 (0)
	Preferred marketed tablet	2 (0)	1 (3)

[a]Parenthetical values are theoretical, showing a "100%" dependency or correlation.

Can we conclude that the "psychological" preference for the color yellow does not carry over to the actual clinical effect? The evidence in this experiment suggests that the color does effect perceived efficacy. However, the small size of the experiment results in weak power, and a 7/3 split in preference is insufficient to show a statistically significant preference. In this example it would not be fair to say that because the color preference results *showed* significance, and the efficacy preference results *did not show* significance, that the two evaluations give different answers.

A further analysis of interest in this experiment would consist of an evaluation of the "correlation" of the results of the two sets of preference data, for color and efficacy. Is there a tendency for a person who prefers the yellow color also to consider the yellow-colored tablet to be more efficaceous? Table 14.3 shows another way of displaying the experimental results. This table includes only persons who expressed a preference for both color and efficacy.

The data in Table 14.3 are too sparse to allow a firm insight into the possible dependence of efficacy and color preference. If the experimental results had been those indicated in parentheses in Table 14.3, this would be strong evidence of dependence; all persons who preferred the yellow tablet for color also preferred the same tablet for efficacy, and vice versa. The statistical test for independence in the 2 × 2 contingency table (Table 14.3) is a χ^2 test if we have a sufficient number of observations (see Secs. 5.2.5 and 15.8). In the present example, the χ^2 approximation is not recommended because of the small sample size; the procedure for Fisher's exact test is suggested (Sec. 15.8.2). If the sample size is large enough, the χ^2 test is calculated exactly as in the test for the equality of two proportions, although the question is different. The question here is: If a person prefers the yellow color, is he or she more likely to believe that the yellow tablet is more efficaceous (and vice versa)? An example where the χ^2 test is appropriate for analyzing data for "independence" is given in Exercise Problem 2 at the end of this chapter.

14.2.2 Monadic Tests

In monadic tests, each subject evaluates only one product during a given time period. These designs can be of two types: (a) *sequential monadic* studies (crossover design) and (b) *monadic* studies. In the former case, the subject evaluates more than one product on distinctly different occasions. This differs from the paired comparison discussed above, where both products are supplied and evaluated concomitantly. Thus a preference decision in the sequential monadic test may have less credibility than a similar decision in the side-by-side paired preference test. However, the sequential monadic test may give a more realistic appraisal of the products under day to day real use conditions.

Since subjects do not make direct comparisons of products in monadic tests, these tests require some kind of quantitative assessment, a *rating scale*. When quantitatively rating a product evaluated on a subjective basis, one has the challenge of transforming descriptive phrases into numerical values in order to make meaningful comparative statements. The rating scales used to quantitate data from consumer tests are similar to those used frequently in animal and human clinical studies. These scales are usually constructed by assigning numbers to a degree of acceptance (like or dislike) of an attribute. For example, if the taste of a syrup were being investigated, one might arbitrarily assign scores as follows:

1 = I do not like the taste

2 = The taste is barely acceptable

3 = The taste is acceptable

4 = I like the taste

5 = The taste could not be better

The subject assigns a score to the product for one or more attributes (color, taste, smell, ease of application, etc.). The scores are then analyzed according to the experimental objectives. Means and standard deviations are obtained, which may be used to assess product differences.

The assignment of scores to verbal statements has been the subject of much research by "psychometricians." The problem is to assign scores in such a manner that the scores are accurate representations of the descriptive statements on some continuous scale, assuming that the statements can be arranged on some continuum according to its perceived psychological meaning. For example, one may be able to show, by using appropriate experiments, that instead of the statements being assigned scores of 1, 2, 3, 4, and 5 in the scale, the statements really would be better represented by scores of 1, 1.5, 2.7, 3.3, and 5, respectively.

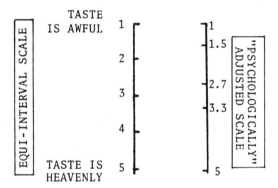

This suggests that the difference between the statement "I like the taste" and the statement "The taste could not be better" is *greater* than the difference between the two statements "I do not like the taste" and "The taste is barely acceptable." The former difference is 1.7 (5 − 3.3) and the latter difference is 0.5 (1.5 − 1). Thus, with the new scale, the statements are not on an equi-interval scale. In the original scale, an improvement of a product from an average of "3" to an average of "4" ("The taste is acceptable" to "I like the taste") would be considered equivalent in magnitude to an improvement from "4" to "5" ("I like the taste" to "The taste could not be better"). With the more scientific scale (psychologically adjusted), the latter improvement of 1.7 is greater than the former (3.3 − 2.7 = 0.6). However, with some care in the choice of descriptive statements, and the use of an equi-interval scale, the conclusions drawn from tests using rating scales should reasonably represent product differences. Often, the rating scale is presented in the guise of a thermometer (Fig. 14.1). Using the "thermometer" scale, the subject can visually choose that point which best represents his or her evaluation. A five- to seven-point scale is generally optimal. More points than this reflect very fine gradations which are difficult to differentiate in subjective evaluations.

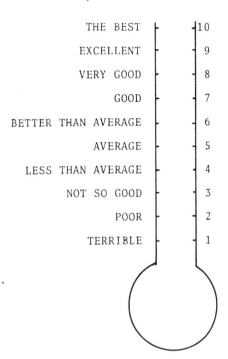

THE BEST — 10

EXCELLENT — 9

VERY GOOD — 8

GOOD — 7

BETTER THAN AVERAGE — 6

AVERAGE — 5

LESS THAN AVERAGE — 4

NOT SO GOOD — 3

POOR — 2

TERRIBLE — 1

Figure 14.1 Thermometer scale to evaluate product effectiveness.

Sequential Monadic (Crossover) Tests

This paired design can be likened to a clinical study where both drugs to be tested cannot be simultaneously evaluated by the same patient. The comparative products are evaluated at separate and distinct points in time. Table 14.4 shows some examples of consumer acceptance tests which can be designed as sequential monadic tests. Table 14.5 shows the results of a test comparing two headache products which were identical except for an advertisement that accompanied the product. Thus any difference perceived by the subjects could be attributed to the effect of the advertised message. The two products were evaluated using a sequential monadic (crossover) design and a thermometer scale, as shown in Fig. 14.1.

If the data in Table 14.5 consisted of the usual objective measurements as are made in clinical trials, the analysis would be identical to that used for a paired-sample t test (Sec. 5.2.3).* The

---

*Treatments are assigned in random order.

Table 14.4   Examples of Consumer Tests
that Can Be Designed as Sequential
Monadic (Crossover) Tests

Comparison of two deodorant formulations

Comparison of alternative shampoo products

Comparison of toothpaste formulations

Comparison of containers

Comparison of hand lotions

---

question that may be raised with data of this sort is whether we can
apply tests that assume normality (continuous measurements) to the
apparently discrete data from the rating scale. With a sufficient
number of observations, the ordinary t test, using the rating scale
results, will give approximately correct probabilities. In their book
Statistical Methods, Snedecor and Cochran describe a test which
they recommend for data of the type shown in this example [1].
The test is the same as the paired t test, except that a small correction is made that reduces the value of the test statistic. After
the differences are calculated for each data pair, the signs of the
differences are changed so as to give the *next* highest *sum* to that
observed. The test is constructed so that the actual sum of the
differences is reduced by a value halfway between the actual sum
and the *next* highest sum. Often, this correction is equal to 1.
Table 14.5 lists the differences (product A minus product B). The
sum of the differences is 18. The next highest sum is 20, obtained
by changing one of the −1 differences to +1. The value of t is
calculated according to Eq. (14.1).

$$t = \frac{|\Sigma\, D| - 1}{s.d.\sqrt{N}} \tag{14.1}$$

where $\Sigma\, D$ is the sum of the differences (18), 1 is the correction
$[(1/2)(20 - 18)]$, N is the sample size (20), and the standard deviation (s.d.) is the standard deviation of the differences. In this
example,

$$t = \frac{18 - 1}{1.683\,\sqrt{20}} = 2.26$$

Table 14.5 Results of a Comparison of Two Headache Products in a Sequential Monadic Design Using a Thermometer Scale

Subject	Score for product A	Score for product B	A - B	Subject	Score for product A	Score for product B	A - B
1	7	8	-1	11	9	8	1
2	3	4	-1	12	5	5	0
3	8	9	-1	13	9	8	1
4	5	5	0	14	7	6	1
5	6	5	1	15	7	8	-1
6	5	3	2	16	7	3	4
7	9	6	3	17	9	8	1
8	8	3	5	18	4	5	-1
9	7	5	2	19	7	6	1
10	8	8	0	20	6	5	1
Sum			10				8

According to Table IV.4, a t value of 2.09 is significant at the 5%
level (19 d.f.). Therefore, the advertising copy for product A can
be considered to be more effective than that for product B with
respect to increasing the perceived efficacy of the product. We can
say that the psychological component (placebo effect) relating to the
efficacy of this remedy has been enhanced for product A relative to
product B.

Monadic Tests

In monadic tests, subjects evaluate only one product. These tests
may be designed to collect data for specific products that may be
used for promotion and advertising or to be part of a data base
consisting of ratings for attributes of products from a similar class
(e.g., acne products, shampoos, etc.). Monadic tests may also be
used to compare two or more products in situations where it is more
expedient to use different subjects for different products. Such
experiments fit into the one-way ANOVA design (see Sec. 8.1).
For data derived from rating scales, the analysis may proceed using
the standard t test or ANOVA, if a sufficiently large number of
subjects are included in the test. Snedecor and Cochran describe
alternative analyses for experiments where the parametric t test and
ANOVA procedures may be considered questionable [2] (see also
Chap. 15). An example of a monadic test in which two dry-skin
lotions were rated by two groups of subjects is shown in Table 14.6.
The average results of the two products can be compared using a
t test, with each variable being analyzed separately. For the attribute "scent," the products were rated as follows:

5 = I like the scent very much

4 = I like the scent

3 = The scent is acceptable

2 = I do not like the scent

1 = The scent is very disagreeable

The test used to compare the two products is a two-independent-
group t test (Sec. 5.2.2). This test is satisfactory for discrete
data such as observed in this study, 20 subjects in each group.
(A nonparametric test based on Fisher's randomization test can be
found in Ref. 3.) The two-sided t test is

$$
t = \frac{|\overline{X}_A - \overline{X}_B|}{S_p \sqrt{(1/N_A + 1/N_B)}}
\tag{6.9}
$$

Table 14.6 Ratings of Two Dry-Skin Lotions by Two Groups of Subjects

	Product A			Product B		
	Scent	Consistency	Effectiveness	Scent	Consistency	Effectiveness
	5	4	4	1	4	4
	5	4	4	4	2	1
	2	3	2	1	2	1
	4	2	2	1	5	5
	3	5	4	2	4	5
	4	3	5	3	1	2
	3	2	1	1	4	5
	1	5	5	1	5	5
	2	5	5	1	1	2
	3	4	2	3	4	3
	4	1	2	1	4	5
	4	3	3	5	3	2
	3	1	1	5	2	2
	4	1	1	4	1	1
	1	2	1	4	4	4
	5	4	3	3	4	3
	3	5	5	4	3	2
	1	5	5	3	2	1
	2	4	5	4	1	2
	5	2	2	3	4	5
Mean	3.2	3.25	3.1	2.7	3.0	3.0
s.d.	1.36	1.45	1.59	1.45	1.38	1.59

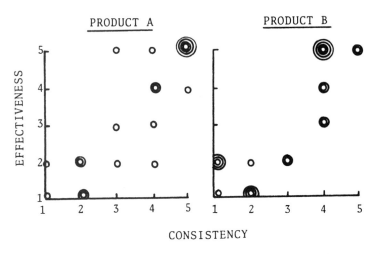

Figure 14.2   Scatter plot of consistency and effectiveness data from
Table 14.6.

In this example, $\overline{X}_A$ = 3.2 and $\overline{X}_B$ = 2.7.   The pooled standard deviation, S_p,* is $\sqrt{(1.853 + 2.116)/2}$ = 1.409. N_A = N_B = 20.
Therefore,

$$t = \frac{3.2 - 2.7}{1.409\sqrt{(1/20 + 1/20)}} = 1.12$$

Although product A was rated somewhat higher than product B for
the attribute "scent," the difference is not significant at the 5%
level (for 38 d.f., t must exceed 2.02, Table IV.4).   Figure 14.2
shows a scatter plot (correlation diagram) of "consistency" and
"effectiveness" for the two products.   There is a clear correlation
between these two variables; the higher the rating for consistency,
the higher the rating for effectiveness.   One may conclude that
effectiveness is dependent on consistency, although one should be
cautious about causal relationships implied by positive correlations.
For further analysis of the data of Table 14.6, see Exercise Problems 5 and 6 at the end of this chapter.

---

*Pooled standard deviation = $\sqrt{(S_A^2 + S_B^2)/2}$ in this example.

14.3 DISCRIMINATION TESTS: THE TRIANGLE TEST

Results of preference tests (Sec. 14.2.1) may be difficult to interpret because of the artificial conditions under which such tests are usually performed. Evaluation of results of these tests may also be problematic if two or more attributes are involved in making the preference decision. In addition, preference tests do not distinguish between the following *two possible situations* when preference of the two products is similar.

1. There exist *two groups of consumers, one of which likes product A and the other likes product B.* In the example illustrating the preference test in Sec. 14.2.1, there may be a segment of the population which prefers a yellow tablet, and another segment which prefers a blue−green tablet. Thus there are markets for both products.
2. Approximately equal preference for both products is indicative of the *inability of the subjects to distinguish the products.* Those subjects who do not give a "no preference" decision are randomly making preferences for one product or the other. The random choices result in an approximately 50−50 split for both products.

These problems of interpretation in preference tests are magnified when the products are identical in appearance, differing, perhaps, only in performance. Designs to estimate the proportion of consumers in the groups described above (i.e., two markets, for "preferers" of each products, and consumers who cannot distinguish the products or who do not care) have been proposed. However, in practice, these designs have been observed to be very sensitive to departures from the assumptions in the statistical model, and are of limited usefulness [4]. A more easily interpretable design which is used to indicate whether or not two products can, indeed, be distinguished is the *triangle test* [5].

The triangle test is applicable, for example, when modifications are made in a formulation, and one wishes to find out if consumers can tell the difference between the original and modified products. As noted above, a preference test may not completely fulfill this objective. If a preference test shows a significant preference for one of the comparative products, one could infer that the products are distinguishable. However, lack of significance in a preference test (approximately equal preference) may indicate either equal preference or indistinguishable products.

The procedure in the triangle test consists of first presenting three apparently identical products to the subject. Two of these three items are the same and one is different. The subject then chooses the single item (product) which he or she thinks is the different, or odd, item. Clearly, in this test, the products should not be obviously distinguishable on the basis of physical appearance. However, subtle differences based on attributes such as color, smell, taste, or efficacy can be tested.

This test has application in a variety of situations. Some examples are:

1. A formulation change, such as the introduction of new flavors, colors, or additives, made with the expectation that the consumer will not be able to detect differences from the original product.
2. Tests to determine if small changes in the product due to instability, as a result of storage, can be detected by the consumer.
3. Situations where both a preference test and a test for distinguishing products is desired. In this case, the triangle test is performed as usual, but a question regarding preference is also included (e.g., "Did you prefer the *odd product* or the other product?").

The design and implementation of the triangle test require special care. If the test involves a "sensory" evaluation, sufficient time must be allowed between the evaluation of the three test products to avoid any carryover effects. Carryover effects may be apparent with strong tasting material, for example. Also, the order of presentation is an important consideration in these tests because of possible psychological (and carryover) effects. Many tests show a differentiation based on the order of presentation. Therefore, the order of presentation should be carefully balanced in triangle tests. A typical balanced design is shown in Table 14.7. One set of three possible orderings includes product A as the odd product. The second set includes product B as the odd product. Assignments of the order of presentation to subjects may be accomplished in various ways. Each group of six subjects could be randomly given products in the orders shown in Table 14.7. Alternatively, the

Table 14.7 Balancing of Order in Triangle Tests

Set I	A B B	B A B	B B A
Set II	A A B	A B A	B A A

entire panel could be divided into six equal-sized groups, with each group being assigned one of the six orders in the table. Thus the test should have a sample size divisible by 6, in order to satisfy the balance constraints in these schemes.

Power considerations should play a part in choosing the sample size for triangle tests. However, similar to many other experiments, sample size is often based more on cost and convenience than statistical considerations. As in other statistical tests, the α level is usually fixed at 5% in triangle tests. The test of the hypothesis in triangle designs is based on the assumption that if the products are, indeed, indistinguishable, the odd product will be chosen correctly one-third of the time, on the average. If the products are indistinguishable, the test can be likened to the process of having a blindfolded subject pick one of three objects out of a hat, two being the same and one different. One-third of the time, the odd object will be chosen (P = 1/3).

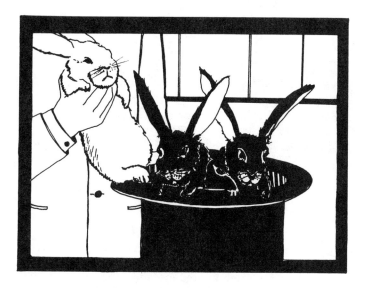

If the products can be distinguished by, at least, some of the subjects, the odd object will be chosen correctly more than one-third of the time. If the products are obviously different (such as would be the case in the example of the yellow and blue—green tablets), we would expect 100% correct choices (in the absence of color-blind subjects). Products to be compared in triangle tests usually have subtle differences. We expect to find less than 100% correct decisions. If less than one-third correct choices are made, we must attribute this result to chance. In an experiment of 12 draws in the example of picking one of three objects from a hat, if the odd object were chosen only three times (25%, 3 of 12), we would not conclude that the proportion of odd objects in the hat is less than one-third. In the triangle test, where we know that the proportion of odd objects is one-third, the only reason for less than one-third correct choices is *chance* or a *faulty* design and/or test procedure. Thus lack of attention to randomization of the order of presentation could result in significantly less than one-third correct choices of the truly indistinguishable objects. For example, if the third product presented tended to be chosen as the odd product, based on psychological factors, *and* the third product was *always one of the two identical products*, there would be less than one-third correct choices, on the average.

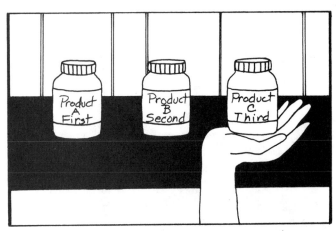

The third one is different!

Table 14.8 shows the results of a triangle test. In this example, a marketed over-the-counter cough syrup with a large and faithful consumer following had to be reformulated because one of the colors in the original formulation had been banned by the FDA. A alternative color system was used in an effort to match the original color. The triangle test was designed to see if consumers could perceive a difference between the original and reformulated product. After the subject had chosen the odd product, a preference was requested. If the products can be differentiated, and the new color is not preferred, another formulation with a different color system would be prepared.

The 18 subjects were told that one product had a different color from the other two products, which were identical. The subject was

Table 14.8   Results of a Triangle Test Comparing Two Products with Different Color Systems

Panelist	Order of presentation	Choice of "odd" product	Preference
1	ABB	A (correct)	A
2	BAB	B (incorrect)	A
3	BBA	A (correct)	A
4	AAB	B (correct)	B
5	ABA	A (incorrect)	B
6	BAA	A (incorrect)	A
7	BAB	A (correct)	B
8	AAB	B (correct)	A
9	ABA	A (incorrect)	A
10	BBA	A (correct)	B
11	BAA	A (incorrect)	A
12	ABB	A (correct)	A
13	BBA	A (correct)	A
14	ABA	B (correct)	B
15	ABB	B (incorrect)	B
16	BAA	A (incorrect)	A
17	BAB	A (correct)	A
18	AAB	B (correct)	B

then instructed to choose the one, "odd" product. An alternative approach would have been not to indicate where the difference existed, but to allow the panelist to examine, to even taste, the products in order to discover on his or her own, where the difference, if detectable, lies.

According to Table 14.8, 11 of 18 subjects correctly chose the odd product. The test of significance is described below. Note that this is a one-sided test. The proportion of correct guesses must *exceed one-third* in order to obtain significance. A significant result means that the panel of subjects can discriminate the products.

$$H_0: \quad P = 1/3 \qquad H_a: \quad P > 1/3$$

We use the normal approximation to the binomial with a continuity correction [Sec. 5.24, Eq. (5.16)]:

$$Z = \frac{|(p - 0.333)| - 1/(2N)}{\sqrt{(0.333)(0.667)/N}}$$

In the present example,

$$Z = \frac{|0.611 - 0.333| - 1/36}{\sqrt{(0.333)(0.667)/18}} = 2.25$$

At the 5% level, a value of Z greater than or equal to 1.65 is needed for significance (Table IV.2). The results of this experiment show that the products probably can be discriminated by some of the consumers. Table IV.11 gives the number of correct guesses needed for significance at the 5% level in the triangle test for panels of sizes 6 to 24.

Eleven of the eighteen panelists noted a preference for product A, the original formulation. However, when considering this result, one would be well advised to discount those preferences where the odd product was not correctly chosen. Although some of the correct choices may have been lucky guesses, one cannot identify which of these were truly discriminatory and which were correct by chance. The test for the preference data is the same as that presented earlier in this chapter (Sec. 14.2.1), using only the results of those who correctly chose the odd product. Of the 11 correct guesses, 6 subjects preferred product A and 5 preferred product B. Clearly, based on these results, one product is not significantly preferred to the other with regard to color.

The decision of what action should be taken as a result of this experiment is not easy. The fact that the products could be distinguished was disturbing to management, although the approximately equal preference was somewhat reassuring regarding the new color. Possible follow-ups to this experiment could involve reformulating with a new color or designing a new test in which the color difference would not be indicated to the participating subjects, as noted above.

KEY TERMS

Attributes
Balanced order
Carryover
Correlation
Discrimination tests
Fisher's exact test
Halo effect
Monadic tests
Multivariate analysis

One-sided tests
Paired comparisons
Preference test
Rating scales
Scatter plot
Sequential monadic
Sign test
Thermometer scale
Triangle test

EXERCISES

1. In a paired preference test, each of 100 subjects was asked to
    make a preference between A and B. Sixty indicated no pref-
    erence, 30 preferred A, and 10 preferred B. Is A significantly
    preferred to B?
2. A new test was performed for preference for color and efficacy
    of the antacid tablet as shown in Tables 14.2 and 14.3. The
    results were as follows:

    Preferred yellow tablet for color and efficacy: 15 patients
    Preferred yellow tablet for color and marketed tablet for efficacy:
        6 patients
    Preferred marketed product for color and yellow tablet for
        efficacy: 8 patients
    Preferred marketed product for color and efficacy: 10 patients

    Test to see if the two attributes (variables) are independent
    using a chi-square test.
3. In a sequential monadic test, the following data resulted from
    the comparison of two acne creams, based on a rating scale.
    The rating scale consisted of five equi-interval points, with a
    rating of 5 meaning very effective and a rating of 1 meaning
    ineffective.

	Score for product:	
Patient	A	B
1	5	3
2	3	3
3	4	5
4	2	4
5	3	4
6	2	4
7	3	2
8	4	5
9	1	3
10	2	3
11	4	4
12	2	5

(a) Perform a t test to determine if the products differ.
(b) Perform the t test with a correction factor as shown in Sec.
     14.2.2.

4. Analyze the data of Table 14.5 as if 20 patients evaluated product A, and 20 different patients evaluated product B (a monadic test). Compare results to that obtained where each patient evaluated both products.

5. Calculate the correlation coefficient for product A for consistency and effectiveness from Table 14.6.

6. Perform a t test for the comparison of consistency of formulas A and B, using the data from Table 14.6.

7. The results of a triangle test showed that 15 of 30 subjects correctly chose the odd product (i.e., the different product). Is this result significant (5% level)? Of the 15 who chose the correct product, 12 preferred product A and 2 preferred product B; 1 had no preference. Is product A significantly preferred? If product A is meant to replace a very good selling product, B, what action would you take?

REFERENCES

1. Snedecor, G. W. and Cochran, W. G., *Statistical Methods*, 7th ed., Iowa State University Press, Ames, Iowa, p. 146, 1980.
2. Snedecor, G. W. and Cochran, W. G., *Statistical Methods*, 7th ed., Iowa State University Press, Ames, Iowa, 1980, Chaps. 8, 15.
3. Siegel, S., *Nonparametric Statistics for the Behavioral Sciences*, McGraw-Hill, New York, 1956.
4. Ferris, G., *Biometrics*, *14*, 39, 1958.
5. *Manual of Sensory Testing Methods*, ASTM Spec. Publ. 434, American Society for Testing and Materials, Philadelphia, 1968.
6. Harris, R. J., *A Primer of Multivariate Statistics*, Academic Press, New York, 1975.

15
Nonparametric Methods

Nonparametric statistics, also known as distribution-free statistics, are methods of testing hypotheses when the nature of the distributions are unknown, and we are not willing to accept the assumptions necessary for the application of the unusual statistical procedures. For most of the statistical tests described in this book, we have assumed that data are normally distributed. This assumption, although never exactly realized, is bolstered by the central limit theorem (Sec. 3.4.2) when we are testing hypotheses concerning the means of distributions. However, occasions arise in which data are clearly too far from normal to accept the assumption of normality. The data may deviate so much from that expected for a normal distribution that to assume normality, even when dealing with means, would be incorrect. In these situations, a data transformation may be used, Chap. 10, or nonparametric methods may be applied for statistical tests. As we shall see, many of the nonparametric tests are easy to compute, and can be used for a quick preliminary approximation of the level of significance when parametric tests may be more appropriate. Although some people believe that any kind of data, no matter what the distribution, can be correctly analyzed using nonparametric methods, a kind of panacea, this is not true. Most nonparametric methods require that the data be continuous and independent, for example. Both of these assumptions are also required for parametric analyses, as exemplified by the normal, t, and F tests.

15.1 DATA CHARACTERISTICS AND AN INTRODUCTION TO NONPARAMETRIC PROCEDURES

Before proceeding, a review of the different kinds of data that are usually encountered in scientific experiments will be useful for the understanding of the applications of nonparametric methods.

Table 15.1   Examples of Nominal Data

Products categorized as acceptable and unacceptable in quality control

Side effects in a clinical study

Males and females in a clinical study

Various descriptions of "feel" of an ointment preparation, or taste of a product (tart, biting, sharp, etc.)

Concomitant diseases or medicaments in a clinical study

---

1. Perhaps the most elementary kinds of data are *categorical* or *attribute* measurements. These are also known as *nominal* observations (i.e., the observation is given a *name*). Thus a person is observed to be a "male" or a "female" or "black," "white," or "yellow." Some other examples are given in Table 15.1. The assignment of a number to such nominal data may be useful to differentiate the categories, perhaps for computer usage. However, actual values, a number assigned to these categories where the numbers have meaning in terms of rank, would not make sense. For example, we could assign the number 1 to a male and 2 to a female, but this does not imply that a female is *larger* (or, for that matter, smaller) than a male. Data that comprise two classes and consist of such attribute measurements may be analyzed using the binomial distribution. As discussed in Chap. 5, chi-square tests may be used to test the significance of differences of the proportion of attributes in comparative groups if the sample size and incidences are sufficiently large. These kinds of data are usually presented in the form of contingency tables, such as the 2 × 2 table for proportions discussed in Chap. 5.

2. The next, perhaps more "sophisticated" level of measurement involves data that can be *ranked* in order of magnitude. That is, we can say that one measurement is equal to, less than, or greater than another. These kinds of ordered data are known as *ordinal* measurements. Continuous variables are ordinal measurements according to this definition, but here, we usually think of ordinal data as arising from some arbitrary scale, as constructed for rating scales. For example, patients receiving antidepressant medication, may be rated according to attributes such as "sociability." A high score will be assigned to a patient performing well on this criterion. If the patient shows characteristics of "withdrawal," a low score will result. Intermediary scores reflect various degrees of response.

Table 15.2   Examples of Ordinal Data

Rating scales for sensory attributes (degree of liking)

Degree of effectiveness of therapeutic agent (pain relief, joint swelling, etc.)

Dichotomization of a continuous variable (underweight and overweight)

Number of anginal attacks in one week

Number of ulcers in skin-diseased patient

These are ordinal measurements. A patient with a score of zero after 1 week of medication, and a score of 3 after 2 weeks of medication can be said to have improved during the period between 1 and 2 weeks of treatment. A score of 3 is *better* than a score of zero. Some examples of this kind of data are shown in Table 15.2. Many nonparametric tests are based on *ranking* data. Certainly, data derived from a continuous distribution, such as the normal distribution, can be ranked in order of magnitude. (Ordinal data, by definition, can be ranked.) The nonparametric tests that will be discussed here, which use ranks for the analysis, require that the data have a continuous distribution. One might question the validity of nonparametric tests using data derived from an arbitrary ordinal rating scale such as that described above. If we understand (or assume) that the rating scale has an underlying continuity, the discreteness and arbitrary nature of the scale can be considered acceptable for nonparametric tests. The condition of the "depressed" patient is a continuum. The condition can vary from one extreme to another with infinitely small gradations, in theory. It is not possible practically to measure the subjective condition with its infinite subtleties, and therefore we substitute an ordered scale that approximates the condition of the patient. Controversy exists regarding the analysis of this kind of data. Some people believe that data derived from rating scales, as described above, should not be analyzed by parametric methods such as the t test. One reason for this position is that the intervals in these rating scales are not equal in terms of the degree of response; that is, the scores do not represent an equi-interval scale. In fact, the scale points do not precisely correspond to the description of the condition. The points are usually arbitrarily defined (see Sec. 14.2.2). Thus there is not an exact correspondence of the numbers on the rating scale to the patients' conditions, as defined by an arbitrary description

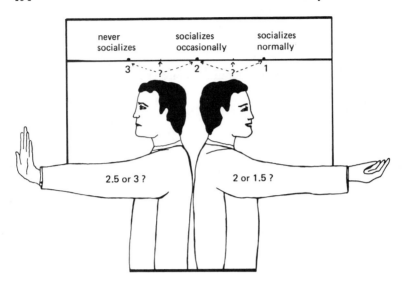

Figure 15.1 Problems with correspondence of a number and a subjective condition.

based on an assumed underlying continuous distribution (Fig. 15.1). For example, if a score of 3 represents "marked improvement" in sociability, 2 represents "moderate improvement," and 1 represents "no improvement," one usually cannot say that the difference between scores of 3 and 2 is equal in magnitude to the difference of 2 and 1. Yet the data analysis of such scores usually treat a difference between 3 and 2 as equivalent to a difference between 2 and 1. Perhaps, if the psychological aspects of depression were known to a sufficient extent, and the observer could discern subtle differences, the scoring system could be shown to be better represented by 3, 2.5, and 0.8 for the conditions corresponding to "marked improvement," "moderate improvement," and "no improvement," respectively.

Although we can and do analyze data from a rating scale using nonparametric methods (as presented below), the typical parametric methods (ANOVA, t tests) are also commonly applied to such data. The use of parametric methods to analyze rating scale data is considered to be acceptable by many statisticians, including members of the FDA. Snedecor and Cochran discuss the analysis of this kind of data using a modified t test [1]. An example of this approach is presented in Sec. 14.2.2.

3. When comparing ages using a "ranking" scale, one person may be said to be older than another without regard to the magnitude

of the difference in age. One can also specify the numerical differences with such data (e.g., one person is *two* years older than another). This is an example of numerical data, often encountered in scientific experiments, where the distances between the values representing experimental outcomes have physical meaning. These data have a precise, better defined meaning than data which are only ranked. Such data are often categorized as *interval* or *ratio* scaled data, depending on whether or not a true "zero point" exists. Age, weight, and concentration are examples of ratio scales. A person who weighs 200 pounds is twice as heavy as one who weighs 100 pounds. Temperature does not have a true zero point (according to the concept above) and is an example of an interval scale. A temperature designated as "zero" is an arbitrary position on the scale and does not represent the lack of temperature. We cannot say that 40° is twice as hot as 20°. Ratio and interval type data are the kinds of numbers that usually are subjected to the typical parametric tests. If these data are not normally distributed, they may be appropriately analyzed using nonparametric methods. One should understand that, in general, nonparametric tests can be applied to most of the data that we usually encounter, including that from continuous data distributions. Hence data that are normally distributed may also be analyzed using these methods. A disadvantage of using nonparametric methods rather than the usual analyses for normally distributed data is that nonparametric methods are less sensitive (i.e., they are less powerful). Nevertheless, some nonparametric methods are surprisingly sensitive and are able to differentiate treatments which are normally distributed with efficiency almost equal to that of the parametric tests.

Nonparametric tests are most effectively used for data which consist of only classified (nominal) variables or ranked variables which are considered to have an underlying continuous distribution. Data derived from continuous distributions are particularly amenable to nonparametric methods when the distributions deviate greatly from normality. A marked disadvantage of the simpler nonparametric techniques is the lack of flexibility of the design and analysis. Elementary designs may be readily analyzed using nonparametric methods, but more complex designs in which interactions and other ANOVA components are present cannot be simply analyzed with these techniques, particularly when sample sizes are small.

Most of the nonparametric methods for data that are not categorical use *ranking* procedures. The observations in the various treatment groups are ranked according to specific procedures, and the ranks that replace the raw data are then analyzed. These analyses use simpler statistical computations than the corresponding parametric analyses. The transformation to ranks results in simple whole or fractional numbers of relatively small magnitude.

15.2 SIGN TEST

The sign test is probably the simplest of the nonparametric tests.
The sign test is a test of the equality of the medians of two comparative groups. This test is used for *paired* data with an underlying continuous distribution, and can be applied to ranked or
higher-level data such as continuous *interval* and *ratio*-type data.
The pairs are matched, and *differences* of the measurements for each
pair tabulated. The differences are then categorized only with regard to the *sign* of the difference. That is, we count the number
of times one treatment has a higher value than the other. *Ties* are
not counted for this test. Ties give no information regarding which
treatment has the higher median value. Theoretically, with continuous variables, there should be no ties.* However, with limited
measuring instruments or the use of a crude rating scale, ties do
occur.
    As noted above, the sign test is a test of equal medians. If
the test shows "significance," we can say that two comparative populations have different medians at the α level of significance. Under
the null hypothesis that the medians of the two comparative distributions are the same, the probability of observing a value for treatment A being larger or smaller than an observation for treatment B
is *one-half*; that is, the probability that an observation for treatment A will be greater than a paired observation for treatment B is
one-half. Having recorded the differences, we compute the proportion of observations where the difference of treatment pairs is positive (or negative), disregarding ties (i.e., zero differences).
    If positive and negative signs are observed to occur with approx-
imately equal frequency, we can conclude that the treatments have a
similar median. If either positive (+) or negative (−) signs predom-
inate, there is evidence that one treatment has a higher median than
the other. The statistical test is based on the binomial distribution.
When applying two treatments to the same person, there are two
possible outcomes: either treatment A is favored or treatment B is
favored. Under the null hypothesis, the probability of A being
favored is one-half; H_0: $P = 0.5$. We compare the observed proportion to one-half (0.5). With N small and $P = 0.5$, the probabilities
of various experimental outcomes can be calculated from the expansion of the binomial [Eq. (3.9)], or from tables of the binomial distribution (Table IV.3). For sample sizes of 6 to 20, inclusive, the
number of positive or negative signs needed for significance at the

---

*With continuous measurements, the probability of two values being
identical is zero.

5% level for the sign test is given in Table IV.12. For sample sizes greater than 20, the normal approximation to the binomial, with a continuity correction, will suffice (see Sec. 5.2.4). The normal approximation test is

$$Z = \frac{|P - 0.5| - 1/(2N)}{0.5/\sqrt{N}} \tag{15.1}$$

where P is the observed proportion and N is the sample size. If Z is greater than 1.96, the treatments differ at the 5% level (two-sided test). The calculation can be simplified as follows:

$$Z = \frac{|\text{number of +'s} - \text{number of -'s}| - 1/2}{\sqrt{\text{number of +'s} + \text{number of -'s}}} \tag{15.2}$$

Remember that ties are discarded and that N, the sample size, does *not* include ties.

Example 1: Because of its simplicity, the sign test may be used for a fast look at data from comparative experiments before applying a more sensitive parametric test such as the t test (if appropriate). This was the case for the data in Table 15.3, which was obtained to

Table 15.3 Paired Data Obtained from the Bioavailability Experiment: Time to Peak Plasma Concentration

Subject	Time to peak (hr) A	B	Difference: B - A
1	2.5	3.5	+1
2	3.0	4.0	+1
3	1.25	2.5	+1.25
4	1.75	2.0	+0.25
5	3.5	3.5	+0
6	2.5	4.0	+1.5
7	1.75	1.5	-0.25
8	2.25	2.5	+0.25
9	3.5	3.0	-0.5
10	2.5	3.0	+0.5
11	2.0	3.5	+1.5
12	3.5	4.0	+0.5

compare the "time to peak" plasma level for two oral formulations of the same drug. These data would usually be analyzed using a more sensitive nonparametric test (see Sec. 15.3) or a t test for paired data (or ANOVA for a crossover design). Values were obtained by administering both drugs to each of 12 persons on two different occasions. Although these data would ordinarily result from a cross-over design, and ANOVA techniques might be more appropriate, for the present purposes, we will consider an example where treat-ments have been assigned in random order. We will, therefore, not analyze "order" effects, and we will assume that no carryover ef-fects are present.

From Table 15.3, tabulation of the differences (B − A) results in nine positive signs and two negative signs. One subject showed no difference between treatments A and B. Referring to Table IV.12, 10 of 11 positive (or negative) signs are needed to obtain signif-icance at the 5% level. Thus, according to the sign test, the differ-ence just misses significance, although product B appears to take a longer time to peak than does product A.

If the differences can be assumed to have a normal distribution, the paired t test would be a more sensitive test than the sign test. For any given, specific example, one could not predict that the t test would result in a "more significant" difference; but on the average, the t test will be more discriminating. In this example, the t test re-sults in a highly significant difference between the two formulations $(t = 3.02$; see Exercise Problem 1).

15.3   WILCOXON SIGNED RANK TEST

For the comparison of two treatments in a paired design, a more sensitive nonparametric test than the sign test is the Wilcoxon signed rank test. In the Wilcoxon test, the magnitude of the difference be-tween the paired results is taken into consideration in addition to the sign. This feature results in a more powerful test. The sign test still retains its advantage for a very quick assessment of the experimental results.

The Wilcoxon test is based on the assumption that the distribu-tions of the comparative treatments are symmetrical. Therefore, we are testing the equality of the means or the medians; the mean and median are equal in a symmetrical distribution.

The initial calculations are the same as in the sign test. We first take differences between the treatment pairs as in Table 15.3. Again, when the values for a treatment pair are equal (a difference of zero), a tie, these data are discarded for purposes of the test. As in the sign test, a zero difference does not contribute informa-tion regarding the differentiation of treatments in the Wilcoxon

Table 15.4   Data from Table 15.3: Ranking Differences
Without Regard to Sign for the Wilcoxon Signed Rank Test

Subject	Value	Rank	Assigned rank	Assigned rank with sign
7	-0.25	1	2	-2
4	0.25	2	2	2
8	0.25	3	2	2
9	-0.5	4	5	-5
10	0.5	5	5	5
12	0.5	6	5	5
1	1.0	7	7.5	7.5
2	1.0	8	7.5	7.5
3	1.25	9	9	9
6	1.5	10	10.5	10.5
11	1.5	11	10.5	10.5

Ranks with positive signs	Ranks with negative signs
2	
2	2
5	5
5	sum = 7
7.5	
7.5	
9	
10.5	
10.5	
sum = 59	

signed rank test. The differences of the untied pairs are then
ranked in order of magnitude, *disregarding sign*. For the data in
Table 15.3, the comparison of the time to peak plasma concentration for two formulations, A and B, the ranking of the absolute values of the differences is shown in Table 15.4. Differences of equal
magnitude (disregarding sign) are given the *average rank*. The
three subjects, 4, 7, and 8, all showed a difference (*absolute value*)
equal to 0.25. Each of the differences are given a rank of 2,
since these are the three smallest differences observed; 2 is the
average of ranks 1, 2, and 3.

After ranking (disregarding sign) is completed, the signs corresponding to the signs of the original differences are reassigned to the ranks. For example, for subject 7 (originally given a rank of 2), the rank is changed to -2, because the difference for this subject was negative. The ranks with *like signs are summed* as shown following Table 15.4. The sum of the positive ranks is 59, and the sum of the negative ranks is 7. These are known as the *rank sums*. Table IV.13 gives the values of the *smaller* of the two rank sums needed for significance at the 5% level for various sample sizes, N (N is the sample size, the number of pairs, less the number of ties). The smaller rank sum must be equal to or less than that designated in Table IV.13 for the two means to be significantly different at the 5% level. In our example, Table IV.13 shows that the means are significantly different. The table shows that a rank sum of 10 or less for the smaller rank sum is significant at the 5% level for N = 11. In our example, the smaller rank sum is 7. Therefore the difference is significant at the 0.05 level (P $\sim$ 0.02) [2]. This test gives very similar conclusions to that obtained by the t test. The Wilcoxon signed rank test is 95% as efficient as a t test for the comparison of normal populations. This means that a sample size of 100 which is analyzed using the Wilcoxon test would have equal sensitivity to a sample size of 95 using the t test. Considering the less restrictive assumptions of the Wilcoxon test compared to the t test, there is much to recommend it.

For sample sizes larger than those shown in Table IV.13, a normal approximation is available to compare two population means using the Wilcoxon signed rank test.

$$Z = \frac{|R - N(N + 1)/4|}{\sqrt{[N(N + 1/2)(N + 1)]/12}} \tag{15.3}$$

where R is the sum of ranks (either the larger or smaller rank sum can be used) and N is the sample size (disregarding ties). This formula works well also for smaller sample sizes. In our example, N = 11 and R = 59.

$$Z = \frac{|59 - 11(12)/4|}{\sqrt{11(11.5)(12)/12}} = 2.31$$

From Table IV.2, P = 0.02, which is very close to the exact probability, if the data are normally distributed.

15.4 WILCOXON RANK SUM TEST (TEST FOR DIFFERENCES BETWEEN TWO INDEPENDENT GROUPS)

The sign test and Wilcoxon signed rank test are nonparametric tests for the comparison of paired samples. These data result from designs where each treatment is assigned to the same person or object (or at least subjects that are very much alike). If two treatments are to be compared where the observations have been obtained from two independent groups, the nonparametric *Wilcoxon rank sum* test (also known as the Mann–Whitney U-test) is an alternative to the two independent sample t test. The Wilcoxon rank sum test is applicable if the data are at least ordinal (i.e., the observations can be ordered). This nonparametric procedure tests the equality of the distributions of the two treatments.

The calculations for the Wilcoxon rank sum test are similar to those for the signed rank test discussed above. First, the observations from both groups are pooled and ranked, regardless of group designation. Identical observations are given a rank equal to the average of the ranks. In this procedure, the signs of the observations are taken into account for ranking. For example, a value of -1 has a lower rank than 0.5, which has a lower rank than 1. After ranking the pooled data, the observations are returned to their respective treatment groups. The observations are then replaced by their corresponding ranks. The *sum of the ranks of the smaller sample* is the basis for the statistical test. If the sample sizes are equal in the two treatment groups, the sum of the ranks in either group can be used as the statistic for the Wilcoxon rank sum test.

Table 15.5 shows tablet dissolution results observed in the original dissolution apparatus and a modification of the apparatus. The objective of this experiment was to compare the performance of the two pieces of apparatus. Twelve individual tablets were used for each "treatment" (apparatus). The amount of drug dissolved in 30 min was determined for each tablet. One tablet assay, determined in the original apparatus, is not included in the results (Table 15.5) because of an overt error during the assay procedure for this tablet.

Note how the ranks are obtained. The original apparatus has the four smallest values, 50, 52, 53, and 54, which are ranked 1, 2, 3, and 4, respectively. The next two highest values are from the modified apparatus, both equal to 55. These values are both given the *average* rank of 5 and 6, equal to 5.5. The next value, 56, from the modified apparatus is given a rank of 7. The next highest value is 57, which occurs twice in the original and once in the modified apparatus. These are each given a rank of 9, the average of the three ranks which these values occupy, 8, 9, and 10, and so on.

Table 15.5   Results of a Dissolution Test Using the Original
Dissolution Apparatus and a Modification: Amount Dissolved
in 30 Minutes

Original apparatus		Modified apparatus	
Amount dissolved	Rank	Amount dissolved	Rank
53	3	58	11
61	14	55	5.5
57	9	67	21
50	1	62	15.5
63	17	55	5.5
62	15.5	64	18.5
54	4	66	20
52	2	59	12.5
59	12.5	68	22
57	9	57	9
64	18.5	69	23
		56	7
Sum of ranks	105.5		170.5

For moderate-sized samples, the statistical test for equality of
the distribution means may be approximated using the normal distribution. This approximation works well if the smaller sample is
equal to or greater than 10. For samples less than size 10, refer
to Table IV.16 for exact significance levels [2]. The normal approximation is

$$Z = \frac{|T - N_1(N_1 + N_2 + 1)/2|}{\sqrt{N_1 N_2 (N_1 + N_2 + 1)/12}} \tag{15.4}$$

where N_1 is the smaller sample size, N_2 is the larger sample size,
and T is the sum of ranks for the smaller sample size. If Z is
greater than or equal to 1.96, the two treatments can be said to be
significantly different at the 5% level (two-sided test). In our
example

$$Z = \frac{|\,105.5 - 11(11 + 12 + 1)/2\,|}{\sqrt{(11)(12)(11 + 12 + 1)/12}} = \frac{26.5}{16.25} = 1.63$$

A value of Z equal to 1.63 is not large enough to show significance in a two-sided test at the 5% level (P = 0.11, Table IV.2). Therefore, these data do not provide sufficient evidence to show that the two different pieces of apparatus give different dissolution results.

One should appreciate, as noted previously, that in ranking tests, *ties* result only because of measurement limitations, because the distributions are assumed to be continuous. Too many ties result in erroneous probabilities with regard to the test of significance. The error is on the "conservative" side. For data with many ties (*more than 10%* of the data results in ties, as is the case in our example) statistical tests will tend to give results that overestimate α (i.e., the α error is larger than it should be). Hence we tend to miss significant differences more often than we should when too many ties appear in the data. A correction for ties is available, but in most applications the difference between the corrected and uncorrected Z value is negligible.

It would also be of interest to compare the two pieces of equipment using the two independent sample t tests in order to see how the conclusions might differ. Of course, in general, one cannot determine what would be expected to occur from a single example. The t test is more efficient than the nonparametric rank sum test if the assumptions for the t test are valid (see Sec. 5.2.4). Similar to the signed rank test, the Wilcoxon rank sum test is very efficient, approximately 95% compared to the corresponding t test. A two-independent-groups t test for the data of Table 15.5 results in a t value of 1.84 with 21 d.f. (P < 0.10):

$$t = \frac{61.3 - 57.45}{5.05\sqrt{1/12 + 1/11}} = 1.84$$

The probability level is somewhat less for the t test compared to the Wilcoxon rank sum test in this example. However, the conclusions are similar for the two statistical procedures.

The tests described above may replace the *paired t test* (use the *sign test* or *signed rank test*) or the *two-independent-groups t test* (use the *rank sum test*) when the assumptions required for the validity of the t tests are questionable. For the comparison of more than two groups, nonparametric tests, analogous to the analysis of variance parametric methods, are available. However, simple nonparametric tests are not available for the analysis of more advanced designs or for tests of interaction. The tests to be described below

can be used to test for treatment effects for a simple one-way or
two-way analysis of variance. These tests are widely used, and
are recommended when ANOVA assumptions regarding normality are
suspect and/or cannot be easily tested. The nonparametric tests
are useful in experiments where the data consist of values derived
from a rating scale with an underlying continuous distribution.

15.5   KRUSKAL–WALLIS TEST
(ONE-WAY ANOVA)

The Kruskal –Wallis test is an extension of the rank sum test to
more than two treatments, and is a test of the *location* of the distributions. Significant differences can be interpreted as meaning
that the averages of at least two of the comparative treatments are
different. The computations and analysis will be illustrated using
an experiment in which data were obtained from a preclinical experiment in which rats, injected with two doses of an experimental compound and a control (a known sedative), were observed for sedation.
The time for the animals to fall asleep after injection was recorded.
If an animal did not fall asleep within 10 min of the drug injection,
the time to sleep was arbitrarily assigned a value of 15 min. The
experimental results are shown in Table 15.6. One data point was
lost from the control group because of an illegible recording,
obliterated in the laboratory notebook.

Table 15.6   "Time to Sleep" for a Control and Two Doses of an
Experimental Compound (min)

Control	Rank	Low dose	Rank	High dose	Rank
8	22	10	26	3	10
1	3.5	5	13	4	12
9	24.5	8	22	8	22
		6	15	1	3.5
9	24.5	7	18.5	1	3.5
6	15	7	18.5	3	10
3	10	15	28	1	3.5
15	28	1	3.5	6	15
1	3.5	15	28	2	7.5
7	18.5	7	18.5	2	7.5
Sum of ranks	149.5		191.0		94.5

The analysis for treatment differences is not dependent on equal numbers of observations per group, although, as in most experiments, equal sample sizes are most desirable (optimal). The analysis consists of first combining all of the data, as in the Wilcoxon rank sum test. To obtain the ranks, one lists all observations in order of magnitude, identifying each value by its group designation. The observations are then reclassified into their original groups, similar to the Wilcoxon rank sum test procedure. The ranks corresponding to each observation are retained and summed for each group as shown in Table 15.6. Note that ties are given the average rank as in the previously described rank sum test. In addition to the usual analysis, we will present a procedure that corrects the analysis for tied observations [3].

The test statistic for the Kruskal—Wallis test, as described below, is approximately distributed as chi-square with $k - 1$ degrees of freedom, where k is the number of treatments (groups) in the experiment. For small sample sizes, tables to determine the treatment rank sums needed for significance are available [3]. The chi-square approximation is good if the number of observations in each group is greater than five. The computation of the chi-square statistic follows:

$$\chi^2_{k-1} = \frac{12}{N(N + 1)} \left(\Sigma \frac{R_i^2}{n_i} \right) - 3(N + 1) \tag{15.5}$$

where

N = total number of observations in all groups combined

R_i = sum of ranks in ith group

n_i = number of observations in ith group

k = number of groups

In our example, $N = 29$, $R_1 = 149.5$, $R_2 = 191$, $R_3 = 94.5$, $n_1 = 9$, $n_2 = 10$, $n_3 = 10$, and $k = 3$. Applying Eq. (15.5), we have

$$\chi^2_2 = \frac{12}{(29)(30)} \left(\frac{149.5^2}{9} + \frac{191^2}{10} + \frac{94.5^2}{10} \right) - 3(29 + 1) = 6.89$$

The value of chi-square with 2 d.f. must be equal to or greater than 5.99 to be significant at the 5% level (Table IV.5). Therefore, the average "time to sleep" differs for at least two of the three treatment groups (control, high dose, and low dose) at the 5% level of significance.

As in the parametric tests, if statistically significant differences among treatments are found, one usually would want to know which treatments are different. For individual (pairwise) comparisons, Table IV.17 tabulates the differences between rank sums needed for significance at the 5% level, given the number of treatments in the design and the sample size [2]. To perform the pairwise treatment comparisons, the number of observations per treatment must be the same. For example, in the case of three treatments, each with a sample size of 10, a difference between the rank sums of two of the treatments (groups) must exceed 92 in order for the two treatments to be considered different at the 5% level. In our example, had the control group had 10 observations instead of nine, we could apply the pairwise test. However, if an additional observation had been included in the control group, the greatest difference between the rank sums of the control group and one of the doses of the experimental drug in this experiment could not exceed 92.* The observed difference between the high and low doses is (191 − 94.5) = 96.5, which exceeds 92. Thus the pairwise comparison criterion shows a significant difference between the high and low doses of the experimental drug ($P < 0.05$), agreeing with the significant chi-square test. For more details concerning multiple comparisons in the Kruskal–Wallis test, see Refs. 2 and 3.

As in the ranking procedures previously described, tied values are given the average rank. A correction for ties can be used which increases the value of chi-square. Therefore, if the null hypothesis is rejected (significant treatment differences), the correction only increases the degree of significance. If chi-square just misses significance, the correction may result in statistically significant differences. The correction is as follows:

$$\text{Correction} = \frac{\chi^2}{1 - \Sigma \, (t_i^3 - t_i)/(N^3 - N)}$$

where t_i is the number of tied observations in group i and N is the total number of observations. The calculations are illustrated

---

*The largest difference between the control and one of the experimental drug doses would occur if the tenth value in the control group were the highest observation. The rank sum of the control group would be increased by 30, resulting in a rank sum of 179.5 (Table 15.6). The difference between the rank sums of the control and high-dose groups would be 179.5 − 94.5 = 85, which is not significant at the 5% level.

below. There are eight groups of ties in the data shown in Table 15.6. For example, there are six values equal to 1. For this group of ties, $t^3 - t$ is equal to $6^3 - 6 = 210$. Another group of ties are the two values equal to 2. There are two values of 2 in the data, and for this group, $t = 2$ and $t^3 - t = 6$. The other ties occurred for values of 3, 6, 7, 8, 9, and 15. The reader can verify that the sum of T (where $T = t^3 - t$) is 378. The correction for chi-square is

$$\frac{6.89}{1 - 378/(29^3 - 29)} = \frac{6.89}{0.984} = 7.00$$

(Note that N = 29 in this example.) The correction for ties is usually very small. Of course, in this example, the correction does not change the conclusion of significant differences among treatment means.

15.6 FRIEDMAN TEST (TWO-WAY ANALYSIS OF VARIANCE)

The Friedman test is a nonparametric test applied to data which is, at least, ranked and which is in the form of a two-way ANOVA design (randomized blocks). This test, which may be applied to ranked or interval/ratio type data, is used when more than two treatment groups are included in the experiment. For two groups in a paired (two-way) design, the rank sum test may be used. In the Friedman test, the treatments are ranked *within each block* (e.g., animal or person), disregarding differences between blocks. The procedure will be illustrated using the data from Table 15.7. These data describe the results of a *validation* experiment to test the performance of four tablet presses, with regard to tablet hardness. The average hardness of 10 tablets was computed for five different tablet products manufactured on four presses. The tablets are a random selection of five typical tablet products. The presses were identically set for the same pressure for each tablet formulation.

The parenthetical values in Table 15.7 are the ranks of the average hardness for each formulation over the four presses. For formulation 1, the lowest value, 6.9, is assigned a rank of 1, and the highest value, 7.5, is assigned a rank of 4. Although no ties occurred in this example, if ties were observed, the average rank would be assigned to the tied observations as discussed in the preceding sections. If one of the presses consistently had the highest (or lowest) rank, one would conclude that the press

Table 15.7   Average Hardness of 10 Tablets for Five
Different Tablet Formulations Prepared on Four Presses[a]

Tablet formulation	Tablet press			
	A	B	C	D
1	7.5 (4)	6.9 (1)	7.3 (3)	7.0 (2)
2	8.2 (3)	8.0 (2)	8.5 (4)	7.9 (1)
3	7.3 (1)	7.9 (3)	8.0 (4)	7.6 (2)
4	6.6 (3)	6.5 (2)	7.1 (4)	6.4 (1)
5	7.5 (3)	6.8 (2)	7.6 (4)	6.7 (1)
R_i	14	10	19	7

[a]Parenthetical values are the within-tablet-press ranks.

(treatment) produced harder (or less hard) tablets than the other presses. In our example, tablet press C had the highest hardness value for all formulations with the exception of formulation 1, where it had the next-to-largest value. The test of significance is an objective assessment of whether or not the data of Table 15.7 provide sufficient evidence to say that tablet press C is, indeed, producing harder tablets than the other presses.

If the sample sizes are sufficiently large, a chi-square distribution can be used to approximate the test of significance. The chi-square test is

$$\chi^2_{c-1} = \frac{12}{rc(c+1)} \left(\Sigma \, R_i^2 \right) - 3r(c+1) \tag{15.6}$$

where

χ^2_{c-1} = the χ^2 statistic with $c - 1$ degrees of freedom

r = number of rows (blocks)

c = number of columns (treatments)

R_i = sum of ranks in ith group (column)

In our example, the chi-square statistic has 3 degrees of freedom:

$$\chi_3^2 = \frac{12}{(5)(4)(4+1)} (14^2 + 10^2 + 19^2 + 7^2) - 3(5)(5) = 9.72$$

A chi-square value of 7.81 or larger is needed for significance at the 5% level (Table IV.5). We can conclude that at least two of the tablet presses differ with regard to tablet hardness. Examination of Table 15.7 shows that tablet press C produces harder tablets than those produced by the other presses. Table IV.18 shows that a difference of 11 is needed for significance (P < 0.05) for individual comparisons between pairs of means for 4 treatments (k = 4) and 5 rows (n = 5). Therefore, press C produces significantly harder tablets than press D with a sum of ranks of 19 and 7, respectively.

For small samples, exact probabilities for the Friedman test are given in *Nonparametric Statistical Methods* [3]. This test also describes a test that corrects chi-square for tied observations.

15.7 RUNS TEST FOR RANDOMNESS

When performing an experiment (or observing a process) where values are observed sequentially, it may be of interest to determine whether the observations are randomly varying about the central value (i.e., the median). If the process is not random, we might expect to see trends in the data, perhaps a consecutive series of high or low values, which are unlikely to occur by chance. The *runs* test is a simple method of investigating the "random" nature of such a process. Tests for runs were introduced in Sec. 12.2.5, the discussion of control charts. A run is a series of *uninterupted, like* observations. For example, suppose that the median weight of 20 tablets, sequentially taken during a batch run, is 200 mg. Twenty consecutive tablets were weighed with the following results:

> The first six tablets weighed more than 200 mg.
> The next five tablets weighed less than 200 mg.
> The next four tablets weighed more than 200 mg.
> The next (remaining) five tablets weigh less than 200 mg.

If we designate tablet weights less than 200 mg by a minus (−), and tablet weights more than 200 mg by a plus (+), the 20 weights can be described by the following sequence:

$$
200 \text{ mg} \longrightarrow \frac{+\ +\ +\ +\ +\ +\qquad\qquad +\ +\ +\ +\qquad\qquad}{\qquad -\ -\ -\ -\qquad\qquad -\ -\ -\ -\ -}
$$

The first six values, +'s, represent a *run*. Each time that a series of like signs change, a new run begins. There are *four* runs in these data: *six* pluses, *five* minuses, *four* pluses, and *five* minuses. If the tablet weights follow a random process, one might suspect that the sequence of values described above is unlikely. It appears that the pluses and minuses come in "bunches." One might guess that the sequence of pluses and minuses could have been due to too-frequent weight adjustments on the tablet press. For example, the first tablets sampled were over the median weight of 200 mg. The tablet press may then have been adjusted down, more than necessary, resulting in too-low tablet weights (the next five tablets were underweight), and so on.

To test for randomness for sample sizes as large as 40, we can refer to Table IV.14. The table gives the lower and upper limits for the number of runs that would be expected to occur in a random process in a sample of size N. An observed number of runs equal to or less than or greater than that shown in Table IV.14 is an indication that the process is not random at the 5% level. The runs test is usually a two-sided test; either too few or too many runs leads to significance (nonrandomness). In some cases, e.g., control charts, only relatively few runs may be considered to suggest problems with a process. In these situations, critical values for a one-sided test as shown in Table IV.14 are appropriate. According to Table IV.14, for a sample size of 20, between 7 and 16 runs would be expected to occur if the null hypothesis of randomness is true. We observed four runs in the sample of 20 tablets (N = 20) in our example. Therefore, we conclude that the process is not random (P < 0.05). The clusters of high and low values are probably due to some malfunctioning of the tableting process.

Consider the following as a further example of an application of the *runs* test. A *standard* is analyzed every twentieth sample in an automated analytical procedure. A record of the readings for the standard in chronological order derived from one day's assay results are shown in Table 15.8. The median value for the data in the table is 0.7985 (the 20th and 21st ordered values are 0.798 and 0.799). As in the previous example, we label values greater than the median as + and values less than the median as −. The sequence of plusses and minuses is as follows (Samples 1 and 2 are below the median; 3 and 4 are above the median, etc.):

$$
\underline{-\ -}\ \underline{+\ +}\ \underline{-}\ \underline{+}\ \underline{-}\ \underline{+}\ \underline{-}\ \underline{+}\ \underline{-\ -\ -}\ \underline{+\ +\ +\ +\ +\ +\ +}\ \underline{-\ -\ -}\ \underline{+\ +\ +\ +\ +}\ \underline{-\ -}
$$

$$
\underline{+\ +\ +}\ \underline{-\ -\ -\ -\ -\ -\ -}
$$

Table 15.8 Readings of a Standard Solution in Chronological Order (Optical Density)

Sample	Reading	Sample	Reading
1	0.795	21	0.796
2	0.796	22	0.797
3	0.804	23	0.795
4	0.801	24	0.802
5	0.792	25	0.800
6	0.816	26	0.801
7	0.791	27	0.802
8	0.819	28	0.820
9	0.796	29	0.788
10	0.815	30	0.780
11	0.782	31	0.813
12	0.795	32	0.804
13	0.798	33	0.801
14	0.800	34	0.793
15	0.800	35	0.790
16	0.802	36	0.791
17	0.799	37	0.784
18	0.805	38	0.791
19	0.820	39	0.788
20	0.802	40	0.794

The runs are underlined in the previous sequence. There are 15 runs. For sample sizes of 40 or more, a normal approximation to the distribution of runs is available, under the null hypothesis that the observed values occur in a random manner.

$$Z = \frac{|r - (N/2 + 1)|}{\sqrt{N(N-2)/4(N-1)}} \qquad (15.7)$$

where r is the number of runs and N is the sample size.

Values of Z equal to or greater than 1.96 are unlikely ($P \leq 0.05$) if the observations are random. In our example $N = 40$ and $r = 15$. Therefore,

$$Z = \frac{|15 - (40/2 + 1)|}{\sqrt{40(40-2)/4(40-1)}} = \frac{6}{3.12} = 1.92$$

The value of Z is not quite large enough for the data to be considered nonrandom at the 5% level. Table IV.14 shows that for a sample of size 40, an observation of between 15 and 26 runs leads to acceptance of the null hypothesis of randomness, agreeing with the conclusion of the normal approximation [Eq. (15.7)]. Had 14 runs been observed, we would have concluded that the data were not random ($P < 0.05$).

15.8   CONTINGENCY TABLES

Chi-square tests for contingency tables (e.g., 2 × 2 tables) are often categorized as nonparametric tests. The analysis of 2 × 2 tables using a chi-square test was described in Sec. 5.2.5. The chi-square test can be applied to nominal or categorical data which cannot be analyzed using the ranking techniques discussed above. These data cannot be ordered (the data are not ordinal or on an interval/ratio scale). Nominal data are usually available in the form of *counts*, such as 25 males and 12 females entered into a clinical study; or the *number* of tablets categorized as acceptable, chipped, cracked, and so on. For large samples, chi-square methods can be used to compare "statistically" the relative frequency of such events which occur in two or more groups. Here we will briefly expand the case of the fourfold table, discussed in Chap. 5, to the analysis of R × C tables, R rows and C columns. We will then examine the case of 2 × 2 tables with small expected frequencies, followed by different tests of hypotheses for four-fold tables.

15.8.1   R × C Tables

In the binomial case, data are dichotomized, resulting in the 2 × 2 table, for example, comparison of success rates of two treatments as shown in Table 15.9. When experiments consist of more than two comparative groups and/or more than two possible outcomes, we are, in general, confronted with an R × C table (Table 15.9).

In the experiments involving contingency tables, we are usually interested in testing group differences with regard to proportions or the distribution of counts in the various outcome categories. Consider the data in the 2 × 3 table in Table 15.9. Two treatments have been compared where the outcomes were categorized as "unsuccessful," "moderately successful," and "successful." Inspection of the data indicates that treatment A has a greater incidence of "successful" events and less "moderately successful" events than treatment B.

Equivalently the hypothesis in contingency tables is often stated in terms of the relationship between rows and columns. "Acceptance"

Table 15.9 Examples of R × C Tables

2 × 2 table
(Fourfold table)

Treatment	Cured	Not cured
A		
B		

2 × 3 table

Treatment	Unsuccessful	Moderately successful	Successful
A	25	10	40
B	27	23	25

R × C table

	Outcome					
Treatment	1	2	3	·	·	C
1						
2						
3						
·						
·						
R						

of the null hypothesis suggests that the rows and columns are independent. For example, in the 2 × 3 contingency table in Table 15.9, lack of rejection of the null hypothesis would be interpreted, in this context, as meaning that the experimental outcomes are independent of the treatment (i.e., the treatments do not differ with respect to the experimental outcome).

The relationship of the rows and columns in an R × C contingency table may be tested by means of the chi-square distribution with (R − 1)(C − 1) degrees of freedom. Note that for a 2 × 2 table, we have 1 d.f., agreeing with the analysis of 2 × 2 tables described in Chap. 5. The chi-square statistic is calculated as

$$\chi^2_{(R-1)(C-1)} = \Sigma \frac{(O - E)^2}{E} \tag{15.8}$$

where O is the observed count and E is the expected count. The summation in Eq. (15.8) is for all R × C cells in the contingency table.

The chi-square test is an approximate test and should be used only when the expected values are sufficiently large. The usually recommended minimum expected values of five for each cell, as described in Sec. 5.2.5, is conservative [1]. If most of the cells have an expected value of five or more, the test should be reliable. If there is doubt about using the chi-square test, the exact test (multinomial) may be computed [4]. The calculations for the exact test solution are usually very tedious.

Table 5.10 shows data from a clinical study in which patients entering the study were categorized according to the severity of disease. Severity was divided into three classes: very severe, moderately severe, and mildly severe. The categorization was made to ensure that the severity of disease was similar for patients in the two treatment groups. Thus the question addressed by these

Table 5.10 Patients Categorized by Severity of Disease Entered into Two Treatment Groups in a Clinical Study

		Very severe	Moderately severe	Mildly severe	Total
Treatment	A	13	24	18	55
	B	19	20	12	51
Total		32	44	30	106

data is: "Is the severity of disease similar for patients entered into the two treatment groups?" or "Is there a relationship between "treatment" and "severity of disease"?" In a sense, this test is a confirmation of the randomization procedure used to assign patients to the two treatment groups. We would expect that, "on the average," the severity would be similar in groups A and B.

The chi-square calculation is similar to that for the fourfold (2×2) table (Chap. 5). The *expected* values for each cell are obtained by multiplying the row and column totals corresponding to the cell, and dividing this result by the grand total (row total × column total/grand total). In the example in Table 15.10, this calculation need be done for only two cells (note the 2 d.f.), because the remaining four expected values can be obtained by subtraction from the fixed row and column totals. The sum of the expected values must equal the row and column totals of the raw data. In the table the expected value for the cell with 13 patients (treatment A, very severe) is $(32)(55)/(106) = 16.60$. For the cell defined by treatment A, moderately severe, the expected value is $(44)(55)/(106) = 22.83$. The expected values are shown in Table 15.11.

The chi-square statistic is calculated according to Eq. (15.8).

$$\chi_2^2 = \frac{(13 - 16.60)^2}{16.60} + \frac{(24 - 22.83)^2}{22.83} + \frac{(18 - 15.57)^2}{15.57}$$

$$+ \frac{(19 - 15.4)^2}{15.40} + \frac{(20 - 21.17)^2}{21.17} + \frac{(12 - 14.43)^2}{14.43} = 2.54$$

Table 15.11   Expected Values for the Data of Table 15.10

		Very severe	Moderately severe	Mildly severe	Total
Treatment	A	16.60	22.83	15.57[a]	55
	B	15.40[a]	21.17[a]	14.43[a]	51
Total		32	44	30	106

[a]Obtained by subtraction from total; see the text (e.g., $55 - 16.60 - 22.83 = 15.57$).

Table 15.12   Number of Successes and Failures
Following Three Treatments

Treatment	Successes	Failures	Total
A	9	6	15
B	8	11	19
C	17	3	20
Total	34	20	54

For significance at the 5% level, a value of 5.99 is needed for chi-
square with 2 degrees of freedom (Table IV.5). Since the observed
chi-square is 2.54, we conclude that there is not sufficient evidence
to show that severity and treatment are related; that is, the two
treatment groups cannot be shown to differ with regard to the distribution of severity of disease.

Another example of an R × C table is shown in Table 15.12.
This differs from the previous example in that we have three treatments each with a dichotomous outcome, rather than two treatments
with three categories of outcome. The analysis tests for differences
among the three treatments. This data is derived from a clinical
study in which three treatments were randomly assigned to 60 patients. Only 54 patients successfully completed the study. Patients were classified as success or failure, depending on their response to treatment.

The analysis proceeds exactly as in the preceeding example.
The value of chi-square with 2 d.f. is 7.76. Since the table chi-
square with 2 d.f. is 5.99, the treatments are significantly different. To test for differences suggested by the data (a posteriori
tests), perform a chi-square test for two treatments (a 1 d.f. test),
but use the chi-square cut-off point for 2 d.f., 5.99, for significance. For example, the chi-square value for the comparison of
treatments B and C is 7.79, and treatments B and C are significantly different (see Exercise Problem 13).

For a further discussion of multiple comparisons and other topics in the analysis of categorical data, the book *Statistical Methods
for Rates and Proportions* by Fleiss [6] is highly recommended.

15.8.2   **Fisher's Exact Test

In the chi-square analysis of 2 × 2 contingency tables, if the expected values are too small, the chi-square test may not be

Table 15.13   Fourfold Table as an Aid to the Calculation of
Fisher's Exact Test

		Column		
		I	II	Total
Row	I	A	C	A + C
	II	B	D	B + D
Total		A + B	C + D	A + B + C + D = N

appropriate. Dichotomous data with small expected values are commonly encountered in pharmaceutical research, particularly in preclinical toxicology studies. For example, in preclinical animal car-
cinogenic studies, when comparing control and treatment groups
with respect to some characteristic that occurs infrequently, the
comparison of the frequencies may not be amenable to a chi-square
analysis. Fisher's exact test for 2 × 2 tables can be used to compute the exact probabilities. This test can be used, for example,
to compare proportions for two independent groups (treatments),
a binomial test, where expected values are very small.

Fisher's exact test makes use of the fact that the probability of
a given configuration in a fourfold table with *fixed margins** can
be computed using the *hypergeometric* distribution. The probability
calculation will be described with reference to the notation in Table
15.13 to help clarify the procedure.

The probability of the values found in Table 15.13, given the
four *fixed* margins, (A + C), (B + D), (A + B), and (C + D), is

---

*Theoretically, Fisher's exact test is appropriate when marginal
totals are fixed. In the example in Table 15.13, this means that
before the initiation of the experiment, we decided to use 12 animals on placebo and 14 animals on drug; a total of five carcinomas
will be observed in both groups. The latter result is clearly not
under our control (although in some experiments, the marginal totals
can be controlled). There exists some controversy whether data,
in which two independent groups are to be compared (as in Table
15.13), where the margins are not fixed, are appropriate for
Fisher's exact test. However, the test is commonly used to analyze
such data.

Table 15.14   Incidence of Carcinoma in Drug- and Placebo-
Treated Animals: Example 1

| | Number of animals with: | | |
	Carcinoma	No carcinoma	Total
Placebo	1	11	12
Drug	4	10	14
Total	5	21	26

$$\frac{(A + B)!(C + D)!(A + C)!(B + D)!}{N!A!B!C!D} \tag{15.9}$$

The numerator of Eq. (15.9) is obtained by multiplying the factorials of the marginal totals.   The denominator is the product of
the factorials of the individual cells of the fourfold table, multiplied
by $N!$, the factorial of the total number of observations.

Table 15.14 shows data typically analyzed using the Fisher's
exact test.   One group of animals was administered a placebo preparation consisting of all components of the drug formulation with the
exception of the active ingredient (placebo group).   Another group
of animals (drug group) was administered the drug formulation.
After a fixed period of time, the incidence of a particular type of
carcinoma was noted.   The probability of the fourfold table shown
in Table 15.14 with fixed margins (12, 14, 5, and 21) is calculated
using Eq. (15.9).

$$\frac{5!\,21!\,12!\,14!}{26!\,1!\,4!\,11!\,10!} = 0.183$$

Thus the probability of the results shown in Table 15.14 are *not*
very unlikely.   However, this is not the entire statistical test.   In
Fisher's test, we compute the probability of the observed configuration *plus* the probabilities of *all less likely* configurations (a cumulative probability).   If the sum of the observed configuration plus
all less likely configurations is *less than* α (0.05, for example), we
conclude that the rows and columns (treatment and carcinoma) are
not independent; that is, the treatments differ with respect to the
incidence of carcinomas.   If the sum of these probabilities exceeds
α (0.05, for example), we accept the null hypothesis of independence, concluding that the evidence is not sufficient to conclude
that the treatments differ.   In the example (Table 15.14), the sum

Table 15.15 Incidence of Carcinoma in Drug- and Placebo-
Treated Animals: Example 2

	Carcinoma present	Carcinoma absent	Total
Placebo	0	12	12
Drug	5	9	14
Total	5	21	26

of probabilities must exceed 0.183. (The probability of the observed table is 0.183.) Therefore, there is insufficient data to show
conclusively that the incidence of carcinoma is greater in the drug
group compared to the placebo group.

To clarify this procedure further, we will work out an example
in more detail based on the data shown in Table 15.15. These data
are similar to that in Table 15.14, except that no carcinomas were
observed in the placebo group and five were observed in the drug
group. Thus the marginal totals are the same in Tables 15.14 and
15.15. The probability of Table 15.15 is calculated as before, using
Eq. (15.9).

$$\frac{5!\,21!\,12!\,14!}{26!\,0!\,5!\,12!\,9!} = 0.0304$$

In order to assess the possible "statistical" significance of this table,
we must compute the probability of all less likely configurations as
discussed above. What constitutes less likely tables is not always
obvious without some "trial and error" calculations. With experience,
good, educated guesses can be made as to what constitutes a less
likely table. If a configuration is mistakenly chosen with a higher
probability than the observed table, the calculation is discarded.
Possible "less likely" tables are shown in Table 15.16 with the probability of each table. The only table with a lower probability than
the observed table (Table 15.15) is the one with all five carcinomas
appearing in the placebo group.

$$\frac{5!\,21!\,12!\,14!}{26!\,5!\,0!\,7!\,14!} = 0.0120$$

The sum of the probabilities of the observed table and all less likely (or equally likely) tables is $0.0304 + 0.0120 = 0.0424$. Therefore,
Table 15.15 is "significant" at the 5% level ($P < 0.05$); the drug
appears to result in an increased incidence of carcinomas.

Table 15.16 Some "Unlikely" Tables with Margins Identical to Table 15.15

	Carcinoma present	Carcinoma absent	Total	Carcinoma present	Carcinoma absent	Total
Placebo	5	7	12	4	8	12
Drug	0	14	14	1	13	14
Total	5	21	26	5	21	26
	Probability = 0.0120			Probability = 0.1054		

Note that Fisher's exact test requires that the probabilities of tables with fixed margins be computed for all possible configurations. If we calculate all possible configurations, the sum of the probabilities of the different tables would be equal to 1. Among all of these probabilities will be the probability of the observed table, in addition to possible probabilities equal to or smaller than that of the observed table. If the sum of these probabilities is less than or equal to 0.05, for example, the treatments are said to be "significantly" different at the 5% level, in the context of the present example.

The computations are often very tedious. For cases where the computations are unduly long and tedious, the use of computer programs or tables to determine significance points in fourfold tables are recommended [5].

15.8.3   Fourfold Tables with Related Samples

The examples of 2×2 contingency tables previously discussed in this chapter and Chap. 5 have involved the comparison of proportions or frequencies in two or more *independent* groups. A similar problem which occurs less frequently in pharmaceutical research is the comparison of two groups where the observations are *related*, also known as matched pairs. For example, Table 15.17 shows the results of two versions of an allergy test, A and B, applied to 50 persons. The test reagents were applied at the same time at different sites for each subject, and either a positive or negative reaction was observed. In this design, the total sample size is specified in advance, but the marginal totals are not fixed. We cannot anticipate the total positive and negative for test B in Table 15.17,

Table 15.17   Frequency of Positive and Negative Reactions to Two Allergy Tests Applied to Two Sites in 50 Persons

		Test B		
		Positive	Negative	Total
Test A	Positive	23	9[a]	32
	Negative	6[a]	12	18
	Total	29	21	50

[a]Patients who were positive on one test and negative on the other test.

for example. In the previous example, the size of the two treatment groups can be fixed in advance. Note that in this example
each person is subjected to both treatments (allergy tests). In the
previous examples of fourfold tables, each person is subjected to a
single treatment and a dichotomous response is observed (e.g.,
cured or *not cured*).

The objective of this experiment is contained in the question:
"Does the proportion of positive reactions for test A differ from
that for test B?" (i.e., H_0: $P_a = P_b$, where P_a and P_b are the
proportion of positive reactions in tests A and B, respectively).
Note that test A has 32 positive reactions (23 + 9), and test B has
29 positive reactions (23 + 6). It can be shown that the statistical
test for the equality of positive reactions for the two tests is equivalent to the test for the equality of the counts in the diagonal cells
designated by an a in Table 15.17 (9 and 6) [6]. The counts (or
proportions) in these two cells represent the *untied* responses
(*positive A* and *negative B*, and *negative A* and *positive B*, 9 and
6, respectively). The counts in the other two cells do not differentiate the two allergy tests. For example, the upper left-hand
cell shows the 23 patients who were positive on *both* tests.

Under the null hypothesis that the probability of a positve reaction is equal for both tests, the diagonal counts, 9 and 6, should
be equal. The test of significance is a binomial test, as in the
paired comparison test (Sec. 14.2.1) or the sign test (Sec. 15.2).
In the latter procedures, the observed proportion is compared to
0.5, the expected proportion if both treatment groups have an equal
probability of being positive. The statistical test in this example
makes use of the normal approximation to the binomial distribution
[Eq. (15.1)].

$$Z = \frac{|\text{observed proportion} - 0.5| - 1/(2N)}{\sqrt{(0.5)(0.5)/N}} \qquad (15.1)$$

If Z is greater than 1.96, the difference is significant at the 5%
level and we conclude that the probability of a positive response is
different for the comparative treatments. (As in other examples
where the normal approximation to the binomial is used, the sample
size should be sufficiently large, approximately 10 for this test.)
The observed proportion in the example in Table 15.17 is 9/15 =
0.60. N = 15, the number of untied pairs. Therefore,

$$Z = \frac{|0.60 - 0.5| - 1/30}{\sqrt{(0.5)(0.5)/15}}$$

Since Z is not equal to or greater than 1.96, the difference is not significant at the 5% level. The difference is not sufficiently large to conclude that the two tests differ with regard to the frequency (proportion) of positive responses. This test is also known as McNemar's test.

The data shown in Table 15.17 can also answer a different question which requires a different analysis. In the previous example, we inquired if the proportion of positive reactions was different in the two tests. Another question that is often relevant to such data is: "Are the allergy tests independent, that is, is the probability of a positive response for test B independent of the outcome for test A?" This question implies that if A and B are independent, there should be an equal proportion of positive results to test A in both patients with a positive test to B *and* in patients with a negative test to B. Table 15.18 shows the *expected results* if, in fact, tests A and B are independent. Note that the expected proportion of positive A's in patients who had a positive test for B is 0.64, 18.56/29. This is the same expected proportion of positive A's as that for patients who had a negative test for B, 13.44/21.

The test for independence is the same chi-square test as that used for the comparison of proportions in two independent samples, although the question to be answered is different (see Sec. 5.2.5). We apply Eq. (15.8):

$$\chi_1^2 = \Sigma \frac{(O - E)^2}{E} \tag{15.8}$$

where O is the observed count and E is the expected count. The expected values for the chi-square test are shown in Table 15.18 (see Sec. 5.2.5 for calculation of expected values). Applying

Table 15.18 Expected Values from Table 15.17 if Allergy Tests A and B are Independent

		Test B		
		Positive	Negative	Total
Test A	Positive	18.56	13.44	32
	Negative	10.44	7.56	18
	Total	29	21	50

Eq. (15.8) to the data of Tables 15.17 and 15.18 (including the
continuity correction discussed in Sec. 5.24), we have

$$\chi_1^2 = \frac{(4)^2}{13.44} + \frac{(4)^2}{18.56} + \frac{(4)^2}{7.56} + \frac{(4)^2}{10.44} = 5.70$$

To obtain significance at the 5% level, a chi-square value of 3.84 is
needed (Table IV.5). Clearly, the test is significant and we conclude that the results of this test warrant rejection of the null hypothesis (i.e., the results of tests A and B are dependent). This
significant result suggests that tests A and B are related; a positive test for A is associated with a positive test for B; and a negative test for A is associated with a negative test for B.

15.8.4 Analysis of Combined Sets of 2 × 2 Tables

Two situations may arise in which the analysis of combined fourfold
tables is needed. Consider a clinical study in which two treatments
are to be compared with regard to a dichotomous variable where the
data is collected from more than one center. Rather than pooling
all the data to form one combined table, the analysis is performed
with the data stratified by center. In a second example, a study
may be performed at a single center, but there may be a variable
within the center which needs further clarification with respect to
interpretation of the results. The data is then stratified by this
variable. Koch and Edwards [7] give an example of a clinical study
at a single center comparing a test drug and placebo in a study of
arthritis. The outcome of the treatment is dichotomized into either
no improvement or (some or marked) improvement. The overall results are shown in Table 15.19. Table 15.20 stratifies Table 15.19

Table 15.19 Fourfold Table for Treatment and
Placebo

| Treatment | Improvement | | Total |
	None	Some or marked	
Active	13	28	41
Placebo	29	14	43
Total	42	42	84

Table 15.20   Table 15.19 with Two Subgroups

Sex	Treatment	Improvement		Total
		None	Some or marked	
Female	Test drug	$n_{111} = 6$	$n_{112} = 21$	$n_{11+} = 27$
Female	Placebo	$n_{121} = 19$	$n_{122} = 13$	$n_{12+} = 32$
Female total		$n_{1+1} = 25$	$n_{1+2} = 34$	$n_1 = 59$
Male	Test drug	$n_{211} = 7$	$n_{212} = 7$	$n_{21+} = 14$
Male	Placebo	$n_{221} = 10$	$n_{222} = 1$	$n_{22+} = 11$
Male total		$n_{2+1} = 17$	$n_{2+2} = 8$	$n_2 = 25$

into two groups, results for males and females. The following discussion summarizes part of their presentation (for more detail, see Ref. 7).

Note that males appear to be less responsive than females to both active drug and placebo. If the distribution of males and females to treatment groups is unbalanced, the experimental results can be biased.

The chi-square test for significance for the data of Table 15.19 is 10.7 with a correction factor, and 12.3 without the correction factor. The Mantel–Haenszel method [8] tests for significance, taking into account the sex-adjusted response (Table 15.20).

If treatments are equally effective, the expected value of n_{111} and n_{211} in Table 15.20 are:

$$E(n_{111}) = m_{111} = \frac{(n_{11+}) \ (n_{1+1})}{n_1}$$

$$E(n_{211}) = m_{211} = \frac{(n_{21+}) \ (n_{2+1})}{n_2}$$

The variances of n_{111} and n_{211} are:

$$\text{Var}(n_{111}) = n_{11+} \, n_{12+} \, n_{1+1} \, n_{1+2} / [(n_1^2)(n_1 - 1)]$$

$$= \frac{(27)(32)(25)(34)}{(59)^2 \, (58)} = 3.63748$$

$$\text{Var}(n_{211}) = n_{21+} \, n_{22+} \, n_{2+1} \, n_{2+2} / [(n_2^2)(n_2 - 1)]$$

$$= \frac{(14)(11)(17)(8)}{(25)^2 \, (24)} = 1.39627$$

The Mantel–Haenszel statistic is calculated as:

$$\frac{[\Sigma_{h=1}^2 (n_{h1+} n_{h2+}/n_h)(p_{h11} - p_{h21})]^2}{\Sigma_{h=1}^2 v_{h11}} \tag{15.9}$$

where $h = 1, 2$ and $p_{hi1} = (n_{hi1}/n_{hi+})$, the proportion of patients in each sex and treatment group who show no improvement.

$$p_{111} = 6/27$$
$$p_{211} = 7/14$$
$$p_{121} = 19/32$$
$$p_{221} = 10/11$$

For the data of Table 15.20, the calculation is:

$$Q_{MH} =$$

$$\frac{[\{(27)(32)/59\}(6/27 - 19/32) + \{(14)(11)/25\}(7/14 - 10/11)\}]^2}{3.63748 + 1.39627}$$

$$= 12.59$$

Q_{MH} is distributed approximately as chi-square with 1 d.f. Therefore, the conclusion is that after adjustment for sex differences, the treatments are significantly different ($P < 0.05$).

This analysis summarizes an elementary but common occurrence in the analysis of clinical studies. For more detail of the application of the Mantel–Haenszel statistic, see Refs. 6 and 7.

KEY TERMS

Attribute
Categorical data
Contingency table (R × C table)
Continuous Data
Distributions
Efficiency
Fisher's exact test
Friedman's test
Hypergeometric distribution
Independence
Interval or ratio scale
Kruskal–Wallis test
Mantel–Haenszel test
McNemar's test

Multinominal distribution
Nominal data
Normal approximation
Ordered data
Ordinal data
Rating scale
Run
Runs test
Sensitive
Sign test
Ties
Wilcoxon rank sum test
Wilcoxon signed rank test

EXERCISES

1. Perform a t test to compare treatments for the data from Table 15.3. Compare the results of this test to the nonparametric test presented in the text.

2. The following data was observed comparing two assays using 12 batches of material:

Batch	Test A	Test B
1	8.1	9.0
2	9.4	9.9
3	7.2	8.0
4	6.3	6.0
5	6.6	7.9
6	9.3	9.0
7	7.6	7.9
8	8.1	8.3
9	8.6	8.2
10	8.3	8.9
11	7.0	8.3
12	7.7	8.8

    (a) Use the sign test to determine if the two tests are different.

    (b) Compare the two tests (A and B) using the t test.

3. Use the Wilcoxon signed rank test to compare the two assay methods to determine if the methods are significantly different for the data in Exercise Problem 2. Use Table IV.13 and the Normal approximation.

4. Blood glucose uptake for corresponding halves of rat diaphragms for compounds A and B are as follows (adapted from Ref. 2):

	Rat								
	1	2	3	4	5	6	7	8	9
A	9	9.5	5.7	3.9	6.7	5	8.6	3	8
B	8	9.7	5.1	3.6	7.1	5	8.4	4.2	7.1

Use a nonparametric procedure to compare the two compounds.

5. Twenty patients were randomly allocated to two treatment groups, 10 patients per group. The following data are the change in serum chloride after treatment.

Treatment A	Treatment B
4.3	6.1
6.2	0.9
4.4	0.7
8.2	0.8
0.5	1.3
2.6	3.1
4.2	1.9
4.1	3.9
5.6	2.1
3.4	0.1

Test for treatment differences using a nonparametric test and a t test.

6. Dissolution is compared for three experimental batches with the following results (each point is the time in minutes to 50% dissolution for a single tablet):

Batch 1: 15, 18, 19, 21, 23, 26
Batch 2: 17, 18, 24, 20
Batch 3: 13, 10, 16, 11, 9

Is there a significant difference among batches?

7. A bioavailability study was conducted in which three products were compared: a standard product and two new formulations, A and B. The peak blood concentrations were as follows:

Subject	Standard	A	B
1	14	12	17
2	12	18	9
3	11	17	8
4	17	15	14
5	20	16	16
6	16	12	13
7	14	11	10
8	16	16	10
9	18	17	19
10	15	10	8
11	22	15	15
12	14	13	14

Use Friedman's test to determine if there is a difference among the three treatments.

8. In a test for pain relief, two drugs are compared where the outcome is 0, 1, or 2, where 0 = no relief, 1 = partial relief, and 2 = complete relief. With drug A, 50 had a score of 0, 50 scored 1, and 75 scored 2. With drug B, 20 had a score of 0, 60 scored 1, and 60 scored 2. Use a chi-square test to compare drugs A and B. How would you interpret a significant effect?

9. The following fourfold table was constructed from data for inspection of 1000 tablets in quality control.
    (a) Are "specks" and "capping" independent?
    (b) Are the proportion of tablets specked and capped different in this batch of tablets?

		Capped	
		Yes	No
Specked	Yes	13	45
	No	18	924

**10. In a preclinical study the following incidence of tumors was observed in control and treated animals.

Controls: 0 of 12 animals
Treated: 5 of 14 animals

Use Fisher's exact test to determine if the incidence is significantly different in the two groups. Compare the results to a chi-square test with continuity correction.

11. The following assay results were observed from sequential readings from a control chart. Using the runs test, determine if these values conform to a "random" sequence. Use a two-sided test. What would be your conclusion if the test were one-sided?

300.1, 300.5, 300.7, 308.2, 304.4, 303.9, 302.1, 303.1, 300.9, 303.4, 305.6, 306.2, 304.1, 306.1, 300.8, 301.3, 304.3, 301.9, 304.2, 302.6

12. Confirm that the corrected χ^2 is 7.0 by computing the correction for ties for the analysis of the data in Table 15.6.

13. For the 3×2 table analyzed at the end of Sec. 15.8.1 (Table 15.12), compute the χ^2 value for the entire table and for the comparison of treatments B and C.

14. Analyze the following data, using the combined data from two centers. Use the Mantel–Haenszel test.

Center I			
	Success	Failure	Total
Drug A	12	6	18
Drug B	9	9	18
Total	21	15	36

Center II			
	Success	Failure	Total
Drug A	14	3	17
Drug B	9	11	20
Total	23	14	37

Are the two treatments significantly different?

REFERENCES

1. Snedecor, G. W. and Cochran, W. G., *Statistical Methods*, 7th ed., State University Press, Ames, Iowa, 1980.
2. Wilcoxon, F. and Wilcox, R. A., *Some Rapid Approximate Statistical Procedures*, Lederle Laboratories, Pearl River, N.Y., 1964.
3. Hollander, M. and Wolfe, D. A., *Nonparametric Statistical Methods*, Wiley, New York, 1973.
4. Sokal, R. R. and Rohlf, F. J., *Biometry*, W. H. Freeman, San Francisco, 1969.
5. Dixon, W. J. and Massey, F. J., Jr., *Introduction to Statistical Analysis*, 3rd ed., McGraw-Hill, New York, 1969.
6. Fleiss, J. L., *Statistical Methods for Rates and Proportions*, Wiley, New York, 1980.
7. Koch, G. G. and Edwards, S., *Statistical Issues in Drug Research and Development* (K. E. Peace, ed.), Marcel Dekker, New York, 1990.
8. Mantel, N. and Haenszel, W., *J. Nat. Cancer Inst.*, 22, 719, 1959.

16
**Optimization Techniques

The optimization of pharmaceutical formulations with regard to one or more attributes has always been a subject of importance and attention for those engaged in formulation research. Product formulation is often considered an art, the formulator's experience and creativity providing the "raw material" for the creation of a new product. Given the same active ingredient and a descritpion of the final marketed product, two different scientists will very likely concoct different formulations. Certainly, human input is an essential ingredient of the creative process. In addition to the *art* of formulation, techniques are available that can aid the scientist's choice of formulation components which will optimize one or more product attributes. These techniques have been traditionally applied in the chemical and foods industries, for example, and in recent years have been applied successfully to pharmaceutical formulations. In this chapter we describe the application of factorial designs (and modified factorials) and simplex lattice designs to formulation optimization.

16.1 INTRODUCTION

The pharmaceutical scientist has the responsibility to choose and combine ingredients that will result in a formulation whose attributes conform with certain prerequisite requirements. Often, the choice of the nature and quantities of additives (excipients) to be used in a new formulation is based on experience, for example, similar products previously prepared by the scientist or his or her colleagues. To break habits based on experience and tradition is difficult. Although there is much to be said for the practical experience of many years, we often become caught in the web of the past. The application of formulation optimization techniques is relatively new to the practice of pharmacy. When used intelligently, with common sense, these "statistical" methods will broaden the perspective of the formulation process.

Although several optimization procedures are available to the pharmaceutical scientist, two frequently used methods will be presented in this chapter. In general, the procedure consists of preparing a series of formulations, varying the concentrations of the formulation ingredients in some systematic manner. These formulations are then evaluated according to one or more attributes, such as hardness, dissolution, appearance, stability, taste, and so on. Based on the results of these tests, a particular formulation (or series of formulations) may be predicted to be optimal. The "proof of the pudding," however, is actually to prepare and evaluate the predicted *optimal* formulation.

If the formulation is optimized according to a single attribute, the optimization procedure is relatively uncomplicated. To optimize on the basis of two or more attributes, dissolution and hardness, for example, may not be possible. The formulation that is optimal for one attribute very well may be different from the formulation needed to optimize other attributes. In these cases, a compromise must be made, depending on the relative importance of each attribute. The final formulation, therefore, is suitably modified to attain an acceptable performance of all relevant attributes, if possible. We will discuss the optimization procedure based on a single attribute. More complex situations may require more complex designs, and the advice of an experienced statistician is recommended in these cases.

16.2 OPTIMIZATION USING FACTORIAL DESIGNS

The basic principles of factorial designs have been presented in Chap. 9. In factorial designs, levels of factors are independently varied, each factor at two or more levels. The effects that can be attributed to the factors and their interactions are assessed with maximum efficiency in factorial designs. Also, factorial designs allow for the estimation of the effects of each factor and interaction, unconfounded by the other experimental factors. Thus, if the effect of increasing stearic acid by 1 mg is to decrease the dissolution by 10%, in the absence of interactions, this effect is independent of the levels of the other factors. This is an important concept. If the levels of factors are allowed to vary haphazardly, as in an undesigned experiment, the observed effect due to any factor is dependent on the levels of the other varying factors. Generalities, or predictions, based on results of an undesigned experiment will be less reliable than those which would be obtained in a designed experiment, in particular, a factorial design.

The optimization procedure is facilitated by construction of an equation that describes the experimental results as a function of the factor levels. A *polynomial* equation can be constructed, in the case of a factorial design, where the coefficients in the equation are related to the effects and interactions of the factors. For the present, we will restrict our discussion to factorial designs with factors at only two levels, called 2^n factorials, where n is the number of factors (see Chap. 9). These designs are simplest and often are adequate to achieve the experimental objectives. Sometimes, use of these smaller designs is imperative, for the sake of economy. Increasing the number of factor levels dramatically increases the number of formulations that are needed to complete the design. With a large number of factors, even designs where factors are restricted to two levels may result in a very large number of formulations to be prepared and tested. In such cases, *fractional* factorial designs may be used. Some information is lost when using fractional factorial designs, but one-half, one-fourth, or less of the formulations are needed compared to those needed to run a full factorial design. A brief description of fractional factorial designs is presented in Sec. 9.5. The theory and construction of these designs are presented in detail in *The Design and Analysis of Industrial Experiments*, edited by O. L. Davies [1].

As noted above, the optimization procedure is facilitated by the fitting of an empirical polynomial equation to the experimental results. The equation constructed from a 2^n factorial experiment is of the following form:

$$Y = B_0 + B_1 X_1 + B_2 X_2 + B_3 X_3 + \cdots + B_{12} X_1 X_2 + B_{13} X_1 X_3$$

$$+ B_{23} X_2 X_3 + \cdots + B_{123} X_1 X_2 X_3 + \cdots \qquad (16.1)$$

where Y is the measured response, X_i is the level (e.g., concentration) of the ith factor, B_i, B_{ij}, B_{ijk}, $\cdots$ represent coefficients computed from the responses of the formulations in the design, as will be described below. (B_0 represents the intercept.)

For example, in an experiment with three factors, each at two levels, we have eight formulations, a total of eight responses. The eight coefficients in Eq. (16.1) will be determined from the eight responses in such a way that each of the responses will be exactly predicted by the polynomial equation. For the present, to illustrate this concept we will look at the problem in reverse. Suppose that we already have an equation to predict the experimental results derived from a factorial design as follows:

$$Y = 5 + 2(X_1) + 3(X_2) + X_3 - 0.6(X_1X_2) - 0.4(X_1X_3)$$

$$+ 0.7(X_2X_3) + 0.12(X_1X_2X_3) \qquad (16.2)$$

From Eq. (16.2), we can reconstruct the original data from the 2^3 experiment. Suppose that the levels (in mg) of the three factors in the design were as follows:

	Low level	High level
X_1 = stearate	0	2
X_2 = colloidal silica	0	1
X_3 = drug	0	5

Based on Eq. (16.2), the formulation with all factors at the low level will have a response of five. All factors are equal to 0, and all terms containing X_1, X_2, or X_3 are equal to 0. If X_1 is at the high level (2 mg), and X_2 and X_3 are at the low level (0), the predicted response is $Y = 5 + 2(X_1) = 5 + 2(2) = 9$. All other terms are equal to 0. If X_1 and X_2 are at the high level, and X_3 is at the low level, the response is

$$5 + 2(X_1) + 3(X_2) - 0.6(X_1X_2) = 5 + 2(2) + 3(1) - 0.6(2(1)) = 10.8$$

The results for all eight combinations (formulations) as predicted from Eq. (16.2) are shown in Table 16.1).

Table 16.1 shows the results of the factorial experiment which were used to construct Eq. (16.2). The practical, more realistic, problem is to construct the polynomial equation, given the experimental results. To solve this problem, we find the solution to eight equations with eight unknowns [the unknowns are the eight coefficients in Eq. (16.2)]. For example, in formulation 1 (Table 16.1),

$$X_1 = X_2 = X_3 = 0$$

Substituting $X_1 = X_2 = X_3 = 0$ into the general equation [Eq. (16.1)] results in

$$Y = B_0 \text{ (all other terms are 0)}$$

Table 16.1   Results of the 2^3 Factorial Experiment Which Led to the Construction of the Polynomial Equation (16.2)

| | Factor level | | | |
Formulation	X_1	X_2	X_3	Predicted response, Y
1	0	0	0	5
2	2	0	0	9
3	0	1	0	8
4	2	1	0	10.8
5	0	0	5	10
6	2	0	5	10
7	0	1	5	16.5
8	2	1	5	16.5

Since the response (Y) for formulation 1 is equal to 5,

$$Y = B_0 = 5$$

This is the simple solution for the first of the simultaneous equations. In the second formulation, X_2 and X_3 are equal to 0 and Eq. (16.1) reduces to

$$Y = B_0 + B_1 X_1 \quad \text{(all other terms are 0)} \tag{16.3}$$

The response, Y, for formulation 2 is 9 (Table 16.1). We can solve for B_1, using Eq. (16.3) ($B_0 = 5$ and $X_1 = 2$)

$$9 = 5 + B_1(2) \qquad B_1 = 2$$

This procedure is continued, until we solve for all coefficients, B_i, B_{ij}, B_{ijk}, and so on.

In the example above, the solution for the coefficients for the polynomial equation is very simple, because the low level of all factors is zero. In general, the solution would be more difficult if the low level of all factors is not equal to zero. However, the general solution for the polynomial coefficients is not difficult for 2^n factorial designs, because of the independence (orthogonality) inherent in factorial designs. The first step in the solution is to code the levels of the factors so that the high level of each factor is +1, and the low level of each factor is -1. This procedure requires a transformation of each of the three variables, X_1, X_2, and X_3 to X'_1, X'_2, and X'_3, respectively, as follows:

> *For X_1, let $X'_1 = X_1 - 1$.* Note that when $X_1 = 2$ (the high level), $X'_1 = +1$, and when $X_1 = 0$ (the low level), $X'_1 = -1$.
> *For X_2, let $X'_2 = 2X_2 - 1$.*
> *For X_3, let $X'_3 = (2X_3 - 5)/5$.*

In general, the formula for the transformation is

$$\frac{X - \text{the average of the two levels}}{\text{one-half the difference of the levels}} \qquad (16.4)$$

After the transformations, the levels of the factors are as shown in Table 16.2 (see also Chap. 9).

Table 16.2 also contains "transformed" values for the interactions, represented by +1 or -1. These values are obtained by multiplying the values in the appropriate columns of X_1, X_2, and X_3. For example, in formulation 1, X_1X_2 is represented by +1, the product of -1 for X_1 and -1 for X_2 [$X_1X_2 = (-1)(-1) = +1$]. $X_1X_2X_3$ is represented by the product of $(-1)(-1)(-1) = -1$, derived from the values in the columns headed by X_1, X_2, and X_3. (See also Chap. 9 to clarify this procedure.) The "total" column contains only the value +1, and is used to calculate the intercept, B_0.

The coefficients for the polynomial equation (16.1) are calculated as the sum of $XY/8$ ($\Sigma XY/2^n$, in general), where X is the value (+1 or -1) in the *column* appropriate for the coefficient being calculated, and Y is the response. An example should make the calculation clear. For the coefficient corresponding to X_1 (B_1), the calculation is performed as follows. We multiply each value in the column headed X_1 (+1 or -1) by the corresponding response, Y. The sum of these products (ΣXY) divided by 8 (2^n) is the coefficient, B_1.

$$[(-1)(5) + (+1)(9) + (-1)(8) + (+1)(10.8) + (-1)(10) + (+1)(10)$$

$$+ (-1)(16.5) + (+1)(16.5)] = \frac{6.8}{8} = 0.85$$

The coefficient, B_2, is calculated using the values (+1 or -1) in the second column, the X_2 column.

Optimization Techniques

Table 16.2 Transformed Levels of Factors Showing Signs to Be Used to Determine Effects and Polynomial Coefficients

Formulation	X_1	X_2	X_3	X_1X_2	X_1X_3	X_2X_3	$X_1X_2X_3$	Total	Y
1[a]	-1	-1	-1	+1	+1	+1	-1	+1	5
2	+1	-1	-1	-1	-1	+1	+1	+1	9
3	-1	+1	-1	-1	+1	-1	+1	+1	8
4	+1	+1	-1	+1	-1	-1	-1	+1	10.8
5	-1	-1	+1	+1	-1	-1	+1	+1	10
6	+1	-1	+1	-1	+1	-1	-1	+1	10
7	-1	+1	+1	-1	-1	+1	-1	+1	16.5
8	+1	+1	+1	+1	+1	+1	+1	+1	16.5

[a]Note that X_1, X_2, and X_3 are at their low levels (0). Transformed values are -1, -1, and -1.

$$[(-1)(5) + (-1)(9) + (+1)(8) + (+1)(10.8) + (-1)(10)$$

$$+ (-1)(10) + (+1)(16.5) + (+1)(16.5)] = \frac{17.8}{8} = 2.225$$

The coefficient for $X_1X_2X_3$ is B_{123}, and is calculated using the values in the column headed by $X_1X_2X_3$ as follows.

$$[(-1)(5) + (+1)(9) + (+1)(8) + (-1)(10.8) + (+1)(10) + (-1)(10)$$

$$+ (-1)(16.5) + (+1)(16.5)] = \frac{1.2}{8} = 0.15$$

All of the coefficients are calculated in this manner. B_0 is the sum of all of the observations, Y, divided by 8 (10.725).* (Note that all of the values in the "total" column are +1; this column is used to obtain B_0 in the same manner as the other coefficients.) The final polynomial equation for predicting the response, Y, is

$$Y = 10.725 + 0.85(X_1) + 2.225(X_2) + 2.525 (X_3) - 0.15(X_1X_2)$$

$$- 0.85(X_1X_3) + 1.025(X_2X_3) + 0.15 (X_1X_2X_3) \qquad (16.5)$$

This equation looks entirely different from Eq. (16.2), which also predicts the responses in this experiment. However, the two equations predict the same response. Equation (16.5) uses the transformed levels of X_1, X_2, and X_3 (+1 or −1), and Eq. (16.2) uses the actual, observed, untransformed values. For example, if X_1 and X_2 are at their high levels, and X_3 is at the low level, we can solve for the response, Y, using Eq. (16.5) and the transformed values +1, +1, and −1 for X_1, X_2, and X_3, respectively.

$$Y = 10.725 + 0.85(+1) + 2.225(+1) + 2.525(-1) - 0.15(+1)(+1)$$

$$- 0.85(+1)(-1) + 1.025(+1)(-1) + 0.15(+1)(+1)(-1) = 10.8$$

The response with X_1 and X_2 at the high level is 10.8, exactly equal to the value obtained from Eq. (16.2), where X_1, X_2, and X_3 are the actual levels, 2, 1, and 0 mg, respectively.

---

*$B_0 = \overline{Y}$.

To reiterate, the reason for the transformation (also called coding) is to allow for easy calculation of the coefficients in the polynomial equation.* The transformation of the high and low factor levels to +1 and -1 also results in easy calculation of the variance of the coefficients. Using the transformed levels, the variance of a coefficient is $\sigma^2/8$ $[\sigma^2/\Sigma (X - \overline{X})^2]$. With an estimate of the variance, S^2, each coefficient can be tested for significance, using a t test. These tests are exactly equivalent to the testing of the effects in the ANOVA of a factorial design as explained in Chap. 9. If, for example, the X_1X_2 interaction were found to be nonsignificant in an ANOVA, the coefficient of X_1X_2, -0.15 in this example, will also be nonsignificant. Usually, when constructing the polynomial equation, only these terms which are statistically "significant" are retained. In the experiment above, an estimate of the standard deviation was available from previous similar experiments; s.d. = 0.32 with 16 d.f. Therefore, the coefficients B_{12} and B_{123} (0.15) are not significant.

$$t = \frac{|0.15|}{0.32/\sqrt{8}} = 1.3 \quad (P > 0.05)$$

Omitting the "nonsignificant" B_{12} and B_{123} terms, the final equation is

$$Y = 10.725 + 0.85(X_1) + 2.225(X_2) + 2.525(X_3)$$

$$- 0.85(X_1X_3) + 1.025(X_2X_3) \tag{16.6}$$

An advantage of the transformation described above is that the omission of the two coefficients, B_{12} and B_{123}, does not affect the values of the remaining coefficients, that is, recalculation of the polynomial equation results in the same coefficients. This result would not occur if Eq. (16.2) were used to describe the data. Equation (16.2) used the untransformed factor levels and would necessitate extensive computations if some terms were omitted, probably requiring use of a computer as a computing aid.

Having derived an equation (16.6) that describes the experimental system based on the results of the experimental formulations, we consider this equation to approximately predict the response within the experimental space. Figure 16.1 shows the space described by this

---

*The coded values also result in orthogonality (independence) of effects.

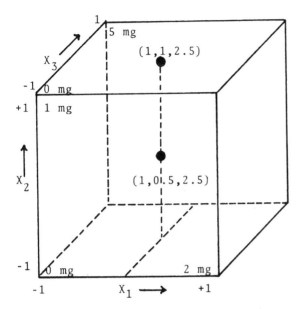

Figure 16.1 Factor space for experiment with factor levels shown in Table 16.1.

design. The *prediction* of the response, Y, at X_1 = 1 mg, X_2 = 1 mg, and X_3 = 2.5 mg is 12.95 [Eq. (16.6)] (see Exercise Problem 1). How do we know that Eq. (16.6) will be a good predictor for responses other than those included in the factorial design? Without actually testing some "extra-design" formulations, we have no way of knowing that the derived empirical equation will be adequate to predict the results of yet-to-be-tested formulations. If the response is "well behaved," the in-between points should be able to be accurately predicted from the response equation.

Usually, it is a good idea to test at least one formulation, not included in the design, as a *check point.* The observed results of the checkpoint formulation can then be compared to the predicted value to test the equation. In our example, a formulation was prepared with X_1 = 1 mg, X_2 = 0.5 mg, and X_3 = 2.5 mg. The transformed values are equal to zero for the three variables (see the transformation equation (16.4). Using Eq. (16.6), the predicted response is 10.725 (only the intercept term is not equal to 0). The actual observation made on this formulation was 10.5, very close to the predicted value. Extrapolation of predicted results outside the factor space, as shown in Fig. 16.1, is not recommended.

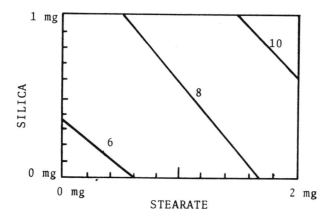

Figure 16.2   Response surface with drug (X_3) constant (low level)
[Eq. (16.6)].

A two-level design can make predictions only in a linear fashion,
usually a gross approximation. If curvature is present, the response may be misrepresented outside the confines of the design.

Once the polynomial-response equation has been established, an
optimum formulation (or a region of optimum formulations) can be
found by various techniques. Sometimes, inspection of the experimental results may be sufficient to choose the desired product. In
the example above, if large values of the response are desirable,
Formulations 7 and 8 may be chosen as "best" (Table 6.1). With
the use of computers (programmable calculators will often do), a
"grid" method may be used to identify optimum regions, and response surfaces may be depicted (see Fig. 16.2). The response
surface is a geometrical representation of the response and the
factor levels, similar to a contour map. For more than two factors,
response surfaces cannot be easily represented in two-dimensional
space. However, one can take slices of the surface, with all but
two factors at fixed levels, as shown in Fig. 16.2. A computer can
calculate the response, based on Eq. (16.1), at many combinations
of the factor levels. The formulation(s) whose response has optimal characteristics based on the experimenter's specifications can
then be chosen. To illustrate the grid method, a very rough grid
with predicted responses based on Eq. (16.6) is shown in Table
16.3.

The experimental system analyzed above is a very simple example, but is a typical approach to the optimization process. More

Table 16.3 Grid Solutions for Responses (Y) Based on Eq. (16.6)

X₁[a]	X₂	X₃	Y	X₁	X₂	X₃	Y	X₁	X₂	X₃	Y
-1	-1	-1	5.3	0	-1	-1	7	+1	-1	-1	8.7
-1	-1	0	7.65	0	-1	0	8.5	+1	-1	0	9.35
-1	-1	+1	10	0	-1	+1	10	+1	-1	+1	10
-1	0	-1	6.5	0	0	-1	8.2	+1	0	-1	9.9
-1	0	0	9.875	0	0	0	10.725	+1	0	0	11.575
-1	0	+1	13.25	0	0	+1	13.25	+1	0	+1	13.25
-1	+1	-1	7.7	0	+1	-1	9.4	+1	+1	-1	11.1
-1	+1	0	12.1	0	+1	0	12.95	+1	+1	0	13.8
-1	+1	+1	16.5	0	+1	+1	16.5	+1	+1	+1	16.5

[a]Transformed values.

sophisticated designs may be used, such as the composite designs to be described below (Sec. 16.3), or fractional factorial designs. The principles are the same. All of these designs have orthogonal properties to allow for clear and simple estimation of the polynomial coefficients.

The polynomial coefficients may be calculated by techniques such as described here, or by using a multiple regression computer program (see App. III). For two-level experiments (2^n factorials), the factor levels should be transformed so that the low level is equal to -1 and the high level equal to $+1$, according to Eq. (16.4). (Experiments with factors at more than two levels should be analyzed with the help of a statistician.) The transformation considerably reduces the complexity of the computations, and aids in the interpretation of the results. Each coefficient may be tested for significance discarding those coefficients that are not significant, although there are no firm rules regarding this procedure. In addition to the statistical criteria, scientific judgment may be used in making decisions about the "significance" of the coefficients. In order to statistically test the coefficients for significance, an estimate of the experimental error is required. This error may be obtained from previous experience, but is best estimated by replicating runs. Replication, however, will result in a large number of experiments, which may be very costly. Replication, accomplished by performing duplicate assays, for example, is usually *not* sufficient. The best procedure for replication consists of preparing each formulation in duplicate (or more), and randomizing the order of the experimental determinations, if all formulations cannot be prepared and tested simultaneously. Methods are available to obtain an estimate of error from an unreplicated factorial experiment (e.g., half-normal plots [2, 3], or from higher-order interactions as discussed in Chap. 9, but these procedures will not be discussed here.

16.2.1 Optimization of a Combination Drug Product

The following example of a 2^2 factorial experiment is another illustration of the technique of "optimization" using factorial designs. In this experiment, a *combination* drug product was tested to obtain the dose of each drug which would result in an optimal response. The product contained two drugs, $A(X_1)$ and $B(X_2)$. The experiment consists of formulating combinations containing each drug at two dose levels. The doses for A were 5 mg and 10 mg; B was chosen at doses of 50 mg and 100 mg. These levels were carefully selected to cover a range of doses which would include an appropriate dose to be chosen as the prime candidate for the final marketed product. The full factorial consists of the four experiments shown in Table 16.4.

Table 16.4 2^2 Factorial Design for the Drug Combination Study

Formulation	Potency (mg)		Potency (transformed)			Response, Y (min)
	A (X_1)	B (X_2)	A (X_1)	B (X_2)	AB (X_1X_2)	
1	5	50	-1	-1	+1	9.7
2	10	50	+1	-1	-1	7.2
3	5	100	-1	+1	-1	8.4
4	10	100	+1	+1	+1	4.1

   The product is a local anesthetic, and the response (Y) is the average time to anesthesia for 12 patients per group. The high and low levels of drug A and drug B are transformed to +1 and −1 [Eq. (16.4)]. For drug A, the transformation is

$$\frac{\text{Potency} - 7.5}{2.5} \quad \text{(high level is 10; low level is 5)}$$

For drug B, the transformation is

$$\frac{\text{Potency} - 75}{25} \quad \text{(high level is 100; low level is 50)}$$

The response equation has the form

$$Y = B_0 + B_1(X_1) + B_2(X_2) + B_{12}(X_1)(X_2) \tag{16.7}$$

The coefficients are computed as described earlier in this section. For example, referring to Table 16.4, B_1 is:

Column A (X_1)	Y	X_1Y
−1	9.7	−9.7
+1	7.2	+7.2
−1	8.4	−8.4
+1	4.1	+4.1
		−6.8/4 = −1.7

(B_1 is the sum of $X_1Y/4 = -1.7$.) The polynomial equation is calculated as

$$Y = 7.35 - 1.7(X_1) - 1.1(X_2) - 0.45(X_1X_2) \tag{16.8}$$

The response, Y, is the time to anesthesia. Formulation 4, which has has the high levels of both drugs, has the shortest time to anesthesia, and formulation 1 has the longest time to anesthesia. Thus, either formulation 1 or 4 would be chosen as optimal if either a long time or a short time to anesthesia is desired. However, an intermediate time might be more desirable. For example, suppose that a time of 5 min is the most desirable time based on considerations such as the administration of the product and the type of conditions that are meant to be treated with the aid of the product. Table 16.5 is a

Table 16.5 Predicted Values of Response to Anesthetic
Combinations of Drugs A and B Based on Eq. (16.8)

		Dose of drug A[a]				
		-1	-0.5	0	+0.5	+1
Dose of drug B[a]	-1	9.7	9.075	8.45	7.825	7.2
	0	9.05	8.2	7.35	6.5	5.65
	+1	8.4	7.325	6.25	5.17	4.1

[a]Coded values of drug potency.

rough grid of the predicted responses based on Eq. (16.8). Based
on a time to anesthesia of approximately 5 min, a formulation containing 0.5 of A and 1 of B would be a candidate. Decoding the values
result in a formulation containing 8.75 mg of A and 100 mg of B.

16.3 COMPOSITE DESIGNS TO ESTIMATE CURVATURE

In general, when looking for optimality, the response equation will
be more reliable if it contains terms that reflect curvature. Physical
systems are less satisfactorily described by empirical equations containing only linear terms. Figure 16.3 shows an example of a single

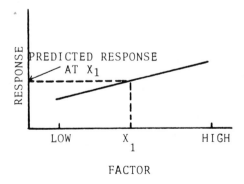

Figure 16.3 Figure showing linear response as a function of a
single variable (factor).

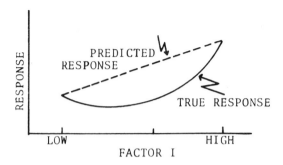

Figure 16.4   Figure showing curved response as a function of a
single variable (factor).

factor, X, at two levels. Clearly, to interpolate the response, Y,
at values of X between the low and high levels requires an assumption of linearity. These predictions would be very much in error if
the response is curved, as shown in Fig. 16.4.

In order to estimate curvature, more than two levels of the factor
must be included in the experiment. The presence of curvature
would be reflected in the presence of terms with a power greater
than 1 (e.g., X_1^2) in the response equation. Such equations are
known as polynomials of order 2, and have the following form for a
two-factor design:

$$Y = B_0 + B_1 X_1 + B_{11} X_1^2 + B_2 X_2 + B_{22} X_2^2 + B_{12} X_1 X_2 + \cdots$$

$$(16.9)$$

Composite designs are effective designs to estimate second-
order terms. These designs have a number of desirable features.
In addition to allowing an estimate of curvature, composite designs
give orthogonal estimates of the polynomial coefficients, and allow
for the possibility of proceding with the experiment in a stepwise
fashion rather than performing the entire experiment at once. The
theory underlying composite designs is beyond the scope of this
book. An excellent description of this optimization procedure can
be found in Chap. 11 of Ref. 1.

Although the following discussion is somewhat more advanced
than the bulk of material presented in this book, for those who are
interested in this subject, an example of a two-factor composite

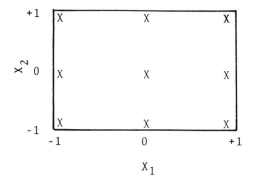

Figure 16.5 Two-factor composite design (3^2 factorial).

design will be presented to illustrate the technique. A two-factor composite design is identical to a 3^2 factorial design, that is, two factors each at three levels, a total of nine combinations (see Table 16.6).

In general, composite designs are not full factorials of the class 3^n, where n is the number of factors. These full factorial designs require a large number of experiments. For example, a 3^n design with three factors requires 27 runs (27 formulations, for example), 3^3. With more than two factors, composite designs consist of the 2^n design, plus *extra-design* points. The extra points include a *center point* and 2n extra points, appropriately chosen to maintain orthogonality of the design [1]. The two-factor composite design is shown in Fig. 16.5.

The coded values -1, 0, and +1 in Table 16.6 for the factor levels represent three *equally spaced* levels of each factor. The coded values in the column headed X_1X_2 are obtained by multiplying the corresponding values in the first two columns (X_1, X_2) as previously described. The values in the columns $X_1^2 - 2/3$ and $X_2^2 - 2/3$ are derived so that the product of corresponding values in any two columns of Table 16.6 sum to zero, resulting in orthogonality (independence) of effects. The special orthogonality obtained by transforming X_i^2 to $X_i^2 - 2/3$ allows for easy calculation of the coefficients and their variances. With this transformation, Eq. (16.9) is modified to

Table 16.6   Orthogonal Composite Design with Two Factors (3^2 Design)

Formulation	Coded level					Response, Y	Predicted response
	X_1	X_2	$X_1 X_2$	$X_1^2 - 2/3$	$X_2^2 - 2/3$		
1	-1	-1	+1	+1/3	+1/3	9.7	9.3
2	-1	0	0	+1/3	-2/3	9.0	9.4
3	-1	+1	-1	+1/3	+1/3	8.4	8.4
4	0	-1	0	-2/3	+1/3	5.3	5.6
5	0	0	0	-2/3	-2/3	4.8	5.0
6	0	+1	0	-2/3	+1/3	3.8	3.3
7	+1	-1	-1	+1/3	+1/3	8.2	8.3
8	+1	0	0	+1/3	-2/3	7.5	6.9
9	+1	+1	+1	+1/3	+1/3	4.1	4.6

$$Y = B_0 + B_1X_1 + B_{11}(X_1^2 - 2/3) + B_2X_2 + B_{22}(X_2^2 - 2/3)$$

$$+ B_{12}X_1X_2 + \cdots \tag{16.10}$$

The data in Table 16.6 consist of the four formulations from Table 16.4 plus five new runs to complete the composite design. The doses of each drug (X_1 and X_2) were chosen at equal intervals. Thus the third dose, in addition to the two doses chosen for the 2^2 factorial, is 7.5 mg for X_1 (A) and 75 mg for X_2 (B). The experiment consists of evaluating the nine combinations of doses, 5, 7.5, and 10 mg for X_1 (A) and 50, 75, and 100 mg for X_2 (B). Note that the *center point* for the composite design is the combination 7.5 mg and 75 mg of X_1 and X_2, respectively.

The results of the nine runs are shown in Table 6.6. The results are shown schematically in Fig. 16.6a. The plane at the bottom of the figure shows the combinations of X_1 and X_2. The vertical "sticks" are the responses at each combination of X_1 and X_2. We will compute an equation of the form of Eq. (16.10) which represents a smooth curved surface based on the experimental data. In general, the equation can be obtained through the use of a multiple regression computer program.

The coefficients can also be calculated by "hand" (calculator) using the coded values in Table 16.6. The sum of the products of the coded values times the responses divided by the sum of the squared coded values in the column of interest gives the coefficient. For example, the coefficient B_{11} in Eq. (16.10) is calculated as follows:

$X_1'^2 =$ $X_1^2 - 2/3$	Y	$(X_1'^2)(Y)$
+1/3	9.7	3.23
+1/3	9.0	3.00
+1/3	8.4	2.80
-2/3	5.3	-3.53
-2/3	4.8	-3.20
-2/3	3.8	-2.53
+1/3	8.2	2.73
+1/3	7.5	2.50
+1/3	4.1	1.37
$\Sigma X_1'^2 = 2$		sum = 6.37

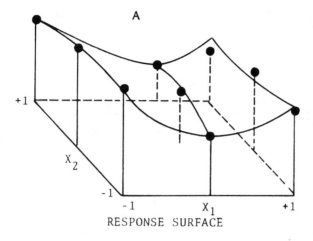

RESPONSE SURFACE

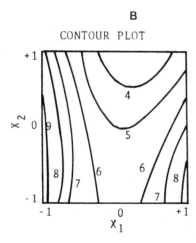

Figure 16.6   Results of composite design experiment from Table 16.6 and response surface computed from Eq. (16.11).

The sum of squared values in the $(X_1^2 - 2/3)$ column is 2. There-fore, the coefficient, B_{11}, is $6.37/2 = 3.18$. The intercept, B_0, is the average of the nine responses, $\overline{Y}$, equal to 6.756. The re-sponse equation is

$$Y = 6.756 - 1.22(X_1) + 3.18(X_1^2 - 2/3) - 1.15(X_2)$$

$$- 0.52(X_2^2 - 2/3) - 0.7(X_1 X_2) \tag{16.11}$$

Note that Eq. (16.11) is not an exact fit to the experimental data, as was the case with the polynomial fit described for factorial de-signs in Sec. 16.2. Had we included three more terms representing various interactions, the equation would exactly fit the data. Equa-tion (16.11) is computed with the assumption that interactions are negligible. The response surface described by Eq. (16.11) is shown in Fig. 16.6b. If this equation does not adequately represent the experimental observations, more terms may be needed in the poly-nomial equation [Eq. (16.9)] to improve the fit.

The contour plot (similar to contour maps) shown in Fig. 16.6b allows the selection of combinations of X_1 and X_2 to satisfy given levels of the response. If a maximum response is desired, the X_1, X_2 combinations are limited to a small area of the $X_1 - X_2$ space. If a response of approximately 5 min is desired, various combina-tions of X_1 and X_2 will satisfy the requirements. The ultimate choice will probably depend on other factors, as well, such as cost, toxicity, and so on.

Use of factorial designs in tablet formulation optimization has been presented by Schwartz et al. [4], Fonner et al. [5], and Lindberg et al. [6]. These papers discuss designs somewhat more complex than that presented here. However, for those interested in pursuing this topic further, these papers and the books *The Design and Analysis of Industrial Experiments* [1] and *Statistics for Experimenters* [3] are recommended.

16.4   THE SIMPLEX LATTICE

Response surfaces and optimal regions for *formulation* characteristics are frequently obtained from the application of simplex lattice de-signs. This class of designs is particularly appropriate in formula-tion optimization procedures where the *total* quantity of the differ-ent ingredients under consideration must be *constant*. For example, suppose that in a liquid formulation, the active ingredient and sol-vent compose 90% of the product. The remaining 10% of the formu-lation consists of preservatives, coloring agents, and a surfactant.

We wish to prepare a formulation with a certain optimal attribute(s) which is dependent on the relative concentrations of preservative, color, and surfactant. In order to determine optimal regions, we vary the concentrations of these three ingredients in a systematic manner, with the restriction that the total concentration of these ingredients is 10%. This approach differs from the previous procedures (Secs. 16.2 and 16.3) in that a constraint is imposed on the total amount of the varying ingredients. In this example, the total amount of the varying components is maintained at 10%.

Implementation of the simplex design consists of preparing various formulations containing different combinations of the variable ingredients. The combinations are prepared in a manner such that the experimental data can be used to predict the responses over the simplex space* in a simple and efficient manner. The combinations (formulations) in a simplex design are chosen to cover the space of interest in a symmetrical manner. The experimental results are used to compute a polynomial (simplex) equation which can be used to estimate the response surface. As is true with all optimization and so-called response surface procedures, extrapolation to combinations outside the range included in the experimental design is not recommended. The equation resulting from the experiment, the simplex equation, is an empirical equation which approximately describes the response pattern in the simplex space. There is no reason to believe that the equation has any physical meaning, other than the fact that the complex response patterns resulting from the varying formulations can often be approximated by simple polynomial equations.

Figure 16.7 representing a two-component system (A and B) is useful to help clarify some concepts of simplex designs. One can consider components A and B to be two solvents, which together comprise the entire solvent system of a drug product. We wish to mix A and B in the correct proportion to optimize the solubility of the drug.

Figure 16.7 is familiar as a solubility phase diagram. This system can also be visualized as an elementary simplex system. The constraint is that the concentrations of A and B must add to 100%. This experiment consists of observing responses (solubility) at three points, *100% A, 100% B* and a *50 − 50 mixture of A and B*, an elementary simplex design. According to Fig. 16.7, the solubilities of the drug at the three simplex points, 100% A, 100% B, and 50% A − 50% B, are 10 mg/ml, 15 mg/ml, and 20 mg/ml, respectively. In the simplex approach, we construct an equation of the form

---

*The simplex space is the region enclosed by the various combinations of ingredients chosen for the experiment. See Fig. 16.8, for example.

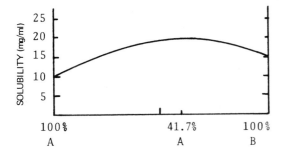

Figure 16.7   Two-component solvent system used to illustrate the simplex approach to optimization.

$$Y = B_1(A) + B_2(B) + B_{12}(A)(B) \qquad (16.12)$$

where Y is the response (solubility in this example), and (A) and (B) are the concentrations (proportions) of A and B, respectively. The coefficients, B_1, B_2, and B_{12}, are calculated from the experimental observations. The response, Y, can then be predicted for all combinations of A and B, where $(A) + (B) = 1.0$ (100%). (The proportion of each component is usually indicated as a decimal rather than as a percentage.) The form of the simplex design allows for easy calculation of the coefficients. In this example, the coefficients are simply calculated as follows:

B_1 = response at (A) equal to 1.0 (100%) = 10

B_2 = response at (B) equal to 1.0 (100%) = 15

B_{12} = 4 (response at 0.5−0.5 mixture of A−B) − (sum of responses at A = 1.0 and B = 1.0)

B_{12} = 4(20) − 2(10 + 15) = 30

The response equation is

$$Y = 10(A) + 15(B) + 30(A)(B) \qquad (16.13)$$

The solution above for the three coefficients is a result of the solution of three simultaneous equations:

With A = 1.0 and B = 0, from Eq. (16.12), $B_1^* = 10$
With A = 0 and B = 1.0, from Eq. (16.12), $B_2 = 15$
With A = 0.5 and B = 0.5, from Eq. (16.12),

$$20 = 0.5B_1 + 0.5B_2 + 0.25B_{12} \text{ or } B_{12} = 4(20) - 2(B_1 + B_2) = 30$$

We will see that in more complex simplex designs, the polynomial coefficients are, similarly, easily calculated as linear combinations of experimental results.

Equation (16.13) exactly predicts the observed points: a fit of a polynomial with three terms to three experimental points. We can always construct an equation with N coefficients which will exactly pass through N points. For example, for the 50−50 mixture,

$$Y = 10(0.5) + 15(0.5) + 30(0.5)(0.5) = 20$$

The *response equation* predicts responses at extra-design points, those formulations not included in the experiment but which lie within the simplex space, 100% A to 100% B in this example. For example, what solubility would be predicted in a solvent system containing 75% A and 25% B? (Note that A + B must equal 100%.) Applying Eq. (16.13), we have

$$Y = 10(0.75) + 15(0.25) + 30(0.75)(0.25) = 16.875$$

See also Fig. 16.7. The entire response may be sketched in by predicting solubilities along the curve, as shown in the figure.

The primary experimental objective in experiments such as that described above may be the determination of the solvent combination that results in maximum drug solubility. The optimum solubility can be computed by calculating the predicted solubility at many solvent combinations so as to clearly define the response over the solvent mixture continuum. This may seem an indirect and tedious approach, but with the ready availability of computers, this is often the most expeditious route. The maximum solubility is predicted to occur at 41.67% A. In this simple example, the maximum can easily be calculated by setting the first derivative of Eq. (16.13) equal to 0 (see Exercise Problem 6).

In general, the simplex design is usually applied to formulation problems in which a mixture of three or more components is to be investigated. The design is conveniently represented by regular-sided figures, which can be visualized for three- or four-component systems. For more than four components, a single figure cannot be

---

*The response, Y, with A equal to 1.0 (100%) is 10.

THREE-COMPONENT SIMPLEX

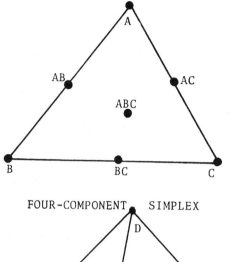

FOUR-COMPONENT SIMPLEX

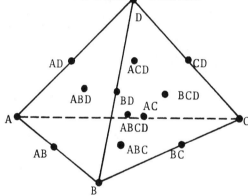

Figure 16.8 Three-component simplex lattice design and four-component simplex lattice design.

conveniently constructed, but can be theoretically conceived as an N-sided figure in $(N - 1)$-dimensional space. For example, Fig. 16.8 shows the three-component system which is represented as an equilateral triangle in two-dimensional space. A regular simplex design for a three-component mixture system consists of six or seven formulations:

Three formulations, one each at each vertex, A, B, and C. These formulations represent formulations with the pure components, A, B, and C, respectively.

Three formulations are prepared with 50 – 50 mixtures of each
   pair of components, AB, AC, and BC.
A *seventh* formulation may be prepared with one-third of each
   component. This lies in the *center* of the design.

A simplex design for four components consists of 15 formulations
shown in Fig. 16.8. The 15 formulations consist of:

Four formulations each with 100% of each of the four pure com-
   ponents
Six fourmulations of 50 – 50 mixtures of component pairs (AB,
   AC, AD, BC, BD, and CD)
Four formulations consisting of one-third mixtures of combina-
   tions of three components (ABC, ABD, ACD, BCD)
A mixture containing 25% of each of the four components (ABCD)

The simplex design is arranged so that the experimental space is
well covered in a symmetrical fashion. In addition, the symmetrical
spacing of the points allows for an easy computation of the response
equation coefficients. The general equation for the response based
on a simplex design contains terms for pure components and all
mixtures of components as follows:

$$Y = B_a(A) + B_b(B) + B_c(C) + \cdots + B_{ab}(A)(B) + B_{ac}(A)(C)$$

$$+ B_{bc}(B)(C) + \cdots + B_{abc}(A)(B)(C) + \cdots \qquad (16.14)$$

where (A), (B), and (C) are the proportions of components A, B,
and C, and (A) + (B) + (C) + $\cdots$ is equal to 1.0.
   The subscripted B's (e.g., B_a) are coefficients which can be
easily calculated from the responses, Y.
   After the coefficients have been calculated, the response equation [Eq. (16.14)] may be used to predict the response of combinations of the N components in the system. With the aid of a computer, responses may be calculated over the simplex space, and
contour diagrams printed (see also Fig. 16.6). The contour plot is
a graphic description of the response surface resulting from data
derived from experimental designs such as the simplex. For the
two-component system (Fig. 16.7), the response surface is simply
the solubility curve. With three components, a three-dimensional
figure would be necessary to show the response surface. A contour plot is a means of illustrating the response on a two-dimensional surface, as is familiar to those who have been exposed to
contour maps. A computer may be programmed to produce two-
dimensional figures, which are slices through the three-dimensional

figure for a three-component system. The slices are taken at a constant concentration of one of the components. In computer outputs, the regions of equal response are indicated by a common symbol, such as a letter or a figure. An example of a contour plot was shown in Fig. 16.6. The contour plot will be discussed further in the example that follows. Examination of the contour plot(s) allows the experimenter to choose formulations which have predicted responses of some specified magnitude.

When constructing an empirical response equation based on a limited number of experimental observations, one should understand that predicted values based on the equation may be in error for several reasons. For example, the empirical equation (or model, as it is often called) rarely exactly defines the experimental system. The equation is an approximation to the system. To understand this important concept, note that the same problem would exist if we had only two points in the experimental space. The empirical equation derived from the two points could only relate the observations by a straight line. In-between points could only be predicted on the basis of the straight-line relationship (see Figs. 16.3 and 16.4).

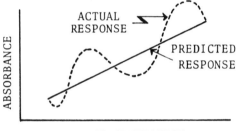

If the true relationship of the X, Y variables were curved, the linear interpolation would be in error. In the simplex design, we use a limited number of points to define a relatively large region of response. Even if the model represented by the empirical equation is a reasonable representation of the true surface, other sources of variation can contribute to error in the prediction equation and predicted responses (e.g., error in measuring the response). Thus, in these systems, we have at least two obvious sources of variability: that due to the empirical model and that due to observational errors.

How can we protect ourselves from inadvertently proceeding with predictions when the derived equation is indeed inaccurate? As insurance against such a possibility, it is a good idea to run one or more extra-design points. These points are not used to estimate the coefficients in the simplex equation [Eq. (16.14)] but will be used as checkpoints. Once the simplex equation is derived, the

result at the extra-design checkpoint(s) is predicted based on the
equation, and its agreement with the observed value assessed. If
the agreement is close, we have increased faith in the predictive
power of the response equation (see Sec. 16.2).

The calculation of the simplex equation coefficients is easily accomplished using the following formulas. These formulas are an
extension of those discussed previously for the two-component system as applied to a three-component system. The general formulas
for calculation of coefficients for an N-component system may be
found in Ref. 6.

$$B_1 = Y_1, \text{ the response at 100\% A} \tag{16.15}$$

$$B_2 = Y_2, \text{ the response at 100\% B}$$

$$B_3 = Y_3, \text{ the response at 100\% C}$$

$$B_{12} = 4(Y_{12}) - 2(Y_1 + Y_2), \text{ where } Y_{12} \text{ is the response at}$$
$$50-50 \text{ AB}$$

$$B_{13} = 4(Y_{13}) - 2(Y_1 + Y_3), \text{ where } Y_{13} \text{ is the response at}$$
$$50-50 \text{ AC}$$

$$B_{23} = 4(Y_{23}) - 2(Y_2 + Y_3), \text{ where } Y_{23} \text{ is the response at}$$
$$50-50 \text{ BC}$$

$$B_{123} = 27(Y_{123}) - 12(Y_{12} + Y_{13} + Y_{23}) + 3(Y_1 + Y_2 + Y_3),$$
$$\text{where } Y_{123} \text{ is the response at } 1/3 \text{ A}, 1/3B, \text{ and } 1/3 \text{ C}$$

The discussion above has been based on an experimental situation
where the components being varied in the simplex design comprise
the entire mixture (100%). In pharmaceutical formulations, a more
common situation is one in which part of the formulation must remain fixed (e.g., drug concentration in a tablet). The remaining
components, which may be varied, therefore do not make up 100%
of the mixture. In addition, the lower limit for the varying components is often not equal to 0. For example, some components must
be present in some minimal quantity in order that a marketable
product can be manufactured. For tablets, some minimal amount of
a lubricating agent may be necessary in order to obtain an acceptable product. These modifications in the simplex design present no problem, however, because we can restrict the treatment
of the simplex to those components which are varied, and with
suitable transformations, treat the data in exactly the same way

as described above. For example, if the components to be varied
make up 60% of the total formulation ingredients, we can appropriately transform the actual percentages of these components so that the
transformed percentages total 100%. In a three-component mixture
containing 20% of each of three components, each component can be
transformed to 33.3% (1/3) for purposes of the simplex analysis.
Transformations can also be made where the components have a
lower limit greater than 0% and an upper limit less than 100%, as
will be explained in the following worked example.

The example presented below is an experiment in which a simplex design was used to obtain a formulation with optimal properties. This example should clarify the concepts and procedures
described above. This experiment was prompted by problems with
tablet hardness for a large-volume marketed product. Although the
reason for the problem was not obvious, the pharmaceutical product
development scientists felt that the cause could be traced to three
components of the tablets, which we will denote as ingredients A,
B, and C. Together, these components consisted of 25% of the original formulation, or 75 mg of the total tablet weight of 300 mg.
A careful evaluation of the product ingredients indicated that the
three components had to be present in an amount equal to at least
10 mg each in order for the tablet to be satisfactorily compressed.
Thus the recommended simplex design to obtain a satisfactory tablet
hardness consisted of varying the three components with the constraint that the sum of the components must be 75 mg, and that
each component be present in an amount equal to at least 10 mg.

In order to apply the simplex equation to be derived from this
experiment in a convenient manner, the actual concentrations used
should be *transformed* such that the minimum concentration (10 mg)
corresponds to 0% and the highest concentration corresponds to
100%.* In our example, the transformation is the same for all three
components because each component is subject to the same restrictions. The minimum quantity is 10 mg and the maximum is 55 mg.
(The other two components, each at 10 mg, make up the 20-mg difference, a total of 75 mg.) The transformation is as follows:

$$\text{Transformed proportion} = \frac{\text{Amount used} - \text{minimum}}{\text{maximum} - \text{minimum}}$$

$$= \frac{\text{Amount used} - 10}{55 - 10} \qquad (16.16)$$

---

*If there are no constraints on the upper and lower limits, the high-
est concentration would ordinarily be 100% and the lowest 0%.

Table 16.7   Results of a Three-Component Simplex System for
Tablet Hardness

Formulation components			Transformed proportion			Average hardness, Y
A	B	C	A	B	C	
55	10	10	1.0	0	0	6.1
10	55	10	0	1.0	0	7.5
10	10	55	0	0	1.0	5.3
32.5	32.5	10	0.5	0.5	0	6.6
32.5	10	32.5	0.5	0	0.5	6.4
10	32.5	32.5	0	0.5	0.5	6.9
25	25	25	0.33	0.33	0.33	7.3
32.5[a]	21.25	21.25	0.5	0.25	0.25	7.2

[a]Extra-design checkpoint.

Thus a formulation prepared with a 50−50 mixture of components A
and B would actually contain 32.5 mg of A, 32.5 mg of B, and 10
mg of C. Note that from Eq. (16.16), if a component is at a con-
centration of 32.5 mg, the transformed proportion is $(32.5 - 10)/(55 - 10) = 0.5$. A formulation with "100%" A would actually contain 55 mg of A, 10 mg of B, and 10 mg of C.

The three-component simplex design was run with one checkpoint, as shown in Table 16.7. The hardness values represent
the average hardness of 20 tablets taken at random from the experimental batches. The simplex coefficients are computed as described previously [Eq. (16.15)], resulting in the following equation:

$$Y = 6.1(A) + 7.5(B) + 5.3(C) - 0.8(A)(B) + 2.8(A)(C)$$

$$+ 2.0(B)(C) + 15(A)(B)(C) \qquad (16.17)$$

For example, the coefficient B_{123} is calculated as follows:

$$27(7.3) - 12(6.6 + 6.4 + 6.9) + 3(6.1 + 7.5 + 5.3) = 15$$

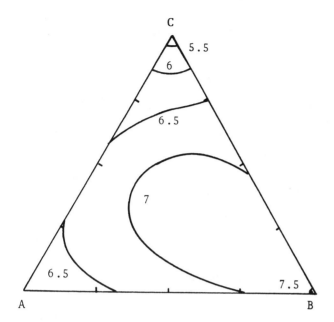

Figure 16.9 Contour plot of three-component simplex system (Table 16.7).

(A), (B), and (C) in Eq. (16.17) are the transformed proportions. The extra-design checkpoint (the final formulation in Table 16.7) has a response of 7.2. The predicted value based on Eq. (16.17) is 7.09, very close to the observed value, 7.2. This is some confirmation of the adequacy of Eq. (16.17) as a predictor of tablet hardness. Figure 16.9 shows a contour plot of the results of the experiment based on Eq. (16.17). Tablets with high hardness are found in the region with relatively larger amounts of component B. If a tablet hardness of 7 or more is satisfactory, the pharmaceutical scientist has a choice of formulations. The final composition may then be dependent on other factors, such as cost or other tablet properties.

16.5 SEQUENTIAL OPTIMIZATION

Sequential optimization was developed as a means to optimize a process in a stepwise fashion. Evolutionary operation (EVOP) uses factorial type designs and usually requires a large number of experiments [8]. A relatively simple approach to sequential optimization is a stepwise application of the simplex procedure [9, 10]. The procedure consists of first generating data from n + 1 experiments where n is the number of independent variables or factors. Based on the n + 1 responses and predetermined rules, one result is eliminated from the set and a new experiment is performed. A decision is made as a result of the most recent experiment, generating another new experiment, and so on, eventually terminating the design at an "optimal" response. Thus each new experiment leads the researcher on a path towards an optimum. The procedure and rules are illustrated in the following example. For further details and illustrations, the reader is encouraged to study Refs. 9–11.

16.5.1   An Example of Sequential Simplex Optimization

This example is based on the presentation by Shek et al. [11] using the simplex procedure to optimize properties of a capsule formulation. They were interested in optimizing dissolution and compaction rates as a function of the factors (or variables) drug, disintegrant, lubricant, and fill weight. In this synthetic example, we will look at a single response, dissolution at 30 minutes, as a function of 3 variables: disintegrant, lubricant, and fill weight.

We start with 4 experiments (we have 3 variables). There are no firm rules regarding the design of these experiments, but principles of good experimental design should prevail. For example, a 1/2 replicate of a 2^3 factorial design can be used for the initial 4 experiments. This requires setting low (−) and high (+) levels for each factor; see Table 16.8.

Table 16.8   Initial Four Experiments for Simplex Experiment

Experiment	Disintegrant	Lubricant	Fill weight	Response
1	+(50)*	−(0.2)	−(100)	37
2	−(0)	+(2.2)	−(100)	58
3	−(0)	−(0.2)	+(400)	46
4	+(50)	+(2.2)	+(400)	40

*Parenthetical value is the amount of ingredient in the formulation.

Let W = vector of worst response

Let S = vector off second worse response

Let B = vector of best response

Let R_w = worst response

Let R_s = second worse response

Let R_b = best response

Let $\overline{P}$ (P – bar) = average vector after elimination of worst response among formulations under consideration

Note that since Formula 2 shows the worst response (the longest dissolution time), $\overline{P}$ is the average of experiments 1, 3, and 4 and is equal to (33.3, 0.87, 300). For example, the first vector element refers to the average disintegrant = (+50 −0 +50)/3 = 33.3.

Procedure:

Step 1. Eliminate W, the vector of the worst response from the data set and compute R [Eq. (16.18) below], the formulation for the new experiment.

$$R = \overline{P} + (\overline{P} - W) \tag{16.18}$$

(33.3, 0.87, 300) + (33.3, −1.33, 200) = (66.6, −0.46, 500)

In this example, we need 66.6 of disintegrant, −0.46 of lubricant and a fill weight of 500. We will interpret this result after the rules are specified and we proceed with the optimization.

If the response from experiment R, R_r, is better than the second-worst response, R_s, but worse than the best response, retain R_r and proceed to Step 1, evaluating a new formulation with the new set of 4 formulations.

If the response to R_r is better than the best response, proceed to Step 2.

If the response to R_r is worse than the second-worst response, go to Step 3.

If the response to R_r is worse than the worst response, go to Step 4.

Step 2. Compute E [Eq. (16.19) below] and evaluate R_e.

$$E = \overline{P} + 2(\overline{P} - W) \tag{16.19}$$

If R_r is better than the response to E, R_e, retain R. If R_e is better than R_r, retain E.

Step 3. Compute C_r [Eq. (16.20) below] and evaluate the response to C_r, R_{cr}.

$$C_r = \overline{P} + 0.5\,(\overline{P} - W) \qquad\qquad (16.20)$$

Retain C_r. However, if R_{cr} is worse than R_s (the next-to-worst response), then set $R_W = R_s$ and $W = S$. (This means that the worst response is set equal to the next-to-worst response.) Set R_{cr} as the next to worst response, i.e., $S = C_r$ and $R_s = R_{cr}$.

Step 4. Compute C_W [Eq. (16.21) below] and evaluate R_{cw}. Retain C_W. However, if R_{cw} is worse than R_s (the next-to-worst response), then set $R_{cw} = R_s$ and $W = S$. (This means that the worst response is set equal to the next-to-worst response.) Set R_{cw} as the next to worst response, i.e., $S = C_W$ and $R_s = R_{cw}$.

Summary of Calculations of New Formulations

1. $R = \overline{P} + (\overline{P} - W)$ $\qquad\qquad (16.18)$

    R_r = The response to Formula R

2. $E = \overline{P} + 2\,(\overline{P} - W)$ $\qquad\qquad (16.19)$

    R_e = The response to Formula E

3. $C_r = \overline{P} + 0.5\,(\overline{P} - W)$ $\qquad\qquad (16.20)$

    R_{cr} = The response to Formula C_r

4. $C_W = \overline{P} - 0.5\,(\overline{P} - W)$ $\qquad\qquad (16.21)$

    R_{cw} = The response to Formula C_W

Although this procedure may appear confusing, if one follows the example, the process will be clarified.

We have already calculated the vector for the first new formulation using Step 1 above: (66.6, −0.46, 500). The response to this formulation will replace the worst formulation, W, which is formulation 2. Unfortunately, we cannot prepare this formulation because of the negative quantity of lubricant. We will make a rule that in such impossible situations we consider the response to this new formulation to be worse than the remaining formulations under consideration (formulations 1, 3, and 4).

This sends us to Step 4 according to our rules. The formulations under consideration are 1, 3, 4, and 5 in Table 16.9. According to Eq. (16.21)

Table 16.9 Sequential Experiments in Optimization Process

Experiment	Disintegrant	Lubricant	Fill weight	Response
1	50	0.2	100	37
2	0	2.2	100	58 $(W_1)^a$
3	0	0.2	400	46 (W_3)
4	50	2.2	400	40
5	66.6	−0.46	500	− (W_2)
6	50	0.20	400	44 (W_4)
7	100	1.54	200	42 (W_6)
8	83.3	2.42	67	43 (W_5)
9	58.4	0.75	316	36
10	8.5	0.07	416	41 (W_7)
11	39	0.56	344	44 (W_8)
12	56.2	0.8	308	35

$^a W_1$ means that this result was eliminated after the first evaluation.

$$C_w = (33.3,\ 0.87,\ 300) - 0.5\ (-33.3,\ 1.33,\ -200)$$
$$= (50,\ 0.20,\ 400)$$

The response, R_{cw}, to C_w is 44. According to Step 4 above, we retain this result. This is shown as experiment 6 in Table 16.9. We now operate on experiments 1, 3, 4, and 6; experiment 3 is the new worst result.

We go to Step 1 and compute our new formulation R from Eq. (16.18):

$$R = (50,\ 0.87,\ 300) + (50,\ 0.67,\ -100) = (100,\ 1.54,\ 200)$$

The response R_r is 42 (represented by experiment 7 in Table 16.9). This is better than the second worst response (44 for experiment 6) and we retain R_r as directed in Step 1 above. We recompute R for the set of experiments 1, 4, 6, and 7:

$$R = (66.7,\ 1.31,\ 233) + (16.7,\ 1.11,\ -167) = (83.3,\ 2.42,\ 67)$$

The response, R_r, is 43. This is worse than the second-to-worst response, 42.

Therefore we go to Step 3:

$$C_r = P + 0.5 (\overline{P} - W)$$

$$C_r = (66.7, 1.31, 233) + 0.5 (-16.7, -1.11, 167)$$

$$= (58.4, 0.75, 316)$$

The new response (experiment 9) is 36.

According to our rules, we go to Step 2:

$$E = \overline{P} + 2 (\overline{P} - W)$$

$$E = (69.5, 1.05, 272) + 2 (-30.5, -0.49, 72)$$

$$= (8.5, 0.07, 416)$$

The response to E is 41. According to Step 2, we retain R in lieu of E because R gave the better response. We compute a new R from Step 1:

$$R = (69.5, 1.05, 272) + (-30.5, -0.49, 72)$$

$$= (39, 0.56, 344)$$

The response is 44. Our new set of 4 experiments is numbers 1, 4, 9, and 11, with number 11 the worst.

We go to Step 4 and compute C_W because the value of R is worse than R_W:

$$C_W = (69.5, 1.05, 272) - 0.5 (30.5, 0.49, -72)$$

$$= (54.2, 0.8, 308)$$

The response was 35 (see experiment 12).

The experiments may continue as described above until repeated experiments do not show improvement. We are searching for an optimal response in the presence of variability. In the present case, a formula containing approximately 55 of disintegrant and 0.75 of lubricant with a fill weight of 300 mg appeared to show minimal dissolution time; the study was stopped after experiment 12.

As with other optimization procedures presented in this chapter, studying details in the literature references is essential to understand the procedure and calculations [8-11].

KEY TERMS

Checkpoint	Multiple regression
Coding	Optimization
Composite designs	Orthogonality
Contour plot	Polynomial equation
Extra-design points	Replication
Factorial designs	Response equation
Fractional factorial designs	Response surface
Grid	Sequential optimization
Independence	Simplex design
Model	Simplex space
Model error	Transformation

EXERCISES

1. Calculate the predicted response from Eq. (16.6) for
    (a) $X_1 = 1$ mg, $X_2 = 1$ mg, $X_3 = 2.5$ mg
    (b) $X_1 = 2$ mg, $X_2 = 1$ mg, $X_3 = 4$ mg
    [Note that Eq. (16.6) uses coded values; see Eq. (16.4).]
    For example, the coded value for $X_1 = 1$ mg is $0 = (1 - 1)/1$.
2. Show that the transformed values of $X_1 = 1$, $X_2 = 0.5$, and
    $X_3 = 2.5$ are all equal to zero for the three variables in Exer-
    cise Problem 1.
3. Calculate the coefficients for the polynomial equation, (16.8).
    The coefficients are calculated from the data in Table 16.4.
4. Show that decoded values of A and B equal to 0.5 and 1, re-
    spectively, are equal to 8.75 mg of A and 100 mg of B, for
    the data of Table 16.4 and Eq. (16.8). Calculate the expected
    response of this combination of A and B using Eq. (16.8).
5. A formulation was to be prepared to optimize dissolution time.
    (The formulation with the dissolution time of approximately
    15 min is "optimal.") Stearic acid and mixing time were varied
    according to a 2^2 factorial design with the following results:

		Stearic acid	
		0.25%	1%
Mixing time (min)	15	10	23
	30	21	25

(a) Construct a polynomial response equation [see Eq. (16.8)].

(b) What concentration of stearic acid and mixing time would you choose for the final product?

**6. Calculate the maximum solubility based on Eq. (16.13), using procedures of calculus. [Hint: Set the first derivative equal to 0 after substituting (1.00 − A) for B.]

7. A total of 100 mg of three components, stearic acid (A), starch (B), and DCP (C), are to be added to a tablet formulation. Dissolution time was measured in a simplex design with the following results:

100% A:	292.0 min
100% B:	5.6 min
100% C:	50.4 min
50% A, 50% B:	25.6 min
50% B, 50% C:	15.6 min
50% A, 50% C:	124.5 min
1/3 A, 1/3 B, and 1/3 C:	37.0 min

(a) Compute the simplex equation coefficients.

(b) Give a combination with very fast dissolution.

(c) Give a combination that has a dissolution time of 90 min.

REFERENCES

1. Davies, O. L., *The Design and Analysis of Industrial Experiments*, Hafner, New York, 1963.

2. Daniel, C., *Technometrics*, *1*, 311, 1959.

3. Box, G. E., Hunter, W. G., and Hunter, J. S., *Statistics for Experimenters*, Wiley, New York, 1978.

4. Schwartz, J. B., Flamholtz, J. R., and Press, R. H., *J. Pharm. Sci.*, *62*, 1165, 1973.

5. Fonner, D. E., Jr., Buck, J. R., and Banker, G. S., *J. Pharm. Sci.*, *59*, 1587, 1970.

6. Lindberg, N.-O., Jonsson, C., and Holmquist, B., *Drug Dev. and Ind. Pharm.*, *11*(4), 931−943, 1985.

7. Gorman, J. W. and Hinman, J. E., *Technometrics*, *4*, 463, 1962.

8. Box, G. E. P. and Draper, N. R., *Evolutionary Operations*, Wiley, New York, 1969.

9. Spendley, W., Hext, G. R., and Himsworth, F. R., *Technometrics*, *4*, 441, 1962.

10. Nelder, J. A. and Mead, R., *Comput. J.*, *7*, 308, 1965.

11. Shek, E., Ghani, M., and Jones, R. E., *J. Pharm. Sci.*, *69*, 1135, 1980.

Appendix I
Some Properties of the Variance

I.1 POOLING VARIANCES

In many statistical procedures, an estimate of the variance is obtained by "averaging" or *pooling* the variances from more than one group of observations. The pooling of variances is appropriate in cases where samples from separate groups or different experiments provide estimates of the *same* variance. Note that we do not pool or average standard deviations. As we have previously noted, the sample variance, $\Sigma (X - \bar{X})^2/(N - 1)$ [Eq. (1.5)], is an unbiased estimate of the true population variance. The standard deviation, estimated from a *sample*, is a *biased estimate* of the true *population* standard deviation. On the average, the sample standard deviation underestimates the population standard deviation. Estimation and properties of the variance are important considerations in both theoretical and applied statistics.

A common example of a procedure where variance estimates from different groups are pooled is the two-sample independent-groups t test for comparison of means discussed in Chap. 5. In this test, the average results of two treatments* (e.g., active drug versus placebo; dissolution behavior of two tablet formulations) are compared. An estimate of the variance of the observations is needed in order to compare the two treatment groups statistically. An important assumption underlying this test is that the variances for each group are equal. The variance is first calculated for each treatment group separately. The variance is more precisely estimated

---

*The word "treatment" in statistics does not necessarily mean treatment in the medical sense. Treatments are conditions or combinations of conditions whose effects on an experimental outcome are to be assessed.

from samples with a larger number of observations, and the pooled variance from both treatment groups is the best estimate of the common variance. For example, suppose that the following variances were observed in a comparative experiment:

Placebo group: N = 25 and the variance $(S^2) = 10$

Drug group: N = 20 and the variance $(S^2) = 15$

Although we assume that the true variance (the population variance) is the same for each group, different variances are observed in the two groups. If the two groups truly have equal variance, the difference in the observed variance is a consequence of random variation, due in part to the particular samples which were chosen, and measurement errors. The pooling procedure, in general, uses a *weighted average*, where the weights are equal to the degrees of freedom [see Eq. (1.2)].

$$S^2 \text{ pooled} = S^2_p = \frac{(24)(10) + (19)(15)}{24 + 19} = 12.21$$

The standard deviation is $3.49(\sqrt{12.21})$. The numbers 24 and 19 are the degrees of freedom for the two groups. If variances are to be pooled from more than two groups, the procedure is the same. Use a weighted average of the group variances, weighting the variance in each group by its number of degrees of freedom.

I.2 COMPONENTS OF VARIANCE

Variability of observations usually arise from more than one source. Hence the variability of observations can often be expressed as the sum of independent sources of error that comprise the total variation. This notion is presented in more detail under the topic of *components of variance* in Sec. 12.4.1. The variance of the average of assay results for three tablets obtained by selecting a single tablet from each of three batches and assaying each tablet is as follows: [*variance* due to mean potency differences among batches (i.e., the batch averages are not identical) + *variance* due to tablet differences within batches* + *variance* due to drug assay]/3. Note

---

*Variation resulting from differences in tablet potency in a randomly chosen sample of tablets which is due to the inherent variability of tablets (a result of the heterogeneity of the tableting process) is also known as "sampling error."

that this is the variance of a mean of three results (a total of three tablets have been assayed from the three batches).   This accounts for the number 3 in the denominator $\left(S_{\overline{X}}^{2} = S^{2}/N\right)$.

Similarly, the variability of individual cholesterol changes, derived from a group of patients, such as shown in Table 1.1, is the sum of the components that contribute to the overall variability: (a) biological variation as reflected in inherent differences between patients, (b) the day-to-day variability within patients (a single person's cholesterol varies from day to day), and (c) the analytical error, among other sources of error.

I.3   VARIANCE OF LINEAR COMBINATIONS OF INDEPENDENT VARIABLES

The variance of linear combinations of variables, where the variables are independent, can be shown to be

$$\text{Variance}(mX_1 \pm nX_2) = m^2 \; \text{variance}(X_1) + n^2 \; \text{variance}(X_2)$$

$$(I.1)$$

where m and n are constants.   This important result can be used to derive the variance of the mean of n independent observations, for example.   Consider m observations of the variable X.   We can represent the observations as $X_1, X_2, X_3, \ldots, X_m$.   The mean is

$$\frac{\Sigma X_i}{m} = \frac{X_1 + X_2 + X_3 + \cdots + X_m}{m}$$

The variance of each X is σ^2.   Therefore, the variance of the mean is

$$\frac{\sigma_1^2 + \sigma_2^2 + \sigma_3^2 + \cdots + \sigma_m^2}{m^2} = \frac{m(\sigma^2)}{m^2} = \frac{\sigma^2}{m}$$

Equation (I.1) also demonstrates that the variance of the difference of two independent observations is the *sum* of their variances.   An example noted by Mandel [1] which illustrates this concept is the timing of a reaction.   A stopwatch is started at the initation of the reaction and stopped at some end point.   The time depends on both the initial and final readings.   If errors in the times are independent, the variance of $t_2 - t_1$, the difference between final and initial readings, is the sum of the variances; that is, the error of the difference of the two readings is larger than the error of either reading alone.   Consider another example where a procedure calls for 10 ml of solution to be removed from a beaker containing 30 ml. Only 10-ml pipettes are available.   The original 30 ml of solution is prepared by pipetting three 10-ml portions into a beaker.   A total of 10 ml is then removed.   The variance of the volume remaining in the solution is calculated as follows:

$$\text{Variance}(P_1 + P_2 + P_3 - P_4) = \sigma^2 P_1 + \sigma^2 P_2 + \sigma^2 P_3 + \sigma^2 P_4$$

where P_i (i = 1, 2, 3, 4) represents the four pipetting steps.   If the variance of a pipetting step is 0.01, the total variance of the remaining solution (with an expected volume of 20 mL) is (4)(0.01) = 0.04.

REFERENCE

1.   Mandel, J., *The Statistical Analysis of Experimental Data*, Interscience, New York, 1964.

Appendix II
Comparison of Slopes and Testing of Linearity: Determination of Relative Potency

A common problem in bioassay, or when comparing the potency of compounds such as in drug screening programs, is the assessment of the relative potency of the comparative drugs. The problems in this analysis consist of (a) obtaining a function of dose and response which is linear, (b) testing the lines for each compound for parallelism (i.e., equality of slopes), and (c) determining the relative potency. We will discuss some elementary concepts for the comparison of two antiinflammatory compounds, a standard drug (St) and an experimental compound (Ex). The experiment consists of measuring the reduction in volume after treatment of initially inflamed paws of two animals at each of three doses for each compound. The results are shown in Table II.1 and plotted in Fig. II.1. The figure shows that the plot of *log* dose versus response is approximately linear. A *transformation* of dose and/or response is often necessary to achieve linearity in dose-response relationships. The response is usually considered to be a linear function of *log* dose (see Chap. 10). Transformations to obtain linearity are desirable because straight-line relationships are more easily analyzed and interpreted than are more complex functions.

How does one determine if the data are represented by a linear function such as a straight line? A known theoretical relationship between X and Y may be sufficient to answer the question. From a statistical point of view, replicate measurements at fixed values of X are needed to test for linearity. Replicate measurements of Y at a fixed X represent S_Y^2 only, a variance estimate which is independent of the functional form of X and Y. If X and Y are truly related by a straight-line function, deviations of the observed values of Y from the fitted line should be due only to the variability of Y. If the relationship between X and Y is not a straight line, the variance as measured by the deviations of Y from the fitted

Table II.1   Results of the Experiment Comparing
Potencies of Two Compounds[a]

| | Dose (mg) | | |
Compound	5	15	45
Standard (St)	0.22	0.51	0.70
	0.27	0.49	0.75
Experimental (Ex)	0.29	0.55	0.76
	0.26	0.54	0.83

[a]Data are relative reduction in paw volume from baseline value.

line will be increased due to "nonlinearity" (see Fig. 7.4b).   To
test for linearity, we compare the variance due to deviations of Y
from the fitted line (deviations from regression) to the variation due
only to Y (the pooled error from the Y replicates, the within mean
square).   The "deviations" mean square is the mean square due to
deviations of the averages of Y (at each X) from the fitted line.

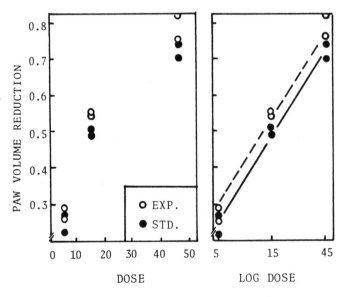

Figure II.1 Plot of dose response data for anti-inflammatory study.

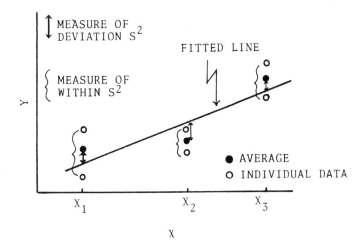

Figure 11.2   ANOVA test for linearity.

The statistical test is an F test obtained from an analysis of variance. The concept of this test is illustrated in Fig. II.2.

To perform the test, a one-way ANOVA is first performed on
the data (Table II.2), duplicate determinations for three doses in
the present example. The ANOVA is computed for each of both the
standard and experimental drugs. For example, the calculations for
the ANOVA for the standard drug follow:

Table II.2   One-Way ANOVA for Data from Standard and
Experimental Drugs

Source	Standard drug			Experimental drug		
	d.f.	SS	MS	d.f.	SS	MS
Between doses	2	0.2307	0.1154	2	0.27053	0.1353
Within (doses)	3	0.0027	0.0009	3	0.00295	0.00098
Total	5	0.2334		5	0.27348	

$$\text{Total SS} = \Sigma \ Y^2 - \frac{(\Sigma \ Y)^2}{N} = 1.674 - 1.4406 - 0.2334$$

$$\text{Between-doses SS} = \frac{0.49^2 + 1.00^2 + 1.45^2}{2} - 1.4406 = 0.2307$$

The within SS is the difference between the total SS and the between SS (see Sec. 8.1).

The between-doses SS is the sum of two components: (a) the SS due to the slope (regression SS) and (b) the SS due to *deviations of the mean values (at each X) of Y from the fitted line*. The *deviation SS* has been discussed above and is shown in Fig. II.2. The easiest way to compute the deviation SS is to divide the between-doses SS into its components as follows. The "regression" SS has 1 degree of freedom and is defined as

$$\text{Regression sum of squares} = b^2 \ \Sigma \ (X - \overline{X})^2 \qquad (\text{II.1})$$

This sum of squares, a result of the slope of the line, will be zero for a line of zero slope ($b = 0$), and will be large for a line with a steep positive or negative slope. For the standard drug, the regression sum of squares is calculated as follows (remember, we are using log dose = X):

$$b = 0.503$$

$$b^2 \ \Sigma \ (X - \overline{X})^2 = 0.503^2 (0.9106) = 0.2304$$

The deviation SS (sometimes called "lack of fit" SS) is equal to the between-doses SS minus the regression SS. Therefore, the deviation SS =

$$0.2307 - 0.2304 = 0.0003$$

The results of this calculation for both standard and experimental drugs are shown in Table II.3.

The test for linearity is an F test (deviation MS)/(within MS). For the standard drug, for example, the F ratio is $0.0003/0.0009 = 0.33$, with 1 and 3 d.f., which is not significant (within MS = 0.0009, Table II.2). There is no evidence for lack of linearity for both lines.

Usually, in these assays, the deviation mean squares are pooled from both products and compared to the pooled error (within MS), testing linearity of both lines simultaneously. The pooled deviation

Table II.3 Regression and Deviations Sum of Squares for Standard and Experimental Drugs[a]

Source	Standard drug d.f.	Standard drug SS	Experimental drug d.f.	Experimental drug SS
Regression	1	0.2304	1	0.2704
Deviations	1	0.0003	1	0.000133
Between doses	2	0.2307	2	0.270533

[a]Degrees of freedom for "regression" in the simple linear regression case is always equal to 1. Degrees of freedom for "deviations" is equal to (number of doses - 2).

MS is (0.000433)/2 with 2 degrees of freedom. The pooled within MS is 0.000942 with 6 degrees of freedom. The F test for linearity is 0.000217/0.00094 = 0.23 (2 and 6 d.f.), which is clearly not significant. The pooling assumes that the error for both drugs is the same, and that both drugs show a linear response versus log dose.

Another assumption in the analysis of the parallel-line assay is that the two lines are parallel. A test of parallelism is equivalent to a test of equality of slopes. The common slope, calculated from all the data combined, is

$$b = \frac{\Sigma \ XY - \Sigma \ X \ \Sigma \ Y/N}{\Sigma \ (X - \overline{X})^2} = 0.5240$$

The regression sum of squares due to the common slope is

$$b^2 \ \Sigma \ (X - \overline{X})^2 = (0.5240)^2 (1.8212) = 0.500$$

The regression sum of squares of the common slope is subtracted from the pooled *regression* sum of squares for the two drugs to obtain the sum of squares attributed to lack of parallelism of the lines. The pooled regression sum of squares is 0.2304 + 0.2704 = 0.5008. The sum of squares for "parallelism" is 0.0008 (0.5008 − 0.5000). The F test has 1 and 6 d.f., using the pooled error term:

$$F_{1,6} = \frac{0.0008}{0.00094} = 0.851$$

Since the F value shows lack of significance at the 5% level, we conclude that the lines appear to be parallel within "experimental error."

The test for parallelism for *two* lines can also be done by using a t test with the same results as the F test. (For the case of two lines, the t is the square root of the F value.) For the t test, we compare the two slopes, using the standard deviation of the difference of the two slopes in the denominator of the t ratio. The slopes are 0.5030 and 0.5449 for the standard and experimental drugs, respectively. The variances in both groups are assumed to be equal.

$$t = \frac{|b_1 - b_2|}{\sqrt{S^2[1/\sum_1 (X - \overline{X})^2 + 1/\sum_2 (X - \overline{X})^2]}} \tag{II.2}$$

$$\frac{|0.5030 - 0.5449|}{\sqrt{0.00094[1/\sum_1 (X - \overline{X})^2 + 1/\sum_2 (X - \overline{X})^2]}}$$

where $\sum_i (X - \overline{X})^2$ represents the sum of squares of the X's for the respective groups. [Note that the variance of a slope equals $S^2/\sum (X - \overline{X})^2$.]

Having satisfied ourselves that the assumptions of the assay have been met (i.e., particularly, linearity and parallelism), we can now estimate the relative potency. The relative potency is the ratio of the potency of the comparative drugs which will give the same response. If the lines are parallel, we can choose any response (Y) to estimate the relative potency; the answer will be the same (see Fig. II.3).

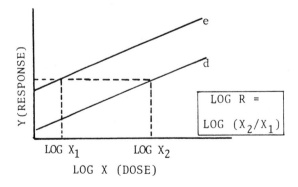

Figure 11.3   Relative potency estimation using parallel dose-response lines; doses equivalent to log X_1 and log X_2 give the same response for products e and d, respectively.

One can show that the log of the relative potency (log R) is equal to

$$\log R = \log \left[\frac{\text{experimental}}{\text{standard}} \right] = \frac{a_e - a_d}{b}$$

where a_e and a_d are the intercepts for the experimental drug and the standard drug, respectively; b is the common slope (0.524, in our example); and (experimental/standard) is the inverse ratio of doses that gives equal response. For the data of Table II.1,

$$a_d = -0.1262 \qquad a_e = -0.0779$$

$$\log R = \frac{-0.0779 - (-0.1262)}{0.5240} = 0.092$$

The relative potency is 1.24; that is, the experimental drug is 1.24 times as potent as the standard. This means that 124 mg of the standard is needed to give the same response as 100 mg of the experimental drug, for example.

Confidence limits can be put on the relative potency based on Fieller's theorem (similar to confidence limits for X at a given Y; see Chap. 7). The procedure is complicated, and the interested reader is referred to the book by Finney, *Statistical Methods in Biological Assay* [1], for details of the computations.

REFERENCE

1. Finney, D. J., *Statistical Methods in Biological Assay*, Hafner, New York, 1964.

Appendix III
Multiple Regression

Multiple regression is a topic of utmost importance in statistics, analysis of variance being a special case of the more general regression techniques. Multiple regression is an extension of linear regression, in which we wish to relate a response, Y (dependent variable), to more than one independent variable, X_i.

Linear regression: $Y = A + BX$

Multiple regression: $Y = B_0 + B_1X_1 + B_2X_2 + \cdots$

The independent variables, X_1, X_2, and so on, generally represent factors which we believe influence the response. Usually, the purpose of multiple regression analysis is to quantitate the relationship between Y and the X_i's by means of an equation, the *multiple regression equation*. For example, tablet dissolution may be measured as a function of several variables, such as level of disintegrant, lubricant, and drug. In this case, a multiple regression equation would be useful to predict dissolution, at given levels of the independent variables.

$$Y = B_0 + B_1X_1 + B_2X_2 + B_3X_3 \tag{III.1}$$

where

Y = some measure of dissolution

X_i = ith independent variable

B_i = regression coefficient for the ith independent variable

Here, X_1, X_2, and X_3 refer to the level of disintegrant, lubricant, and drug. B_1, B_2, and B_3 are the coefficients relating the X_i to

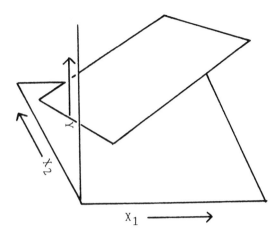

$X_1 \longrightarrow$

Figure III.1 Representation of the multiple regression equation response, $Y = B_0 + B_1 X_1 + B_2 X_2$, as a plane.

the response. These coefficients correspond to the slope (B) in linear regression. B_0 is the intercept. This equation cannot be simply depicted, graphically, as in the linear regression case. With two independent variables (X_1 and X_2), the response surface is a plane (Fig. III.1). With more than two independent variables, it is not possible to graph the response in two dimensions.

Data suitable for multiple regression analysis can be obtained in different ways. Optimal efficiency and interpretation are obtained by using data from "designed" experiments. In designed experiments, the independent variables are carefully chosen and deliberately controlled at preassigned levels. For example, in the dissolution experiment noted above, we may be able to fix the levels of disintegrant, lubricant, and drug according to a factorial design (as described in Chap. 9). Table III.1 illustrates a 2^3 factorial design. These data correspond to the eight combinations in the 2^3 design which can be used to construct a multiple regression equation. The procedure for fitting data from a factorial design to a regression equation is given in Sec. 16.2.

The form of the equation and the number of independent variables necessary to define the response adequately depend on a knowledge of the system being investigated. In the example above, there are three independent variables (factors), but interactions of factors may also be needed to define the response. In multiple regression equations, interactions may be represented by "cross-product" terms, such as $(X_1 X_2)$ or $(X_1 X_2 X_3)$. We usually include

Table III.1   Factorial Design to Be Used as the Source for a
Multiple Regression Equation

		Disintegrant Low level		Disintegrant High level	
		Drug		Drug	
		Low level	High level	Low level	High level
Lubricant	Low level				
	High level				

only those terms in the equation which probably have a meaningful
effect on the response. Suppose, in our example, that the three
factors and the lubricant X drug interaction are related to the response, dissolution. We would include terms for X_1, X_2, X_3, and
X_2X_3 in the model.

$$Y = B_0 + B_1X_1 + B_2X_2 + B_3X_3 + B_{23}X_2X_3$$

Data for multiple regression fits are often obtained from undesigned
experiments where the levels of the independent variables are not
controlled. This less desirable alternative is often a consequence of
convenience or cost considerations. Sometimes, the circumstances
are such that we have no choice; we get the data in any way that
we can. For example, suppose that tableting pressure, temperature,
and humidity all affect some particular quality of a finished tablet.
Tablets may be conveniently selected for inspection during the manufacturing process, at which time measurements of the pressure, temperature, and humidity are made. After collecting a sufficient quantity of data, these variables may be related to tablet quality using
multiple regression techniques.

$$Y = B_0 + B_1(\text{tablet press pressure}) + B_2(\text{temperature})$$
$$+ B_3(\text{humidity})$$

In this example, we have no control of the variables; their values
are a matter of "happenstance." We take the values as they come.
A significant disadvantage of making conclusions based on data of
this sort is that a correlation exists among the independent variables,

which can be eliminated (or controlled) in a designed experiment. The result of this correlation is that the effects of the variables cannot be clearly separated. What we attribute to one variable, temperature for example, has a component due to humidity and pressure as well. With data derived from a designed experiment, such as the factorial design noted above, the regression equation can be constructed so that the effects of different factors and interactions are represented by the coefficients (B_j) and are independent of other factors.

The computations to determine the coefficients in multiple regression analysis are very tedious, and without the use of computers, analysis of undesigned experiments of reasonable size are virtually impossible. Manipulations of large matrices are often performed in the solution of these problems. Regression equations for orthogonal (designed) factors are much easier to compute. However, with easy access to computers, hand analysis should be done only as a learning tool to gain insight into the analytical process. We will not discuss computational methods in the general multiple regression model. However, because of the importance of multiple regression in optimization procedures discussed in Chap. 16, some further introductory concepts will be presented here.

The technique of fitting a linear model to data consisting of N observations of a response, Y, and one or more independent variables, X_i, is applicable when the number of observations is equal to or greater than the number of parameters to be estimated (the coefficients are the parameters in multiple regression). In simple linear regression, we estimate two parameters in the usual case, the intercept and the slope. Given two X, Y points, the line (slope and intercept) is unambiguously fixed. With more than two points, the best straight line is considered to be that line which minimizes the sum of the squared deviations of the observed values from the fitted least squares line. Multiple regression is just an extension of this procedure. If there are N parameters (coefficients) in the regression model, N observations will result in an exact fit to the model. For example, an equation with six coefficients will be exactly fit to six appropriate experimental values (with certain mathematical restrictions). With more than N observations, the coefficients, B_j, are calculated to minimize the squared deviations of the observations from the least squares regression fit (the same concept as in simple linear regression).

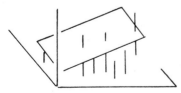

The relationship of the independent variables and the dependent variable in the multiple regression model must be *linear in the coefficients*, B_i, in order to obtain the regression equation by the usual procedures [1]. The general form of the regression equation is given by Eq. (III.1).

$$Y = B_0 + B_1 X_1 + B_2 X_2 + B_3 X_3 \qquad\qquad (III.1)$$

The X_i's can be "nonlinear" functions such as X^2, log X, or 10^X. However, the coefficients, B_i, cannot be in this nonlinear form. Thus

$$Y = B_1 X_1 + B_2 X_2 + B_3 X_1^2 + B_4 X_1 X_2 \qquad \text{is linear in } B_i$$

$$Y = B_0 + B_1 X_1 + X_2^{B_2} \qquad\qquad \text{is not linear in } B_i$$

The basic problems in multiple regression analysis are concerned with estimation of the error and the coefficients (parameters) of the regression model. Statistical tests can then be performed for the significance of the coefficient estimates.

When many independent variables are candidates to be entered into a regression equation, one may wish to use only those variables that contribute "significantly" to the relationship with the dependent variable. In designed experiments (e.g., factorial designs) the significance of each factor can be determined using analysis of variance, or, equivalently, by testing the regression coefficients for significance. In an undesigned experiment, where the data come from "uncontrolled" combinations of the variables, the independent variables will inevitably be more or less correlated. Thus, if dissolution is to be related to tablet weight, drug content, and tablet hardness, based on production records, we are obliged to fit an equation with the available data, and some correlation will exist between drug content and weight, for example. This lack of independence presents special problems when deciding which variables are relevant, contributing significantly to the regression relationship. If two of the X variables, X_i and X_j, are highly correlated, inclusion of both in the regression equation will be redundant. Therefore, there may be some X variables which appear to contribute to the regression but which are correlated to other X variables. We must then make a choice regarding their inclusion in the final regression equation. Draper and Smith note: "There is no unique statistical procedure for doing this," and some degree of arbitrariness must be used in making choices [1]. Two methods used to help make such decisions are made possible through the use of computers. One method involves regression fits using all possible combinations of the independent variables (2^k regressions, where k is the number of independent variables). For two independent variables, X_1 and X_2, the four possible regressions are:

1. $Y = B_0$
2. $Y = B_0 + B_1X_1$
3. $Y = B_0 + B_2X_2$
4. $Y = B_0 + B_1X_1 + B_2X_2$

The best equation may then be selected based on the fit and the number of variables needed for the fit. The multiple correlation coefficient, R^2, is a measure of the fit. R^2 is the sum of squares due to regression divided by the sum of squares without regression. For example, if R^2 is 0.85 when three variables are used to fit the regression equation, and R^2 is equal to 0.87 when six variables are used, we probably would be satisfied using the equation with three variables, other things being equal. The inclusion of more variables in the regression equation cannot result in a decrease of R^2.

Another method of selecting variables to be included in the regression equation is the popular stepwise procedure, which is considered a better method than the "all possible regressions" approach. Independent variables (X_i) are entered into the equation, one at a time, starting with the independent variable that is most highly correlated to the dependent variable, Y. As each new variable is considered, its inclusion is based on a preassigned statistical test related to its correlation with the dependent variable, as well as its correlation to those independent variables already included in the regression equation.

Probably the biggest pitfall in multiple regression techniques lies in the interpretation of the coefficients. Draper and Smith discuss this problem, and the answer is by no means simple [1].

Interpretation of the meaning of the coefficients in multiple regression equations is much more clear in a designed (orthogonal) experiment. As we have noted previously, in a factorial experiment, the levels of the factors can be controlled, so that the effects of the factors can be independently evaluated. Techniques to describe and optimize pharmaceutical systems by fitting experimental data to regression models using designed experiments are discussed in Chap. 16.

An application of regression analysis to physical properties of finished tablets, with compression pressure and various tablet components as independent variables can be found in Ref. 2. In this paper, the authors considered five independent variables for inclusion in the regression equation. They suggested the following equation as a predictor of dissolution:

$$Y = 69.91 - 37.3X_5 - 17.48X_2 + 4.24X_3$$

where

Y = dissolution

X_5 = magnesium stearate level

X_2 = compression pressure

X_3 = starch disintegrant

Magnesium stearate and compression pressure decrease dissolution (negative coefficient). Starch increases dissolution. The authors discuss possible mechanisms for these effects.

Multiple regression equations that relate variables such as those described above are empirical relationships. We do not encounter real systems that can be described so simply, theoretically. The multiple regression equation is a "model" of a real system which must be recognized as being only an approximation of reality. How good an approximation the equation is can be evaluated only by seeing how the equation performs as a predictor of the response in new situations, where the levels of the independent variables are changed. Also, particularly in undesigned systems, placing physical interpretation on the signs and magnitude of the coefficients can be hazardous. As noted previously, the coefficients can give insights into the mechanisms of a process, but great caution is needed before making definitive judgments on this basis. Problems similar to those discussed for prediction in linear regression apply here as well. Error (variability) in the estimation of the coefficients, extrapolating to areas outside the levels of the variables in the experiment, and the choice of an incorrect model all adversely affect the reliability of the predicted value.

In addition to its use as a predictive equation, the regression equation may also be used to help obtain combinations of ingredients that will give a desired (e.g., optimum) response. This process is discussed in Chaps. 9 and 16. For those readers who are interested in a more advanced, in-depth discussion of regression, the excellent book by Draper and Smith, *Applied Regression Analysis*, is recommended [1].

REFERENCES

1.   Draper, N. R. and Smith, H., *Applied Regression Analysis*, 2nd ed., Wiley, New York, 1981.
2.   Bohidar, N. R., Restaino, F. A., and Schwartz, J. B., *Drug Dev. Ind. Pharm.*, 5, 175, 1979.

Appendix IV
Tables

Table IV.1   Random Numbers

44	17	50	92	09	79	27	71	05	07	76	21	95	93	04
83	50	39	13	89	83	45	72	40	94	78	62	93	55	62
28	79	77	81	43	04	54	23	14	80	49	98	32	70	27
55	29	62	11	00	62	65	76	31	83	08	22	02	35	53
88	93	30	81	50	24	43	07	88	45	96	24	60	78	89
46	00	76	13	83	31	98	15	30	74	17	76	73	31	40
99	05	78	83	75	79	52	47	39	12	70	33	42	30	45
24	88	59	45	16	73	64	63	03	16	04	43	81	66	97
14	90	27	33	43	46	37	68	94	35	12	72	70	43	54
50	27	98	87	19	20	15	73	00	94	52	85	80	22	26
55	47	03	77	04	44	22	78	84	26	04	33	46	09	52
59	29	97	68	60	71	91	38	67	54	13	58	18	24	76
48	55	90	65	72	96	57	69	36	10	96	46	92	42	45
66	37	32	20	30	77	84	57	03	29	10	45	65	04	26
68	49	69	10	82	53	75	91	93	30	34	25	20	57	27
83	62	64	11	12	67	19	00	71	74	60	47	21	92	86
06	90	91	47	68	25	49	33	74	02	16	29	35	65	16
33	23	97	78	26	78	26	45	40	19	61	29	53	73	09
47	15	40	15	02	82	06	93	20	01	67	38	02	37	90
79	65	14	62	16	34	96	02	75	82	46	75	43	89	36

Table IV.2   Cumulative Normal Distribution:
Cumulative Area Under the Normal Distribution (Less Than or Equal to Z)

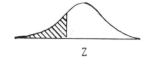

Z	Area	Z	Area	Z	Area	Z	Area
−3.25	0.0006	−1.50	0.0668	0.25	0.5987	2.00	0.9772
−3.20	0.0007	−1.45	0.0735	0.30	0.6179	2.05	0.9798
−3.15	0.0008	−1.40	0.0808	0.35	0.6368	2.10	0.9821
−3.10	0.0010	−1.35	0.0885	0.40	0.6554	2.15	0.9842
−3.05	0.0011	−1.30	0.0968	0.45	0.6736	2.20	0.9861
−3.00	0.0013	−1.25	0.1056	0.50	0.6915	2.25	0.9878
−2.95	0.0016	−1.20	0.1151	0.55	0.7088	2.30	0.9893
−2.90	0.0019	−1.15	0.1251	0.60	0.7257	2.35	0.9906
−2.85	0.0022	−1.10	0.1357	0.65	0.7422	2.40	0.9918
−2.80	0.0026	−1.05	0.1469	0.70	0.7580	2.45	0.9929
−2.75	0.0030	−1.00	0.1587	0.75	0.7734	2.50	0.9938
−2.70	0.0035	−0.95	0.1711	0.80	0.7881	2.55	0.9946
−2.65	0.0040	−0.90	0.1841	0.85	0.8023	2.60	0.9953
−2.60	0.0047	−0.85	0.1977	0.90	0.8159	2.65	0.9960
−2.55	0.0054	−0.80	0.2119	0.95	0.8289	2.70	0.9965
−2.50	0.0062	−0.75	0.2266	1.00	0.8413	2.75	0.9970
−2.45	0.0071	−0.70	0.2420	1.05	0.8531	2.80	0.9974
−2.40	0.0082	−0.65	0.2578	1.10	0.8643	2.85	0.9978
−2.35	0.0094	−0.60	0.2743	1.15	0.8749	2.90	0.9981
−2.30	0.0107	−0.55	0.2912	1.20	0.8849	2.95	0.9984
−2.25	0.0122	−0.50	0.3085	1.25	0.8944	3.00	0.9987
−2.20	0.0139	−0.45	0.3264	1.30	0.9032	3.25	0.9994
−2.15	0.0158	−0.40	0.3446	1.35	0.9115		
−2.10	0.0179	−0.35	0.3632	1.40	0.9192	Z	Area
−2.05	0.0202	−0.30	0.3821	1.45	0.9265		
−2.00	0.0228	−0.25	0.4013	1.50	0.9332	1.282	0.90
−1.95	0.0256	−0.20	0.4207	1.55	0.9394	1.645	0.95
−1.90	0.0287	−0.15	0.4404	1.60	0.9452	1.960	0.975
−1.85	0.0322	−0.10	0.4602	1.65	0.9505	2.326	0.99
−1.80	0.0359	−0.05	0.4801	1.70	0.9554	2.576	0.995
						3.090	0.999
−1.75	0.0401	0	0.5000	1.75	0.9599		
−1.70	0.0446	0.05	0.5199	1.80	0.9641		
−1.65	0.0495	0.10	0.5398	1.85	0.9678		
−1.60	0.0548	0.15	0.5596	1.90	0.9713		
−1.55	0.0606	0.20	0.5793	1.95	0.9744		

Table IV.3 Individual Terms of the Binomial Distribution for
N = 2 to 10 and P = 0.2, 0.5, and 0.7

These tables may be used for P = 0.8 and P = 0.3 as follows. Use
the table with P = 0.2 to obtain terms for P = 0.8; and use the table
with P = 0.7 to obtain terms for P = 0.3. For example, for the
probability of 5 (X' = 5) successes in 8 trials (N = 8) for P = 0.8,
look in the table for P = 0.2, N = 8, and X = N − X' = 8 − 5 = 3.
This is equal to 0.147.

	P = 0.2								
	N								
X	2	3	4	5	6	7	8	9	10
0	0.64	0.512	0.410	0.328	0.262	0.210	0.168	0.134	0.107
1	0.32	0.384	0.410	0.410	0.393	0.367	0.336	0.302	0.268
2	0.04	0.096	0.154	0.205	0.246	0.275	0.294	0.302	0.302
3		0.008	0.026	0.051	0.082	0.115	0.147	0.176	0.201
4			0.002	0.006	0.015	0.029	0.046	0.066	0.088
5				*	0.002	0.004	0.009	0.017	0.026
6					*	*	0.001	0.003	0.006
7						*	*	*	0.001
8							*	*	*
9								*	*
10									*

Table IV.3 (Continued)

	P = 0.5								
	N								
X	2	3	4	5	6	7	8	9	10
0	0.250	0.125	0.0625	0.031	0.016	0.008	0.004	0.002	0.001
1	0.500	0.375	0.250	0.156	0.094	0.055	0.031	0.018	0.010
2	0.250	0.375	0.375	0.313	0.234	0.164	0.109	0.070	0.044
3		0.125	0.250	0.313	0.313	0.273	0.219	0.164	0.117
4			0.0625	0.156	0.234	0.273	0.273	0.246	0.205
5				0.031	0.094	0.164	0.219	0.246	0.246
6					0.016	0.055	0.109	0.164	0.205
7						0.008	0.031	0.070	0.117
8							0.004	0.018	0.044
9								0.002	0.010
10									0.001

	P = 0.7								
	N								
X	2	3	4	5	6	7	8	9	10
0	0.090	0.027	0.008	0.002	0.001	*	*	*	*
1	0.420	0.189	0.076	0.028	0.010	0.004	0.001	*	*
2	0.490	0.441	0.265	0.132	0.060	0.025	0.010	0.004	0.001
3		0.343	0.412	0.309	0.185	0.097	0.047	0.021	0.009
4			0.240	0.360	0.324	0.227	0.136	0.074	0.037
5				0.168	0.303	0.318	0.254	0.172	0.103
6					0.118	0.247	0.296	0.267	0.200
7						0.082	0.198	0.267	0.267
8							0.058	0.156	0.233
9								0.040	0.121
10									0.028

*P < 0.0005.

Table IV.4   t Distributions

Two-sided:	40%	20%	10%	5%	1%
One-sided:	20%	10%	5%	2.5%	0.5%
d.f.:	$t_{0.80}$	$t_{0.90}$	$t_{0.95}$	$t_{0.975}$	$t_{0.995}$
1	1.38	3.08	6.31	12.71	63.66
2	1.06	1.89	2.92	4.30	9.92
3	0.98	1.64	2.35	3.18	5.84
4	0.94	1.53	2.13	2.78	4.60
5	0.92	1.48	2.02	2.57	4.03
6	0.91	1.44	1.94	2.45	3.71
7	0.90	1.42	1.89	2.36	3.50
8	0.89	1.40	1.86	2.31	3.36
9	0.88	1.38	1.83	2.26	3.25
10	0.88	1.37	1.81	2.23	3.17
11	0.88	1.36	1.80	2.20	3.11
12	0.87	1.36	1.78	2.18	3.05
13	0.87	1.35	1.77	2.16	3.01
14	0.87	1.35	1.76	2.14	2.98
15	0.87	1.34	1.75	2.13	2.95
16	0.86	1.34	1.75	2.12	2.92
17	0.86	1.33	1.74	2.11	2.90
18	0.86	1.33	1.73	2.10	2.88
19	0.86	1.33	1.73	2.09	2.86
20	0.86	1.33	1.72	2.09	2.85
25	0.86	1.32	1.71	2.06	2.79
30	0.85	1.31	1.70	2.04	2.75
40	0.85	1.30	1.68	2.02	2.70
60	0.85	1.30	1.67	2.00	2.66
120	0.85	1.29	1.66	1.98	2.62
∞	0.84	1.282	1.645	1.96	2.576

Table IV.5   Short Table of Chi-Square Distributions

χ^2

Probability	Degrees of freedom												
	1	2	3	4	5	6	7	8	9	10	15	20	30
0.99	6.63	9.21	11.3	13.3	15.1	16.8	18.5	20.1	21.7	23.2	30.6	37.6	50.9
0.975	5.02	7.38	9.35	11.1	12.8	14.45	16.0	17.5	19.0	20.5	27.5	34.2	47.0
0.95	3.84	5.99	7.81	9.49	11.1	12.6	14.1	15.5	16.9	18.3	25.0	31.4	43.8
0.90	2.71	4.61	6.25	7.78	9.24	10.6	12.0	13.4	14.7	16.0	22.3	28.4	40.3

Table IV.6A Upper 5% Values of the F Distribution

For degrees of freedom not included in the table, interpolate using the reciprocal of degrees of freedom. For example, $F_{1,60}$ is between 4.08 and 3.92. $1/40 = 0.025$; $1/120 = 0.0083$; $1/60 = 0.0167$, which is halfway between $1/120$ and $1/40$. Therefore, $F_{1,60} = 4.00$.

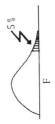

Degrees of freedom in denominator	Degrees of freedom in numerator												
	1	2	3	4	5	6	7	8	9	10	20	40	∞
1	161	200	216	225	230	234	237	239	241	242	248	251	254
2	18.5	19.0	19.2	19.2	19.3	19.3	19.4	19.4	19.4	19.4	19.4	19.5	19.5
3	10.1	9.55	9.28	9.12	9.01	8.94	8.89	8.85	8.81	8.79	8.66	8.59	8.53
4	7.71	6.94	6.59	6.39	6.26	6.16	6.09	6.04	6.00	5.96	5.80	5.72	5.63
5	6.61	5.79	5.41	5.19	5.05	4.95	4.88	4.82	4.77	4.74	4.56	4.46	4.37
6	5.99	5.14	4.76	4.53	4.39	4.28	4.21	4.15	4.10	4.06	3.87	3.77	3.67
7	5.59	4.74	4.35	4.12	3.97	3.87	3.79	3.73	3.68	3.64	3.44	3.34	3.23
8	5.32	4.46	4.07	3.84	3.69	3.58	3.50	3.44	3.39	3.35	3.15	3.04	2.93
9	5.12	4.26	3.86	3.63	3.48	3.37	3.29	3.23	3.18	3.14	2.94	2.83	2.71
10	4.96	4.10	3.71	3.48	3.33	3.22	3.14	3.07	3.02	2.98	2.77	2.66	2.54
11	4.84	3.98	3.59	3.36	3.20	3.09	3.01	2.95	2.90	2.85	2.65	2.53	2.40
12	4.75	3.89	3.49	3.26	3.11	3.00	2.91	2.85	2.80	2.75	2.54	2.43	2.30

5%

F

Table IV.6A (Continued)

Degrees of freedom in denominator	Degrees of freedom in numerator												
	1	2	3	4	5	6	7	8	9	10	20	40	∞
13	4.67	3.81	3.41	3.18	3.03	2.92	2.83	2.77	2.71	2.67	2.46	2.34	2.21
14	4.60	3.74	3.34	3.11	2.96	2.85	2.76	2.70	2.65	2.60	2.39	2.27	2.13
15	4.54	3.68	3.29	3.06	2.90	2.79	2.71	2.64	2.59	2.54	2.33	2.20	2.07
16	4.49	3.63	3.24	3.01	2.85	2.74	2.66	2.59	2.54	2.49	2.28	2.15	2.01
17	4.45	3.59	3.20	2.96	2.81	2.70	2.61	2.55	2.49	2.45	2.23	2.10	1.96
18	4.41	3.55	3.16	2.93	2.77	2.66	2.58	2.51	2.46	2.41	2.19	2.06	1.92
19	4.38	3.52	3.13	2.90	2.74	2.63	2.54	2.48	2.42	2.38	2.16	2.03	1.88
20	4.35	3.49	3.10	2.87	2.71	2.60	2.51	2.45	2.39	2.35	2.12	1.99	1.84
25	4.24	3.39	2.99	2.76	2.60	2.49	2.40	2.34	2.28	2.24	2.01	1.87	1.71
30	4.17	2.21	2.92	2.69	2.53	2.42	2.33	2.27	2.21	2.16	1.93	1.79	1.62
40	4.08	3.23	2.84	2.61	2.45	2.34	2.25	2.18	2.12	2.08	1.84	1.69	1.51
120	3.92	3.07	2.68	2.45	2.29	2.18	2.09	2.02	1.96	1.91	1.66	1.50	1.25
∞	3.84	3.00	2.60	2.37	2.21	2.10	2.01	1.94	1.88	1.83	1.57	1.39	1.00

Table IV.6B   Short Table of Upper 1% Values of the F Distribution

Degrees of freedom in denominator	Degrees of freedom in numerator								
	1	2	3	4	5	7	10	15	20
2	98.49	99.00	99.17	99.25	99.30	99.36	99.39	99.44	99.45
3	34.12	30.82	29.46	28.71	28.24	27.67	27.23	26.87	26.69
4	21.20	18.00	16.69	15.98	15.52	14.98	14.54	14.19	14.02
5	16.26	13.27	12.06	11.39	10.97	10.45	10.05	9.72	9.55
6	13.74	10.92	9.78	9.15	8.75	8.26	7.87	7.56	7.40
8	11.26	8.65	7.59	7.01	6.63	6.19	5.82	5.52	5.36
10	10.04	7.56	6.55	5.99	5.64	5.21	4.85	4.56	4.41
15	8.68	6.36	5.42	4.89	4.56	4.14	3.80	3.52	3.36
20	8.10	5.85	4.94	4.43	4.10	3.70	3.37	3.09	2.94
30	7.56	5.39	4.51	4.02	3.70	3.30	2.98	2.70	2.55
40	7.31	5.18	4.31	3.83	3.51	3.12	2.80	2.52	2.37
60	7.08	4.98	4.13	3.65	3.34	2.95	2.63	2.39	2.20
100	6.90	4.82	3.98	3.51	3.20	2.82	2.51	2.22	2.06
8	6.63	4.60	3.78	3.32	3.02	2.64	2.32	2.04	1.87

Table IV.7   Upper 5% Points in the Studentized Range

					Number of treatments, k						
d.f. (error)	2	3	4	5	6	7	8	9	10	15	20
2		8.33	9.80	10.89	11.73	12.43	13.03	13.54	13.99	15.65	16.77
4		5.04	5.76	6.29	6.71	7.06	7.35	7.60	7.83	8.67	9.24
5	3.64	4.60	5.22	5.67	6.03	6.33	6.58	6.80	6.99	7.72	8.21
6	3.46	4.34	4.90	5.31	5.63	5.89	6.12	6.32	6.49	7.14	7.59
8	3.26	4.04	4.53	4.89	5.17	5.40	5.60	5.77	5.92	6.48	6.87
10	3.15	3.88	4.33	4.66	4.91	5.12	5.30	5.46	5.60	6.12	6.47
12	3.08	3.77	4.20	4.51	4.75	4.95	5.12	5.27	5.40	5.88	6.21
14	3.03	3.70	4.11	4.41	4.64	4.83	4.99	5.13	5.25	5.72	6.03
16	3.00	3.65	4.05	4.34	4.56	4.74	4.90	5.03	5.15	5.59	5.90
18	2.97	3.61	4.00	4.28	4.49	4.67	4.83	4.96	5.07	5.50	5.79
20	2.95	3.58	3.96	4.24	4.45	4.62	4.77	4.90	5.01	5.43	5.71
24	2.92	3.53	3.90	4.17	4.37	4.54	4.68	4.81	4.92	5.32	5.59
30	2.89	3.48	3.84	4.11	4.30	4.46	4.60	4.72	4.83	5.21	5.48
40	2.86	3.44	3.79	4.04	4.23	4.39	4.52	4.63	4.74	5.11	5.36
60	2.83	3.40	3.74	3.98	4.16	4.31	4.44	4.55	4.65	5.00	5.24
120	2.80	3.36	3.69	3.92	4.10	4.24	4.36	4.47	4.56	4.90	5.13
∞	2.77	3.32	3.63	3.86	4.03	4.17	4.29	4.39	4.47	4.80	5.01

Table IV.7A Values of t' for Dunnett's Comparison of Several
Treatments and a Control (α = 0.05)

	Number of treatments					
d.f.	2	3	4	5	6	7
5	3.03	3.39	3.66	3.88	4.06	4.22
6	2.86	3.18	3.41	3.60	3.75	3.85
7	2.75	3.04	3.24	3.41	3.54	3.66
8	2.67	2.94	3.13	3.28	3.40	3.51
9	2.61	2.86	3.04	3.18	3.29	3.39
10	2.57	2.81	2.97	3.11	3.21	3.31
11	2.53	2.76	2.92	3.05	3.15	3.24
12	2.50	2.72	2.88	3.00	3.10	3.18
13	2.48	2.69	2.84	2.96	3.06	3.14
14	2.46	2.67	2.81	2.93	3.02	3.10
15	2.44	2.64	2.79	2.90	2.99	3.07
20	2.38	2.57	2.70	2.81	2.89	2.96
24	2.35	2.53	2.66	2.76	2.84	2.91
30	2.32	2.50	2.62	2.72	2.79	2.86
40	2.29	2.47	2.58	2.67	2.75	2.81
60	2.27	2.43	2.55	2.63	2.70	2.76
120	2.24	2.40	2.51	2.59	2.66	2.71
∞	2.21	2.37	2.47	2.55	2.62	2.67

Table IV.8   Dixon's Criteria for Rejecting Outliers

		Significance level	
k		5%	1%
3	$r_{10} = (X_2 - X_1)/(X_k - X_1)$ if smallest	0.941	0.988
4	value is suspected;	0.765	0.889
5	$= (X_k - X_{k-1})/(X_k - X_1)$ if largest	0.642	0.780
6	value is suspected	0.560	0.698
7		0.507	0.637
8	$r_{11} = (X_2 - X_1)/(X_{k-1} - X_1)$ if	0.554	0.683
9	smallest value is suspected;	0.512	0.635
10	$= (X_k - X_{k-1})/(X_k - X_2)$ if	0.477	0.597
	largest value is suspected		
11	$r_{21} = (X_3 - X_1)/(X_{k-1} - X_1)$ if	0.576	0.679
12	smallest value is suspected;	0.546	0.642
13	$= (X_k - X_{k-2})/(X_k - X_2)$ if	0.521	0.615
	largest value is suspected		
14	$r_{22} = (X_3 - X_1)/(X_{k-2} - X_1)$ if	0.546	0.641
15	smallest value is suspected;	0.525	0.616
16	$= (X_k - X_{k-2})/(X_k - X_3)$ if	0.507	0.595
17	largest value is suspected	0.490	0.577
18		0.475	0.561
19		0.462	0.547
20		0.450	0.535
21		0.440	0.524
22		0.430	0.514
23		0.421	0.505
24		0.413	0.497
25		0.406	0.489

Table IV.9 Critical Values of T for a Two-Sided Test at the 5% Level of Significance (Test for Outliers)

Sample size	T	Sample size	T
3	1.155	15	2.549
4	1.481	16	2.585
5	1.715	17	2.620
6	1.887	18	2.651
7	2.020	19	2.681
8	2.126	20	2.709
9	2.215	25	2.822
10	2.290	30	2.908
11	2.355	35	2.979
12	2.412	40	3.036
13	2.462	50	3.128
14	2.507	100	3.383

Table IV.10   Factors for Determining Upper and Lower 3σ Limits for Mean ($\overline{X}$) and Range (R) Charts; and for Estimating σ from $\overline{R}$

Sample size of subgroup, N	A: Factor for $\overline{X}$ chart	Factors for range chart		$\sigma = \dfrac{\overline{R}}{d_2}$
		D_L for lower limit	D_U for upper limit	d_2
2	1.88	0	3.27	1.128
3	1.02	0	2.57	1.693
4	0.73	0	2.28	2.059
5	0.58	0	2.11	2.326
6	0.48	0	2.00	2.534
7	0.42	0.08	1.92	2.704
8	0.37	0.14	1.86	2.847
9	0.34	0.18	1.82	2.970
10	0.31	0.22	1.78	3.078
15	0.22	0.35	1.65	3.472
20	0.18	0.41	1.59	3.735

Example: If $\overline{X}$ = 100 and $\overline{R}$ (the average range) = 5, and N = 6, the upper and lower limits for the $\overline{X}$ chart are

$$\overline{X} \pm A\overline{R} = 100 \pm 0.48(5) = 100 \pm 2.4 = (102.4, 97.6)$$

The upper limit for the range chart is $D_U\overline{R} = 2.0(5) = 10$. The lower limit for the range chart is $D_L\overline{R} = 0(5) = 0$.

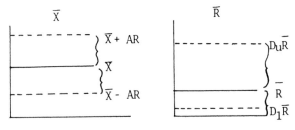

For samples of size 4, $\sigma = \dfrac{\overline{R}}{2.059}$

If $\overline{R} = 5$, $\sigma = \dfrac{5}{2.059} = 2.43$

Table IV.11 Number of Correct Guesses Needed for Significance in the Triangle Test

Panel size	Correct guesses for significance	
	5% Level	1% Level
6	5	6
7	5	6
8	6	7
9	6	7
10	7	8
11	7	8
12	8	9
13	8	9
14	9	10
15	9	10
16	9	11
17	10	11
18	10	12
19	11	12
20	11	13
21	12	13
22	12	14
23	12	14
24	13	15

Table IV. 12   Number of Positive or
Negative Signs Needed for Significance for
the Sign Test

Sample size	Number of positive or negative signs for significance[a]	
	5% Level	1% Level
6	6	—
7	7	—
8	8	8
9	8	9
10	9	10
11	10	11
12	10	11
13	11	12
14	12	13
15	12	13
16	13	14
17	13	15
18	14	15
19	15	16
20	15	17

[a]This is a two-sided test.   Choose positive
or negative signs, whichever is larger.

Table IV.13   Values Leading to
Significance for the Wilcoxon Signed
Rank Test (Two-Sided Test)

Sample size, N	5% Level[a]	1% Level
6	0	—
7	2	—
8	3	0
9	5	1
10	8	3
11	10	5
12	13	7
13	17	10
14	21	13
15	25	16
16	30	19
17	35	23
18	40	28
19	46	32
20	52	37

[a]If the smaller rank sum is less than or
equal to the table value, the comparative
groups are different at the indicated level
of significance.

Table IV.14 Critical Values for Number of Runs at the 5% Level of Significance

Sample size, N	Two-sided test Lower number[a]	Upper number	One-sided test Lower number
10	2	9	3
12	3	10	3
14	3	12	4
16	4	13	5
18	5	14	6
20	6	15	6
22	7	16	7
24	7	18	8
26	8	19	9
28	9	20	10
30	10	21	11
32	11	22	11
34	11	24	12
36	12	25	13
38	13	26	14
40	14	27	15

[a]If the number of runs is less than or equal to the lower number or greater than or equal to the upper value, the sequence is considered nonrandom at the 5% level of significance. The sample size (N) is the number of values above and below the median. For odd-size samples where one value is the median, use the next smaller sample size for the critical values.

Table IV.15 Probability of Getting at Least One Run of Given Size for N Samples

N	5% Level	1% Level
10	5	—
20	7	8
30	8	9
40	9	10
50	10	11

Table IV.16   Critical Values for Wilcoxon Rank Sum Test[a] ($\alpha = 0.05$)

Size of larger sample	Size of smaller sample (M)						
	M = 3	4	5	6	7	8	9
M	5, 16	11, 25	18, 37	26, 52	37, 68	49, 87	63, 108
M + 1	6, 18	12, 28	19, 41	28, 56	39, 73	51, 93	66, 114
M + 2	6, 21	12, 32	20, 45	29, 61	41, 78	54, 98	68, 121
M + 3	7, 23	13, 35	21, 49	31, 65	43, 83	56, 104	71, 127
M + 4	7, 26	14, 38	22, 53	32, 70	45, 88	58, 110	74, 133
M + 5	8, 28	15, 41	24, 56	34, 74	46, 94	61, 115	77, 139
M + 6	8, 31	16, 44	25, 60	36, 78	48, 99	63, 121	79, 146
M + 7	9, 33	17, 47	26, 64	37, 83	50, 104	65, 127	82, 152
M + 8	10, 35	17, 51	27, 68	39, 87	52, 109	68, 132	85, 158
M + 9	10, 38	18, 54	29, 71	41, 91	54, 114	70, 138	88, 164
M + 10	11, 40	19, 57	30, 75	42, 96	56, 119	72, 144	90, 171
M + 15	13, 53	24, 72	36, 94	50, 118	66, 144	84, 172	104, 202
M + 20	16, 65	28, 88	42, 113	58, 140	76, 169	96, 200	118, 223
M + 25	18, 78	32, 104	48, 132	66, 162	86, 194	108, 228	132, 264

[a]From Wilcoxon, F. and Wilcox, R. A., *Some Rapid Approximate Statistical Procedures*, Lederle Laboratories, 1964.

If rank sum of smaller sample is equal to or lower than smaller numbers in table or equal to or larger than larger number, groups are significantly different at 0.05 level.

Table IV.17   Critical Difference for Significance
(α = 0.05) Comparing All Possible Pairs of Treatments
for Nonparametric One-Way ANOVA[a]

N (for each treatment)	Number of treatments				
	3	4	5	6	7
3	15	23	30	37	45
4	24	35	46	57	69
5	33	48	63	79	96
6	43	63	83	104	125
7	54	79	105	131	158
8	66	96	128	160	192
9	79	115	152	190	229
10	92	134	178	223	268
11	106	155	205	257	309
12	121	176	233	292	352
13	136	199	263	329	397
14	152	222	294	368	444
15	169	246	326	408	492
16	186	271	359	449	542
17	203	296	393	492	593
18	221	323	428	536	646
19	240	350	464	581	700
20	259	378	501	627	756
21	278	406	538	674	814
22	298	435	577	723	872
23	319	465	617	773	932
24	340	496	657	824	994
25	361	527	699	875	1056

[a]From Wilcoxon, F. and Wilcox, R. A., *Some Rapid
Approximate Statistical Procedures*, Lederle Laboratories,
1964.

Table IV.18 Critical Differences for Significance
(α = 0.05) Comparing All Possible Pairs of Treatments
for Nonparametric Two-Way ANOVA[a]

N (for each treatment)	Number of treatments				
	3	4	5	6	7
3	6	8	10	13	15
4	7	10	12	15	18
5	8	11	14	17	20
6	9	12	15	18	22
7	9	13	16	20	24
8	10	14	17	21	25
9	10	14	18	23	27
10	11	15	19	24	28
11	11	16	20	25	30
12	12	16	21	26	31
13	12	17	22	27	32
14	13	18	23	28	34
15	13	18	24	29	35
16	13	19	24	30	36
17	14	19	25	31	37
18	14	20	26	32	38
19	14	20	27	33	39
20	15	21	27	34	40
21	15	21	28	35	41
22	16	22	29	35	42
23	16	22	29	36	43
24	16	23	30	37	44
25	17	23	31	38	45

[a]From Wilcoxon, F. and Wilcox, R. A., *Some Rapid
Approximate Statistical Procedures*, Lederle Laboratories, 1964.

Answers to Exercises

CHAPTER 1

1. (a) Tablet hardness, blood concentration of drug, creatinine in urine
    (b) Number of patients with side effects, bottles with fewer than 100 tablets, white blood cell count
    (c) Any continuous variable, rating scale
    (d) Race, placebo group in clinical study, number of bottles of syrup that are cloudy

2. None (This is a simple linear transformation; the C.V. is unchanged.)

3.

Interval	Frequency
-99.5 to -83.5	1
-83.5 to -67.5	2
-67.5 to -51.5	10
-51.5 to -35.5	16
-35.5 to -19.5	26
-19.5 to -3.5	34
-3.5 to +12.5	33
12.5 to 28.5	24
28.5 to 44.5	8
44.5 to 60.5	2

4. -10.27

5. Approximately 82% between 95 and 105 mg $(0.91-0.09)$; approximately 9% above 105 mg

6. (a) Mean $= -12.65$, $S = 31.68$; (b) $\overline{X} = -7$, $S = 30.48$ (read data in columns). Differences probably not significant. The last set is more precise but the standard deviations are virtually identical (the variability is probably not different in the two sets of data).

7. Median $= -16 = (-13 - 19)/2$; range $= 46$ to $-64 = 110$

8. (a) Median $= -16$ as in Problem 7; range $= 100$ to $-64 = 164$
   (b) Mean $= -8.5$, $S = 40.09$, $S^2 = 1607$

10. Probably not unbiased

11. $\sigma = \sqrt{2/3} = 0.816$, $\overline{S} = 0.793$

13. $\sqrt{\Sigma(X - \overline{X})^2/(N - 1)} = \sqrt{(0.0001 + 0 + 0.0001)/2} = 0.01$. The s.d. of 2.19, 2.20, and 2.21 is also 0.01. If a constant is added to each value (the constant added here is 1), the s.d. is unchanged. Standard deviation depends on differences among the values, not the absolute magnitude.

14. (a) 101.875; (b) 4.79; (c) 22.98; (d) $4.79/101.875 = 0.047$; (e) 14; (f) 101.5

15. $\Sigma N_i X_i^2 = 1(90.5)^2 + 6(70.5)^2 + \cdots + 16(29.5)^2 + 3(49.5)^2$

   $= 137,219$

   $\Sigma N_i X_i = 1(-90.5) + 6(-70.5) + \cdots + 16(29.5) + 3(49.5)$

   $= -1658$

   $\Sigma N_i = 156$

   $S^2 = [137,219 - (-1658)^2/156]/155 = 771.6$

   $S = 27.78$

16. 16.167, 9.865, 7.009

CHAPTER 2

1.

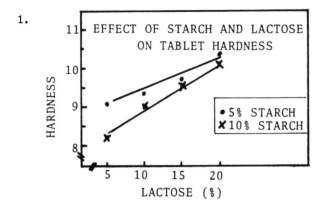

2.

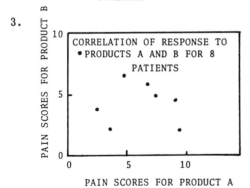

3.

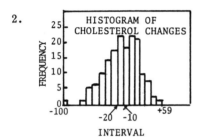

4.

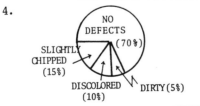

PIE CHART FOR TABLET DEFECTS

5.

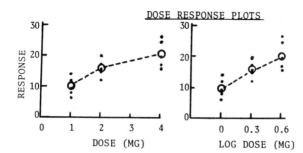

DOSE RESPONSE PLOTS

6.

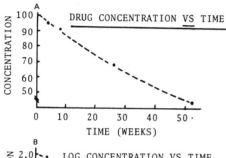

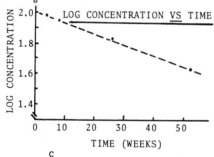

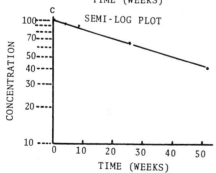

7.

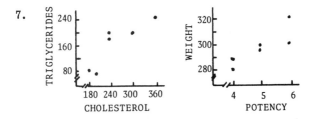

CHAPTER 3

1. Larger sample, more representative, blinded, less bias, etc.

2. All patients with disease who can be treated by antibiotic

3. Preference for new formulation among 24 panelists; number of broken tablets in sample of 100; race of patients in clinical study

4. 50,000 specked, but 20,000 are also chipped. Therefore, 30,000 are only specked. Probability of spek or chip is 0.06 (60,000 tablets have either a speck or a chip).

5. (a) P(A and B) = P(A|B)P(B). Let A = high blood pressure and B = diabetic. Then P(A and B) = (0.85)(0.10) = 0.085.
   (b) If independent, P(A) = P(A|B); 0.25 ≠ 0.85; they are not independent.

6. $(0.75)^2(0.25)^2 = 0.035163 \times 6 = 0.21094$. There are 6 ways of choosing 2 patients out of 4 $\binom{4}{2}$.

7. $(0.6)^3(0.4)^3 = 0.013824 \times 20 = 0.276$. There are 20 ways of choosing 3 patients out of 6 $\binom{6}{3}$.

8. 0.3697

9. (a) Approximately 0.8; (b) 0.2

10. Z = (170 − 215)/35 = −1.29; probability = approximately 0.10

11. Z = (60 − 50)/5 = 2, P(X ≤ 60) = 0.977; Z = (40 − 50)/5 = −2, P(X ≤ 40) = 0.023; P(40 ≤ X ≤ 60) = 0.977 − 0.023 = 0.954

12. Not necessarily; the patient may have a cholesterol value in the extremes of the normal distribution.

13. $Z = (137 - 140)/2.5 = -1.2$, probability $\leqslant Z = 0.115$; $Z = (142 - 140)/2.5 = 0.8$, probability $\leqslant Z = 0.788$; $P(137 \leqslant Z \leqslant 142) = 0.788 - 0.115 = 0.673$

14. $Z = (280 - 205)/45 = 1.67$; probability $= 0.952$; probability $Z > 280 = 1 - 0.952 = 0.048$

15. There are 36 equally likely possibilities, of which one is 2.

16. Yes! The order of heads and tails is not considered in the computation of probability.

17. $P(0 \text{ defects}) = \binom{20}{0} (0.01)^{0}(0.99)^{20} = 0.818$; $P(1 \text{ defect}) = \binom{20}{1}(0.01)^{1}(0.99)^{19} = 0.165$; $P(0 \text{ or } 1 \text{ defect}) = 0.818 + 0.165 = 0.983$

18. $\binom{10}{1} (0.5)^{1}(0.5)^{9} = 0.0098$

19. $\binom{4}{2} (0.01)^{2}(0.99)^{2} = 0.00059$. The probability is small; and two of four cures can be considered unlikely. The probability of this event plus equally likely or less likely events (three of four and four of four cures) is close to 0.00059. Thus we conclude that the new treatment is effective.

20. $\sqrt{(0.01)(0.99)20} = 0.445$; $\sqrt{(0.01)(0.99)/20} = 0.022$ (Problem 17) $\sqrt{(0.01)(0.99)4} = 0.199$; $\sqrt{(0.01)(0.99)/4} = 0.0497$ (Problem 19)

21. $S = \sqrt{(0.5)(0.5)/20} = 0.112$; $Z = (0.75 - 0.5)/0.112 = 2.24$; $P(Z > 2.24) = 1 - 0.988 = 0.012$

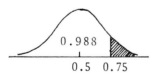

$$0.988$$
$$0.5 \quad 0.75$$

Drug is a promising candidate. The probability of observing such a large response is small if the true proportion of responses is 50%.

22. $P(0 \text{ defects}) = 0.99^{30} = 0.7397$; $P(1 \text{ defect}) = (30)(0.01)(0.99)^{29} = 0.2242$; $P(0 \text{ or } 1 \text{ defect}) = 0.7397 + 0.2242 = 0.9639$; $P(\text{more than 1 defect}) = 1 - 0.9639 = 0.0361$

CHAPTER 4

1. Starting at the upper left corner,* going down in Table IV.1. Even numbers to A. Patients assigned to A: 1, 2, 3, 5, 6, 8, 13, 14, 15, 16, 17, and 19.

2. Start as in Problem 1. If the number is 1 to 3, assign to A; 4 to 6, assign to B; 7 to 9, assign to C; do not count zeros.

Patient	Random number	Treatment
1	4	B
2	8	C
3	2	A
4	5	B
5	8	C
6	4	B
7	9	C
8	2	A
9	1	A
10	5	B
11	5	B
12	5	B
13	4	B
14	6	B (8 B's)
15	8	C
16	3	A
17	9	C
18	3	A
19	8	C
20	8	C
21	9	C (8 C's)

Remaining patients (22, 23, 24) given A

(May also randomize in groups of three; e.g., the first three patients are B, C, A —random numbers 4 and 8 refer to B and C.)

3. Start as above in Table IV.1. Use two-digit numbers between 1 and 30: 28, 24, 14, 6, 17, 29.

---

*We start at the upper left and read down for convenience and for the purpose of illustration. Otherwise, the starting point should be random.

5. Placebo: 1, 2, 4, 5, 7, 8, 9, 10, 12, 18; Drug: 3, 6, 11, 13, 14, 15, 16, 17, 19, 20

6. Take 20 tablets at a specific time every hour, all at the same time each hour (e.g., on the hour). Take 20 tablets each hour, but randomize the time the 20 are taken; e.g., first hour, take the sample at 5 min past the hour; second hour, take at 25 min past the hour; etc. Take tablets, one every 3 min during each hour. Take tablets at random times during each hour.

7. (See also Problem 3) 44, 8, 28, 55, 88

10. $\overline{X} = 300.7$

CHAPTER 5

1. $Z = (49.8 - 54.7)/2 = -2.45$; $P = 0.0071$

2. $103 \pm 2.58(2.2)/\sqrt{10} = 103 \pm 1.8 = 101.2$ to 104.8

3. (a) $5.95 \pm 2.57(0.16)/\sqrt{6} = 5.95 \pm 0.17$
   (b) $0.024 \pm 1.96\sqrt{(0.024)(0.976)/500} = 2.4 \pm 1.34\%$
   (c) $(0.83 - 0.50) \pm 1.96\sqrt{(0.83)(0.17)/60 + (0.50)(0.50)/50} = 0.33 \pm 0.17$

4. (a) $Z = |498 - 502|/(5.3/\sqrt{6}) = 1.85$; not significant, $\alpha = 0.05$; two tailed test
   (b) $t = (5.08 - 4.86)/\sqrt{0.095(2/5)} = 1.13$; not significant at 5% level
   (c) $t = 4/\sqrt{(15.2)/6} = 2.51$; $t_5 = 2.57$; just misses significance at 5% level; two-tailed test

5. (a) 0.098, larger
   (b) 0.350 and 0.261, average s.d. = 0.305, pooled s.d. = 0.308

6. (a) $\overline{X} = 10.66$, s.d. = 0.932
   (b) $\overline{X} = 9.66$, s.d. = 0.4695. $t_{18} = 1/(0.738\sqrt{2/10}) = 3.03$; difference is significant
   (c) Approximate test: $Z = (0.7 - 0.2)/\sqrt{(0.45)(0.55)(2/10)} = 2.24$; significant. Chi-square test with correction = 3.23; not quite significant
   (d) $0.45 \pm 1.96\sqrt{(0.45)(0.55)(1/20)} = 0.45 \pm 0.22$

7. Paired t test; 3 d.f.; $\alpha = 0.05$; two tailed test
   (a) $t = 0.07/\sqrt{0.0039/4} = 2.23$; not significant
   (b) $0.07 \pm 3.18(0.0627)/\sqrt{4} = 0.07 \pm 0.10$

8. (a) Paired t test, 11 d.f.; $t = 0.5/(0.612/\sqrt{12}) = 2.83$; significant at 5% level
   (b) $0.5 \pm 2.2(0.612)/\sqrt{12} = 0.5 \pm 0.39$

9. 9/60 and 6/65 = 15/125 = 0.12; 80/1000 and 57/1000 = 137/2000 = 0.0685

10. $t = (16.7 - 15)/(3.87/\sqrt{10}) = 1.39$; 10% level, one-sided test, this is significant

11. Chi-square $= (3.5)^2(2/12 + 2/88) = 2.32$; not significant

12. $Z = (|0.05 - 0.028| - 1/400)/\sqrt{(0.028)(0.972)/200} = 1.67$; not significant. $0.05 \pm 1.96 \sqrt{0.95(0.05)/200} = 0.05 \pm 0.03$
   $10 \pm 1.96\sqrt{(0.95)(0.05)(200)} = 10 \pm 6$

13. (a) $50 \pm 1.96\sqrt{(0.01)(0.99)(5000)} = 50 \pm 13.79$ in 5000 for 1,000,000 tablets; $10,000 \pm 2758$
   (b) $(0.01 - 0.02)/\sqrt{(0.02)(0.98)/5000} = -5.05$; $P \ll 0.001$; very unlikely
   (c) $1.96\sqrt{(0.01)(0.99)/N} = 0.001$, $N = (1.96)^2(0.99)(0.01)/10^{-6}$ $= 38,032$

14. Chi-square $= (4.5)^2(1/35.45 + 1/24.55 + 1/29.55 + 1/20.45) = 3.07$; not significant at 5% level. $(40/60 - 25/50) \pm 1.96$ $\sqrt{(0.67)(0.33)/60 + (0.5)(0.5)/50} = 0.167 \pm 0.183$

15. $Z = (|0.75 - 0.5| - 1/80)/\sqrt{(0.5)(0.5)/40} = 3.0$; $P < 0.05$

16. $Z = (|0.45 - 0.20| - 1/40)/\sqrt{(0.8)(0.2)/20} = 2.51$; $P < 0.05$
   $0.45 \pm 2.58\sqrt{(0.45)(0.55)/20} = 0.45 \pm 0.287$

17. Chi-square $= (3.5)^2(1/13.85 + 1/86.15 + 1/13.15 + 1/81.85) = 2.10$; not significant

18. $(1.8)^2(1/7.2 + 1/7.8 + 1/52.8 + 1/57.2) = 0.98$

19.

80	920
57	943

   = 2 × 2 table

   $\chi^2 = 11^2(1/68.5 + 1/931.5 + 1/68.5 + 1/931.5) = 3.79$; just misses significance at 5% level

20. $F_{9,9} = 0.869/0.220 = 3.94$, $P < 0.10$ (Table IV.6). This is a two-sided test. A ratio of 3.18 is needed for significance at the 10% level.

21. Correct $\chi^2 = 3.79$; D'agostino = 2.04

22. $\chi^2 = 28.6135 - 20.8591 = 7.75$ ($P < 0.05$)

CHAPTER 6

1. $2(5/10)^2(1.96 + 0.84)^2 + 0.25(1.96)^2$ = approximately 5 per group

2. $2(5/10)^2(1.96 + 0.84)^2$ = approximately 4 per group

3. $[(0.8 \times 0.2 + 0.9 \times 0.1)/(0.1)^2](1.96 + 1.28)^2$ = approximately 263 per group

4. $[(0.5 \times 0.5 + 0.5 \times 0.5)/(0.2)^2](1.96 + 1.28)^2$ = approximately 132 per group

5. $(1.96)^2(0.5 \times 0.5)/(0.15)^2$ = approximately 43
   $(1.96)^2(0.2)(0.8)/(0.15)^2$ = approximately 28

6. $(10/10)^2(1.96 + 2.32)^2 + 2$ = approximately 21 tablets

7. (a) $Z_\beta = (3/5)\sqrt{19/2} - 1.96 = -0.11$; power is approximately 46%
   (b) $Z_\beta = (3/5)\sqrt{49/2} - 1.96 = 1.01$; power = 84%

8. $(10/3)^2(1.96 + 1.28)^2$ = approximately 117

9. $Z_\beta = (0.2/0.25)\sqrt{10} - 1.96 = 0.57$; power is approximately 71%

10. $2(12/10)^2(1.96 + 1.65)^2 + 0.25Z_\alpha^2$ = approximately 39

11. $Z_\beta = (15/40)\sqrt{16} - 1.96 = -0.46$; power = approximately 0.32

12. $(1.96)^2(0.90)(0.10)/(0.05)^2 = 138.2$ = approximately 139

13. $N = 2(5/6)^2(1.96 + 1.28)^2 + 0.25(1.96)^2 = 15.5$ = approximately 16

14. 23 tablets per formulation

CHAPTER 7

1. (a) $b = 40/10 = 4$; $a = 12 - (4)(3) = 0$
   (b) $S_{Y.x}^2 = (164 - 16 \cdot 10)/3 = 1.33$; $S_b^2 = 1.33/10 = 0.133$;
      $t = 4/\sqrt{0.133} = 10.95$, significantly different from 0
   (c) $|4 - 5|/\sqrt{0.133} = 2.74$; d.f. = 3; not significant, 3.18 needed for significance
   (d) 3 hr; $Y = 4X = 12 \pm 3.18\sqrt{1.33}\ \sqrt{1/5 + 0/10} = 10.36$ to 13.64. 5 hr; $Y = 4X = 20 \pm 3.18\ \sqrt{1.33}\ \sqrt{1/5 + 4/10}$ = 17.16 to 22.84
   (e) $Y = 4(20) = 80 \pm 3.18\sqrt{1.33}\ \sqrt{1 + 1/5 + (20 - 3)^2/10}$ = 80 ± 20.1
   (f) $b = \Sigma\ Xy/\Sigma\ X^2 = 220/55 = 4$

2. (a) $a = -0.073$; $b = 0.2159$

    (b) $S_{Y.x}^2 = 0.003377$; $S_a^2 = 0.001848$; $t = -1.69$ (3 d.f.); not significant; may be due to interfering impurity

    (c) $C = 7.98$; confidence limits are 7.43 to 8.64; see Eq. (7.17)

3. (a) $b = 27/41.2 = 0.655$, $a = 100 - 0.655(200.4) = -31.3$

    (b) $Y = -31.3 + 0.655(200) = 99.74$

    (c) $99.74 \pm 3.18\sqrt{0.102} \, \sqrt{1/5 + (200 - 200.4)^2/41.2} = 99.74 \pm 0.46$

4. (a) 0.9588

    (b) $t_{10} = 10.7$; r is significantly different from 0 at 5% level

5. $r = 0.6519$; $t_8 = 1.84/0.76 = 2.43$, significant at 5% level

6. $r = -0.93135$; $t_7 = 6.77$, significant at 5% level

7. $r = 0.2187$; $F = 6.54/1.067 = 6.135$

    $r_{ds} = (6.135 - 1)/\sqrt{(6.135 + 1)^2 - 4(0.2187^2)6.135} = 0.728$

    $t_8 = 0.728\sqrt{8} / \sqrt{1 - 0.728^2} = 3.00$; $P < 0.05$; drug B is less variable

8. $Y = -3.90082 + 0.99607 X$; predicted values: 0.10049 ($X = \ln 5$); 0.20043 ($X = \ln 10$), 0.49928 ($X = \ln 25$), 0.99584 ($X = \ln 50$), 1.98626 ($X = \ln 100$).

9. (a) $C = 2.5482 - 0.01209 t$; (b) 24.66 mos; (c) 23.27 mos; (d) 23.55 mos.

10. $a = 0.5055$

CHAPTER 8

1. For significance at the 5% level, t (8 d.f.) ≥ 2.31 (two-sided test) A vs. B: $t = (101.2 - 99.4)/S_p\sqrt{1/5 + 1/5} = 2.84$ ($P < 0.05$); $S_p = 1.0$.   A vs. C: $t = (101.6 - 101.2)/(1.58\sqrt{1/5 + 1/5}) = 0.40$.   B vs. C: $t = (101.6 - 99.4)/(1.67\sqrt{1/5 + 1/5}) = 2.08$
    The ANOVA showed no significant differences

2.

Source	d.f.	MS	F
Between treatments	2	0.167	0.039
Within treatments	3	4.33	

Treatments are not significantly different.

3. Pooled error term from ANOVA table (Table 8.3) = 2.10
   A vs. B: $t = 1.8/\sqrt{2.10(2/5)} = 1.96$
   A vs. C: $t = 0.44$
   B vs. C: $t = 2.40$ ($P < 0.05$)
   Pooled error results in different values of t. This is appropriate if F is significant and/or tests are proposed a priori (use pooled error, i.e., WMS).

4. (a) H_0: $\mu_1 = \mu_2 = \mu_3 = \mu_4$; H_a: $\mu_i \neq \mu_j$; $\alpha = 0.05$
   (b) Fixed

   (c)

Source	d.f.	MS	F
Between analysts	3	2.89	5.78 ($P < 0.05$)
Within analysts	8	0.50	

   $LSD = 2.31\sqrt{0.5(2/3)} = 1.33$
   A differs from B, C, and D; B differs from C and D
   (d) Tukey test: $4.53\sqrt{0.5/3} = 1.85$; only analysts A and C differ at 5% level
   Scheffé test: $\sqrt{0.5(3)4.07(1/3 + 1/3)} = 2.02$; none of the analysts differ at 5% level

5. H_0: $\mu_i = \mu_j$; H_a: $\mu_i \neq \mu_j$; $\alpha = 5\%$

   (a)

Source	d.f.	MS	F
Between clinics	6	16.425	8.21 ($P < 0.05$)
Within clinics	13	2	

   (b) Yes
   (c) Fisher's LSD method (for example) at the 5% level
   $LSD = 2.16\sqrt{2(1/3 + 1/3)} = 2.49$
   Clinic 1 $\neq$ clinics 2, 5, 7; clinic 2 $\neq$ clinics 3, 5, 6; clinic 3 $\neq$ clinics 5, 7; clinic 4 $\neq$ clinic 5; clinic 5 $\neq$ clinics 6, 7; clinic 6 $\neq$ clinic 7
   For comparisons to clinic 7, $LSD = 2.16\sqrt{2(1/3 + 1/2)} = 2.79$

6. (a) Drugs fixed; (b) Machines fixed; (c) formulations fixed; (d) Machines random; (e) Clusters chosen at random

7. H_0: $\mu_1 = \mu_2 = \mu_3$; $\alpha = 0.05$

Source	d.f.	MS	F
Between batches	2	115.2	10.26 ($P < 0.05$)
Within batches	12	11.24	

   t test shows that batch 3 is different from batches 1 and 2; e.g., batch 1 vs. batch 3: $t_{12} = (20.33 - 11.8)/\sqrt{11.24(1/6 + 1/5)}$

8. (a)

Source	d.f.	MS	F
Row	5	1679.0	
Column	2	8.22	0.34 (P > 0.05)
Error	10	23.96	

(b)

Source	d.f.	MS	F
Row	5	52.99	
Column	2	26.06	5.37 (P < 0.05)
Error	10	4.86	$(F_{2,10} = 4.10$ for $\alpha = 0.05)$

(c) Averages of drugs are: placebo $= -0.33$, drug 1 $= -3.67$, and drug 2 $= -4.17$. Tukey test: $3.88\sqrt{4.86/6} = 3.49$; therefore, drug 2 is different from placebo. Newman-Keuls test: Drugs 1 and 2 different from placebo (P < 0.05). Dunnett test: Drug 1 and drug 2 different from control (P < 0.05).

9. (a) If the six presses comprise all of the presses, the presses are fixed.
Hours are fixed (i.e., each hour of the run is represented).

Source	d.f.	MS	F
Hour	4	11.95	6.76 (P < 0.05)
Presses	5	2.45	1.38 (P > 0.05)
Error	20	1.77	

(b) Presses are not significantly different (5% level)
(c) "Hours" are significantly different.
(d) Assume no interaction.
(e) Use Tukey test: $4.23\sqrt{1.77/6} = 2.30$; hour 3 is significantly different from hours 1, 2, and 5.

10.

Source	d.f.	MS	F
Rows	2	7.06	2.05
Columns	2	16.89	4.91 (P < 0.05)
Interaction	4	3.03	0.88
Within	9	3.44	

$(F_{2,9} = 4.26$ for significance at 5% level.)

"Presses" are significant. "Interaction" is not significant. Interaction means that differences between presses depend on the hour at which tablets are assayed.

11. Average results: A = 2.90, B = 6.50, C = 6.07
    If "sites" are random, use CR as error term.

    $5.04\sqrt{22.66/24}$ = 4.90 (no significant differences)

    If "sites fixed," use within error.

    $3.4\sqrt{3.215/24}$ = 1.24 (A is lower than B and C)

CHAPTER 9

1. ANOVA table:

Source	d.f.	MS	F
Stearate	1	1.56	5.21
Mixing time	1	1.82	6.1
Stearate × mixing time	1	0.72	2.41

Mixing time and stearate are significant at 5% level. Interaction is not significant.

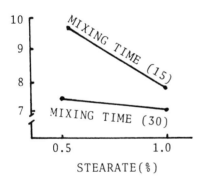

2. Low starch, low stearate   Low starch, high stearate

        0.475   0.487
        0.421   0.426
        ─────   ─────
    Av. = 0.448   Av. = 0.4565

    High starch − low starch = 0.4565 − 0.4480 = 0.0085

3. ANOVA:

Source	d.f.	MS	F
a	1	0.66	14.0*
b	1	0.06	1.3
ab	1	0.03	—
c	1	7.41	158**
ac	1	0.10	—
bc	1	3.25	69**
abc	1	0.01	—

$*P < 0.05; **P < 0.01.$

Error $= (0.03 + 0.10 + 0.01)/3 = 0.047$; d.f. $= 3$

(a)   a, c, bc

(b)

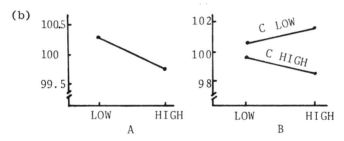

(c)   When C is low, as B is increased, recovery is increased.
        When C is high, as B is increased, recovery is decreased.

4. Synergism (or antagonism) would be evidenced by a significant
    AB interaction. If the effects are additive, we would expect
    an increase of 12 for the AB combination beyond placebo (4 from
    A and 8 from B). This is close to the observed increase of 14
    (35 − 21) for AB. The combination of A and B work better than
    either one alone, but the evidence for synergism is not strong.

5. Weigh (1), ab, ac, bc: empty, a and b together, a and c
    together, b and c together.

Source	d.f.	MS	F
A	1	2014	21.3**
B	1	356	3.8
AB	1	14	0.2
C	1	45	0.5
AC	1	741	7.9*
BC	1	121	1.3
ABC	1	36	—

Source	d.f.	MS	F
D	1	5704	60.5**
AD	1	114	1.2
BD	1	226	2.4
ABD	1	128	–
CD	1	0.02	0
ACD	1	27	–
BCD	1	10	–
ABCD	1	271	–
	15	9806	

Estimate of error = 94.3

**P $<$ 0.01
*P $<$ 0.05

AC interaction is significant: at low C, the A effect is
52.2 − 43.3; i.e., changing from low to high level of A has
little effect when C is at the low level. At high C, the A
effect is 62.4 − 26.4.

CHAPTER 10

1. 1.00, 1.11, 1.60, 1.64, 1.74, 1.80, 2.06, 2.16, 2.30, 2.34,
    2.36, 2.57, 2.70, 2.90, 2.90, 2.99, 3.10, 3.12, 3.18, 3.66

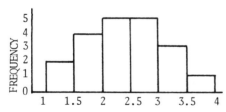

2. log Y = -0.127 + 1.068 log X
    log 47 = -0.127 + 1.068 log X
    log X = 1.685
    X = 48.4 mg

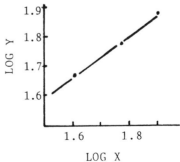

3. $\overline{R}$ = 1.066, S = 0.281; (0.066)/(0.089) = 0.75 (not significant at
    5% level). The t test for log B − log A is identical except for
    sign as the t test for log A − log B. This example shows the
    problem of using ratios. The average of A/B is not (in gen-
    eral) the reciprocal of B/A.

4. (62 − 54)/(62 − 47) = 8/15 = 0.533. This is an outlier accord-
    ing to the Dixon test. We probably should not omit this value
    without further verification. The outlier could be due to
    analytical error and/or the presence of tablets with unusual
    high potency.

5. Winsorized, 50.7; using all values, 51.4

6. t = [2.8 − 0.6]/[1.732 $\sqrt{1/5 + 1/5}$] = 2.01
    (Note the difference between the variances of the two groups.)

    Use a square-root transformation:

    Process 1: mean = 1.4363, s.d. = 0.960

    Process 2: mean = 0.6, s.d. = 0.548

    t = [1.4363 − 0.6]/[0.782 $\sqrt{1/5 + 1/5}$] = 1.69

CHAPTER 11

1. (b) $t = \dfrac{107.2 - (-3.05)}{\sqrt{1983.9(1/20 + 1/20)}} = 7.83 \ (t^2 = F)$

2.
Source	d.f.	MS	F	
Subjects	11	5.19		
Treatment	1	0.04	0.005	Treatments are not
Order	1	2.04	0.25	significantly different.
Error	10	8.04		

3.
Source	d.f.	MS	F	
Subjects	11	16.41		
Treatments	1	155	13.19	(P < 0.01)
Order	1	177	9.96	(P < 0.05)
Error	10	11.75		

$(22.3 - 17.3) \pm 2.23\sqrt{11.75(1/12 + 1/12)} = 5 \pm 3.12$

Grizzle analysis: Residual effect $= \dfrac{(245)^2 + (230)^2}{12} - \dfrac{(475)^2}{24}$

$$= 9.375;$$

within MS $= 17.11$; $F_{1,10} = 9.375/17.11 = 0.55$; not significant at 5% level

4. $\overline{A/B} = 1.334$, $S^2 = 0.238$; $t = (1.334 - 1.0)/\sqrt{0.238(1/12)} = 2.37$; $P < 0.05$

5. $\overline{\log X} = 0.0954265$; antilog $= 1.246$; $S^2 = 0.0309$; $t = 1.88$ (not significant; assume no order effect); $0.0954 \pm 2.20\sqrt{0.031(1/12)} = -0.016$ to 0.207; antilogs: 0.96 to 1.61

6. Two-way ANOVAS:

Source	Placebo d.f.	Placebo MS	Active d.f.	Active MS	Combined ANOVA d.f.	Combined ANOVA MS
Patients	5	2.866	5	2.742	10	2.804
Weeks	3	1.055	3	7.264	3	3.91
Patients × weeks	15	0.956	15	0.897	30	0.926
Drugs	1	. . . .			1	15.1875
Drugs × weeks	3	. . . .			3	4.41

For "drugs," $F_{1,10} = 15.1875/2.804 = 5.416$ ($P < 0.05$); for "drugs × weeks," $F_{3,15} = 4.41/0.926 = 4.76$ ($P < 0.05$).
From the accompanying plot and the F test for interaction, the active effect increases with time while the placebo is relatively constant.

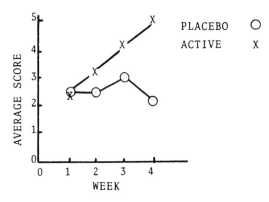

PLACEBO ○
ACTIVE X

7. $N = 2\,(55/60)^2\,(1.96 + 1.28)^2 + 1 \overset{=}{\sim} 19$

8. $|-4.75 + 7.6|/(3.433\,\sqrt{1/8 + 1/9}) = 1.71$ ($P > 0.05$)

CHAPTER 12

1. $\bar{X} = 9.95$; limits are $9.95 \pm 1.88(0.10) = 9.95 \pm 0.19$
   $\bar{R} = 0.10$; for $N = 2$, limits are 0 to $(3.27)(0.10) = 0.33$

2. $\sigma = \sqrt{0.02(0.98)/1000} = 0.004427$; $3\sigma = 0.0133$; $0.02 \pm 3\sigma = 0.0067$ to 0.0333

3. $\bar{X}$ control chart is centered at 47.6 with limits $47.6 \pm 1.02(1.2) = 47.6 \pm 1.22$. R chart has a target of 1.2 with lower limit of 0 and upper limit of $2.57(1.2) = 3.1$ (see Table IV.10)

4. $p = 1\%$; accept if 0 or 1 rejects. Probability 0 rejects = $0.99^{100} = 0.366$. $P(1 \text{ reject}) = 0.370$; $P(\text{batch rejected}) = 1 - 0.736 = 0.264$

5. $\bar{X} = 10.02$; limits: $10.02 \pm 0.31(0.38) = 10.02 \pm 0.12$
   $\bar{R} = 0.38$; limits: lower is $0.22(0.38) = 0.08$; upper is $1.78(0.38) = 0.68$
   Many means are out of limits. Either find cause or, if not possible use moving average if means are well within official limits.

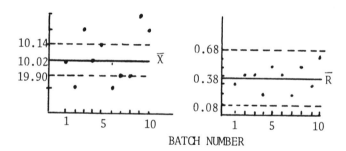

BATCH NUMBER

6. $p = 50/100,000 = 0.005 = $ probability of reject; $q = 0.9995$; therefore, probability of passing batch $= 0.9995^{100} = 0.951$

7.
Source	d.f.	MS
Between	3	483.3
Within	8	87.83

Between-analyst component $= (483.3 - 87.83)/3 = 131.8$; within-analyst component $= 87.83$
Three analysts perform four assays:

$$S^2 = \frac{4(131.8) + 87.83}{12} = 51.3$$

Four analysts perform two assays:

$$S^2 = \frac{2(131.8) + 87.83}{8} = 43.9$$

Cost is \$24 for both procedures. The latter procedure (four analysts) is more precise.

8. Limits are $399.6 \pm 1.02(3.48) = 3.99.6 \pm 3.55$

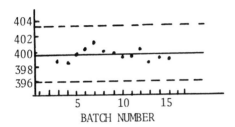

9. $\overline{X} = 10.21,\ \overline{R} = 0.24,\ \overline{S} = \sqrt{0.052} = 0.23$
    Limits for $\overline{X} = 10.21 \pm 1.88(0.24) = 10.21 \pm 0.45$
    Limits for $\overline{R} = 0$ to $3.27(0.24) = 0$ to 0.78

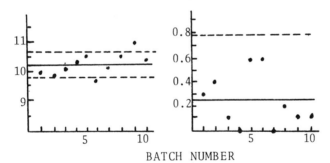

10. $N = 4$; limit $= 2.28\ \overline{R} = 2.28\ (12.5) = 28.5$ (0 is lower limit)

11. 6.25 vs. 3.8

CHAPTER 13

1. $\overline{R} = 3.375$; upper limit $= 3.375 \times 2.57 = 8.7$

2. $\overline{X} = 106.5$; $\overline{R} = 5.4$; limits $= 106.5 \pm 1.02(5.4) = 106.5 \pm 5.5$

3. $S_1^2 = 15.67$; $S_2^2 = 2.83$; $S_3^2 = 3.94$

    $\overline{S}^2 = 7.48$

    $\chi_2^2 = 72.440 - 61.958 = 10.482$ (P < 0.05)

4. $\overline{R} = 2.38$; upper limit = $2.38 \times 3.27 = 7.78$

5. $\overline{X} = 102.4$; $\overline{R} = 3.3$; limits = $102.4 \pm 3(3.3)/1.128 = 102.4 \pm 8.8$

CHAPTER 14

1. $\dfrac{(0.75 - 0.50) - 1/80}{\sqrt{(0.5)(0.5)/40}} = 3.00$; P < 0.05; yes

2.

		Preference for efficacy		
		Yellow	Marketed	Total
Preference	Yellow	15 (12.38)	6 (8.62)	21
for color	Marketed	8 (10.62)	10 (7.38)	18
	Total	23	16	39

$\chi^2 = (2.5)^2(1/12.38 + 1/8.62 + 1/10.62 + 1/7.38) = 2.65$; not significant at 5% level

3. (a) $t = 0.833/(1.4\sqrt{1/12} = 2.06$
    (b) $t = (10 - 1)/(1.4\sqrt{12}) = 1.86$
    Neither test is significant at 5% level.

4. $t_{18} = (6.8 - 5.9)/(1.83\sqrt{1/20 + 1/20}) = 1.56$ (P > 0.05); the paired test showed significance (P < 0.05).

5. $0.837 = r$

6. $\dfrac{3.25 - 3.00}{1.42\sqrt{1/20 + 1/20}} = 0.56$ (not significant)

7. $\dfrac{|0.5 - 0.33| - 1/60}{\sqrt{(1/3)(2/3)/30}} = 1.74$ (P < 0.05, one-sided test); yes

CHAPTER 15

1. $t = 0.583/0.6685\sqrt{1/12} = 3.02$; P < 0.05; parametric t test shows significance

2. (a) 9 of 12 comparisons are higher for B: not significant
   (b) $t = 0.5/(0.61\sqrt{1/12}) = 2.83$; $P < 0.05$

3. Σ Ranks for A = 11 (or 67); Σ ranks for B = 67; N = 12, $\alpha = 0.05$

$$Z = \frac{|67 - 12(13)/4|}{\sqrt{12(12.5)(13)/12}} = 2.20; \; P < 0.05$$

4. Use the Wilcoxon signed-rank test. $\Sigma R = 13.5$ (or 22.5); $P > 0.05$ (not significant)

5. Use the Wilcoxon rank sum test.

$$Z = \frac{|74 - 10(10 + 10 + 1)/2|}{\sqrt{10(10(10 + 10 + 1)/12}} = 2.34; \; P < 0.05$$

$$t = \frac{4.35 - 2.09}{\sqrt{3.816(1/10 + 1/10)}} = 2.59; \; P < 0.05$$

6. Use the Kruskal–Wallis test. Sum of ranks = 63.5, 40.5, and 16.

$$\chi_2^2 = \frac{12}{15(16)} (1133.3) - 3(15 + 1) = 8.67; \; P < 0.05$$

There is a significant difference (batch 3 has lowest dissolution).

7. Sum of ranks = 31, 21.5, and 19.5.

$$\chi_2^2 = \frac{12}{36(3 + 1)} (31^2 + 21.5^2 + 19.5^2) - 3(12)(4) = 6.29;$$

$P < 0.05$

The standard has the highest C_{max} (standard is greater than B, $P < 0.05$; see Ref. 2).

8.

	0	1	2	Total
A	50 (38.9)	50 (61.1)	75 (75)	175
B	20 (31.1)	60 (48.9)	60 (60)	140
Total	70	110	135	315

$\chi_2^2 = 11.69$; $P < 0.01$. The distribution of scores for A and B is different.

9.

		Capping		
		Yes	No	Total
Specks	Yes	13 (1.8)	45 (56.2)	58
	No	18 (29.2)	924 (912.8)	942
	Total	31	969	1000

(a) $\chi_1^2 = 73.7$ (corrected); $P \ll 0.01$; not independent

(b) $Z = \dfrac{|0.714 - 0.5| - 1/126}{\sqrt{0.5(0.5)/63}} = 3.27$; $P < 0.01$

The difference is significant at the 1% level.

10. The probability of the fourfold table is 0.0304:

$$\frac{12!\,5!\,14!\,21!}{0!\,12!\,5!\,9!\,26!} = 0.0304$$

The only least likely table has five tumors in the controls and zero tumors in the treated group. This table has a probability of 0.01204. Therefore, the probability of the given table + more unlikely tables is 0.0304 + 0.01204 = 0.0421. The χ^2 test (corrected) is equal to 3.98, which is equal to P = 0.0460.

11. The median is 303.25. There are nine runs. According to Table IV.14, fewer than 6 or more than 15 runs are needed for significance at the 5% level. Therefore, the sequence is not significantly nonrandom for both one- and two-sided tests.

14. $\chi^2 = 5.44$ (P < 0.05)

CHAPTER 16

1. (a) $X_1' = 0$; $X_2' = 1$; $X_3' = 0$; $Y = 10.725 + 2.225 = 12.95$

   (b) $X_1' = 1$; $X_2' = 1$; $X_3' = 0.6$; $Y = 15.36$

2. See Eq. (16.4). $X_1' = (1 - 1)/1 = 0$; $X_2' = (0.5 - 0.5)/0.5 = 0$; $X_3' = (2.5 - 2.5)/2.5 = 0$

3. $Y = (9.7 + 7.2 + 8.4 + 4.1)/4 + (-9.7 + 7.2 - 8.4 + 4.1)X_1/4$
$+ (-9.7 - 7.2 + 8.4 + 4.1)X_2/4 + (9.7 - 7.2 - 8.4 + 4.1)$
$X_1X_2/4 = 7.35 - 1.7X_1 - 1.1X_2 - 0.45X_1X_2$

4. $A' = (8.75 - 7.5)/2.5 = 0.5$; $B' = (100 - 75)/125 = 1.0$;
$Y = 7.35 - 1.7(0.5) - 1.1(1) - 0.45(0.5) = 5.725$

5. $Y = 19.75 + 4.25(St) + 3.25(M) - 2.25(M)(St)$. Note: M and St are coded. One possibility is $(St) = -0.23$ and $(M) = -1$. This is equivalent to 15 min of mixing and 0.539% stearate, for a 15-min dissolution time.

6. $Y + 10A + 15B + 30AB$; let $B = 1 - A$. $Y = 10A + 15(1 - A) + 30A(1 - A) = -30A^2 + 25A + 15$; $dY/dA = -60A + 25 = 0$;
$A = 0.417 = 41.7\%$

7. (a) $Y = 292A + 5.6B + 50.4C - 492.8AB - 186.8AC - 49.6BC$
$+ 54.6ABC$

(b) 100% B is 5.6 min. Combinations between 50 and 100% B and 0 and 50% A may give a fast dissolution (e.g., 0.6 of B and 0.4 of A = less than 2 min).

(c) There are many combinations. For example, 35% of A and 65% of C results in a dissolution of approximately 92 min.

Index